Differential Diagnosis of Common Complaints

Second Edition

ROBERT H. SELLER, MD

Professor of Medicine and Professor of Family Medicine
State University of New York at Buffalo
School of Medicine and Biomedical Sciences

W.B. SAUNDERS COMPANY
A Division of Harcourt Brace & Company
Philadelphia ○ London ○ Toronto ○ Montreal ○ Sydney ○ Tokyo

W. B. SAUNDERS COMPANY
A Division of Harcourt Brace & Company

The Curtis Center
Independence Square West
Philadelphia, Pennsylvania 19106

Library of Congress Cataloging-in-Publication Data

Seller, Robert H.

Differential diagnosis of common complaints / Robert H. Seller.—2nd ed.

p. cm.

Includes bibliographical references and index.

ISBN 0–7216–3327–7

1. Diagnosis, Differential.   I. Title.   [DNLM: 1. Diagnosis, Differential.   WB 141.5 S467d]

RC71.5.S45 1993   616.07′5—dc20

DNLM/DLC   92–11626

Differential Diagnosis of Common Complaints   ISBN 0–7216–3327–7

Printed in the United States of America.

Last digit is the print number: 9   8   7   6   5   4

To Our Patients

ACKNOWLEDGMENTS

Sharon Murphy, Assistant Librarian, Information Services Department, generously assisted me in the literature reviews and Wende Birkbeck graciously typed material for the second edition. I wish to thank my faculty colleagues at the School of Medicine at the University of Buffalo for reviewing each chapter.

PREFACE

The purpose of the second edition of *Differential Diagnosis of Common Complaints* remains the same as the first—to help physicians accurately and efficiently diagnose common complaints. This book emphasizes a clinical approach to diagnosis rather than one that relies largely on diagnostic studies. Most medical school curricula, texts, and continuing education courses deal with diseases. Patients, however, usually come to their physicians complaining of headache, backache, or fatigue—not migraine, spinal stenosis, or depression. To address this reality, the book is organized around common presenting complaints, the patients' symptoms rather than their diseases. The 34 symptoms reviewed account for more than 80 per cent of the chief complaints with which physicians are confronted. The physician who has mastered the differential diagnosis of these symptoms will be able to diagnose accurately nearly all the problems seen in a typical medical practice.

Each chapter deals with a different common complaint. The chapters are organized to approximate the problem-solving process that most physicians use to make a diagnosis. Initially, the presenting symptom suggests several diagnostic possibilities. Then this diagnostic list is further defined and reduced by additional, more specific, historical findings; by the patient's physical findings; and then by the results of diagnostic studies. The index lists all complaints, symptoms, and diagnoses mentioned in the text.

The second edition was revised to include suggestions by colleagues and students who like the book's clinical orientation and practical approach to differential diagnosis. New chapters have been added: Breast Lumps, Swelling of Legs, and Voiding Disorders and Incontinence. Each chapter has been revised to include new information with emphasis on the latest clinical and diagnostic studies. The format of each chapter has remained the same:

Introduction. Includes relevant definitions as well as a list of the most common causes of the symptom.

Nature of the patient. Identifies those conditions that are most prevalent within a particular patient subgroup (children, elderly, premenopausal, diabetic, hypertensive, immunocompromised, and the like).

Nature of symptom. Further identifies conditions by amplifying additional characteristics of the symptoms (how, when, where, radiation, acute/chronic, and so on).

Associated symptoms
Precipitating and aggravating factors
Ameliorating factors
Physical findings
Diagnostic studies
Less common diagnostic considerations

Selected references. Most articles represent an approach to differential diagnosis of problems rather than a review of a specific disease.

A concise summary table is located at the end of each chapter. These tables summarize the salient differential diagnostic features of each of the most common clinical entities that cause a particular complaint.

The text does not deal extensively with pathophysiology or therapy except in situations in which this information is particularly useful in the diagnostic process. The most useful diagnostic studies for differential diagnosis are reviewed. The text concentrates on the most likely diagnoses and common illnesses that include many serious illnesses. It also notes when there is a need to rule out extremely serious diagnostic possibilities.

Clinicians and students may use this book for general information about the many causes of common chief complaints. They can also use it as a reference text when treating a patient who has a specific symptom (such as facial pain, shortness of breath, or fever) when the diagnosis is not apparent.

Differential Diagnosis of Common Complaints was written to be useful. I hope you find it so. . . . Remember the adage "If you don't think about it, you will never diagnose it."

CONTENTS

1
Abdominal Pain in Adults 1

2
Abdominal Pain in Children 19

3
Backache 29

4
Belching, Bloating, and Flatulence 45

5
Breast Lumps 53

6
Chest Pain 61

7
Colds, Flu, and Stuffy Nose 75

8
Constipation 83

9
Cough 95

10
Diarrhea 105

11
Dizziness/Lightheadedness and Vertigo 117

12
Earache 127

13
Facial Pain 137

14
Fatigue 149

15
Fever 161

16
Headache 169

17
Heartburn and Indigestion 185

18
Insomnia 195

19
Menstrual Irregularities 203

20
Menstrual Pain 225

21
Nausea and/or Vomiting Without Abdominal Pain 233

22
Pain in the Foot 243

23
Pain in the Lower Extremity in Adults 251

24
Pain in the Lower Extremity and Limp in Children 267

25
Pain in the Upper Extremity 273

26
Palpitations 289

27
Shortness of Breath 297

28
Skin Problems 307

29
Sore Throat 333

30
Swelling of Legs 343

31
Urethral Discharge and Dysuria 351

32
Vaginal Discharge and Itching 361

33
Voiding Disorders and Incontinence 371

34
Weight Gain and Weight Loss 379

INDEX 389

Chapter 1

Abdominal Pain in Adults

The most common causes of abdominal pain are discussed here, with special attention given to the acute abdomen and recurrent abdominal pain. The term *acute abdomen* is medical jargon that refers to any acute condition within the abdomen that requires immediate surgical attention. It must be noted that acute abdominal pain may be of non-abdominal origin and does not always need surgery. The majority of patients who consult a physician for abdominal pain do not have an acute abdomen, although their chief complaint may be a sudden or acute onset of abdominal pain. In studies involving analysis of large series of patients presenting to emergency rooms with acute abdominal pain, NSAP (nonspecific abdominal pain) was the most common diagnosis. Most patients with this symptom probably have gastroenteritis.

The common causes of abdominal pain include *gastroenteritis, gastritis, peptic ulcer disease, reflux esophagitis, irritable bowel syndrome, dysmenorrhea, salpingitis, appendicitis, cholecystitis, cholelithiasis, intestinal obstruction, mesenteric adenitis, diverticulitis, pancreatitis, ureterolithiasis, incarcerated hernias, gas entrapment syndromes,* and *ischemic bowel disease* (particularly in the elderly). All the aforementioned conditions can present with an acute or sudden onset of abdominal pain, many can cause recurrent abdominal pain, and a few require surgical intervention. Any acute abdominal condition requires the physician to make an early, precise diagnosis, since in many instances prognosis depends on prompt initiation of therapy (particularly surgical therapy). The more serious the problem, the more urgent the need for an accurate diagnosis.

The examiner can best establish a complete and accurate diagnosis by noting carefully age and sex, past medical history, precipitating factors, location of the pain itself and of radiated discomfort, associated vomiting, altered bowel habits, chills and fever, and findings yielded on physical examination, particularly of the abdomen. **Abdominal pain without other symptoms or signs is rarely a serious problem.**

The physician must be particularly aware of the conditions that cause abdominal pain and that usually require surgical intervention. According to one large study, the most common conditions requiring surgical intervention are *appendicitis, cholecystitis,* and *perforated peptic ulcer.* Others include *acute intestinal obstruction, torsion of a viscus or ovary, perforation of a viscus, tumors, ectopic pregnancy, dissecting* and *ruptured aneurysms, mesenteric occlusion,* and *embolizations* and *infarctions of the bowel.*

Several authors warn against the practice of "pattern matching" in the diagnosis of acute abdominal surgical conditions; they have found that typical findings occur in only 60 to 70 per cent of patients. This means that if physicians attempt to match acute problems with patterns or stereotypes of the disease, they will fail to make the correct diagnosis in 30 to 40 per cent of cases. Therefore, to improve diagnostic accuracy, physicians must know the standard and typical presentations and must also be aware of the subtleties involved in the differential diagnosis. The "best test" method is more accurate than "pattern matching" in establishing the diagnosis.

The "best test" method involves elicitation of specific information that correlates well with the correct diagnosis. This method suggests that when a specific symptom or physical sign is noted, its presence is highly useful in establishing the correct diagnosis. For instance, the finding of pain in the right upper quadrant most frequently suggests *cholecystitis.* Likewise, if pain is aggravated by movement, it most frequently indicates *appendicitis* but also suggests *perforated peptic ulcer* to a lesser degree. A "best test" question used to differentiate the most common causes of abdominal pain—nonspecific abdominal pain and appendicitis—is whether the pain is aggravated by coughing or movement. The pain of appendicitis is aggravated by movement or coughing, whereas the pain of nonspecific abdominal pain is not. Abdominal pain that is aggravated by movement or coughing is probably due to peritoneal inflammation. "Best test" signs that are helpful in differential diagnosis include the presence of a *palpable mass* in diverticular disease, *hyperactive bowel sounds* in small bowel obstruction, *reduced bowel sounds* in perforation, and *involuntary guarding* in the right lower quadrant with appendicitis. The validity of "best test" findings has been supported by retrospective studies in which the diagnosis is known.

NATURE OF PATIENT

In elderly patients, it is often difficult for the physician to elicit an accurate description of the nature of the pain. These patients may be unable to distinguish new symptoms from pre-existing complaints and concomitant illnesses. Many present late in their illnesses, often after treating themselves for indigestion or constipation. In contrast to the high frequency of appendicitis, cholecystitis, and perforated ulcers in most general surgical series, the most common causes of acute surgical abdomen in patients over 70 years of age are *strangulated hernias* (45 per cent) and other forms of *intestinal obstruction (25 per cent)*.

It must be remembered that cancer is a common cause of abdominal pain in the elderly. In a study of patients over the age of 50 years presenting with nonspecific abdominal pain, 10 per cent had cancer. The majority of these patients with cancer had large bowel cancer. *Colonic cancer* is almost as common as perforated peptic ulcer, pancreatitis, and renal colic in patients over age 50. Cancer should be strongly suspected if the patient is older than 50 years and has had previous bouts of unexplained abdominal pain, if the present abdominal pain has lasted at least 4 days, and if constipation is present.

Elderly patients also have a higher frequency of uncommon causes of surgical abdomen, including *ruptured aortic aneurysm, acute mesenteric infarction,* and *inflammatory diverticular disease.*

The person's age also offers clues to diagnosis in other groups of patients. *Appendicitis* has its peak incidence in the second decade, although it can occur in patients older than 60 years as well as in infants. The incidence of *cholecystitis* increases with age.

Cholecystitis is more common in whites than in blacks, more prevalent in females than in males, and more common in women who take birth control pills or estrogens than in those who do not. Drugs that increase cholesterol saturation also increase the incidence of *cholelithiasis*. They include clofibrate (Atromid), conjugated estrogens, and estrogen-progestin combinations.

Nonspecific abdominal pain is an imprecise diagnosis, yet it is the most common diagnosis given to patients presenting to an emergency room with abdominal pain as their chief complaint. This diagnosis is most common in patients under the age of 40 years.

Irritable colon seems to be most common in young women, particularly those who have young children. This frequency has been attributed to the life pressures to which these women are subjected. Symptoms of irritable colon are also more frequent in others under stress, including children. The abdominal pain from an irritable colon may be a vague discomfort or pain in the left lower quadrant, right lower quadrant, or midabdomen. It occasionally radiates to the back. This pain may be relieved by defecation and may be associated with other well-recognized symptoms of irritable colon—mucus in the stool, constipation alternating with diarrhea, and small marble-like stools.

Surgical emergencies of gynecologic origin are more common in women of reproductive age, and include *pelvic inflammatory disease with abscess, ectopic pregnancy, hemorrhage from an ovarian cyst,* and *adnexal* or *ovarian torsion.*

Peptic ulcer pain is most common between ages 30 and 50 years but may occur in teenagers and, rarely, in young children. It is considerably more common in men than in women. This diagnosis should not be entirely disregarded in women, however, because there is a significant incidence of perforated peptic ulcer among them that may be a result of the physician's failure to consider peptic ulcer in the diagnosis. Although only 15 per cent of patients with ulcer symptoms are older than 60 years, 80 per cent of deaths due to ulcers occur in this group, since ulcer disease in the elderly is more likely to run a virulent course.

Acute intestinal obstruction occurs in all age groups. In the elderly, intestinal obstruction is usually caused by *strangulated hernias* or *cancer.* However, in any patient who presents with severe abdominal pain and has a history of abdominal surgery, adhesions are the most likely cause of intestinal obstruction.

Pancreatitis occurs most frequently in alcoholics and in patients with gallstones. *Sigmoid volvulus* is more common in males, the mentally retarded, and those with parkinsonism; *cecal volvulus* is more common in females. *Gallstone ileus* causes small bowel obstruction more often in the elderly and in women. *Mesenteric adenitis* is more common in children. *Peptic esophagitis* is more common in obese patients. The incidence of *diverticulitis* increases with age; this disorder is more common after age 60.

NATURE OF PAIN

Colicky or crampy pain that begins in the midabdomen and progresses to a constant pain in the right lower quadrant suggests *appendicitis.* Other conditions that may begin in a crampy or colicky manner and progress to a more constant pain include *cholelithiasis* and *cholecystitis* (which tend to localize in the right upper quadrant), *intestinal obstruction,* and *ureterolithiasis.* The latter condition involves excruciating pain that frequently radiates to the groin, testes, or medial thigh.

A constant, often annoying burning or gnawing pain that is located in the midepigastrium and is occasionally associated with posterior radiation is seen with *peptic ulcer.* Peptic ulcer pain may be worse at night, although this is unusual. It is not ordinarily made worse by recumbency. The pain of peptic ulcer in the elderly may be vague and poorly localized. Because of a lack of classic symptoms, an occasional absence of prior symptoms, and a confusing picture of abdominal pain, perforation associated with peritonitis is more common in the elderly. It is particularly important to note that pain induced by percussion in the epigastrium may be the only physical finding suggesting ulcer disease in a person complaining of typical peptic ulcer pain. Likewise, severe exacerbation of pain that occurs when the physician percusses over the right upper quadrant strongly suggests the presence of an *inflamed gallbladder.*

The diagnosis of abdominal pain due to an *irritable colon* is fairly easy to make: the pain is usually dull, crampy, and recurrent. It is often associated with constipation that alternates with diarrhea, small stools, and mucus in the stools. In addition, moderate pain may be elicited when the physician palpates the colon. In the elderly, however, severe diverticulitis may exist with similar symptoms.

Most abdominal pain, even when severe, usually develops over several hours. When the onset of severe abdominal pain is abrupt, it suggests *perforation, strangulation, torsion, dissecting aneurysms,* or *ureterolithiasis.* The most severe abdominal pain occurs with dissecting aneurysms and with ureterolithiasis. The pain of a dissecting aneurysm is often described as a "tearing" or "ripping" sensation and often radiates into the legs and through to the back. Patients with such pain usually present in profound shock. Individuals with the excruciating pain of ureterolithiasis may be writhing in agony but do not experience cardiovascular collapse. This pain is usually unilateral in the flank, groin, or testicle and is often associated with nausea and occasional vomiting.

LOCATION OF PAIN

The location of the pain is one of the "best tests" for determination of a diagnosis (Fig. 1–1). Right upper quadrant pain is most frequently seen in *cholecystitis, cholelithiasis,* and leaking *duodenal ulcer* (Fig. 1–2). Another clue to gallbladder disease is the radiation of right upper quadrant pain to the inferior angle of the right scapula. Right upper quadrant pain is also seen in patients with *hepatitis* or *congestive heart failure.* In the latter group, the pain is thought to be due to swelling of the liver that results in distention of Glisson's capsule. Less severe right upper quadrant pain may be seen in patients with a *hepatic flexure syndrome* (gas entrapment in the hepatic flexure of the colon). If questioned carefully, these patients will admit to experiencing relief with the passage of flatus.

A gnawing, burning, midabdominal to upper abdominal pain suggests a condition with a peptic etiology—*ulcer, gastritis,* or *esophagitis.* Burning epigastric pain that radiates to the jaw is frequently seen in patients with peptic esophagitis.

Left upper quadrant pain is most frequently seen in patients with *gastroenteritis* or *irritable colon* and less commonly in those with splenic flexure syndrome, splenic infarction, or pancreatitis. The pain from splenic flexure syndrome can be located in the left upper quadrant or in

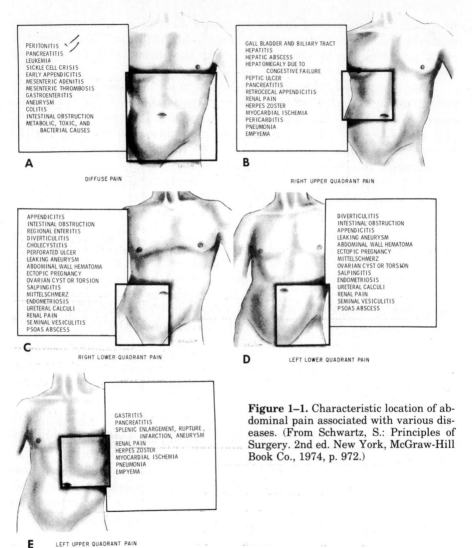

Figure 1–1. Characteristic location of abdominal pain associated with various diseases. (From Schwartz, S.: Principles of Surgery. 2nd ed. New York, McGraw-Hill Book Co., 1974, p. 972.)

the chest; therefore, it is also part of the differential diagnosis of chest pain. These pains tend to arise when the individual is bending over or wearing a tight garment, and they frequently are relieved by the passage of flatus.

Other causes of both right and left upper quadrant pain include supradiaphragmatic conditions with inflammation of the diaphragm, such as pneumonia, pulmonary embolism, pleurisy, and pericarditis.

Right lower quadrant pain is most commonly seen with *muscle strain, appendicitis, salpingitis,* and *diverticulitis* (Fig. 1–3). Diverticulitis pain is more common in the left lower quadrant, however. Less

Leaking duodenal ulcer; Acute cholecystitis; Appendicitis with high appendix; Pleurisy.

Figure 1–2. Tenderness and rigidity in right hypochondrium. (From Cope, Z.: Early Diagnosis of the Acute Abdomen. 13th ed. London, Oxford University Press, 1968, p. 43.)

common causes of right lower quadrant pain include ileitis, pyelone-phritis, obturator hernia, carcinoma of the cecum, and colonic obstruction in patients with a competent ileocecal valve.

Other causes of right or left lower quadrant pain include ureteroli-thiasis, salpingitis, ruptured ovarian cyst, ovarian torsion, ectopic pregnancy, and obturator hernia. The pain of salpingitis usually is unilateral, although it may present bilaterally.

Left lower quadrant pain suggests *irritable colon* and *diverticulitis*.

Common causes of central abdominal pain include early *appendicitis, small bowel obstruction, gastritis,* and *colic* (Fig. 1–4).

Tender & rigid area

Appendicitis: Leaking duodenal ulcer; Pyelitis; Acute pancreatitis; Regional ileitis (exacerbation); inflamed ileocœcal glands; inflamed Meckel's diverticulum; Cholecystitis (low gall-bladder); Biliary peritonitis.

Figure 1–3. Tenderness and rigidity in the right iliac region. (From Cope, Z.: Early Diagnosis of the Acute Abdomen. 13th ed. London, Oxford University Press, 1968, p. 45.)

THINK OF . . . Acute appendicitis (earliest stage); Acute obstruction of small gut ; Acute gastritis or simple intestinal colic ; Acute pancreatitis. EXCLUDE . . . coronary thrombosis ; tabetic crisis ; herpes zoster.

Figure 1–4. Acute central abdominal pain without any other symptom. (From Cope, Z.: Early Diagnosis of the Acute Abdomen. 13th ed. London, Oxford University Press, 1968, p. 38.)

PRECIPITATING OR AGGRAVATING FACTORS

The pain of *appendicitis* is aggravated by motion or coughing, as is the pain of *peritonitis*, regardless of its cause. The pain of *gastritis* is worsened by most foods, particularly alcoholic beverages. *Peptic ulcer* pain usually begins an hour or so after eating and is generally relieved by eating. If epigastric pain occurs primarily or is worsened in the recumbent position, *peptic esophagitis* should be suspected. The pain of *salpingitis* and *endometriosis* is often worse during or before menstruation. Although patients may find that this pain is not exacerbated by limited movement in bed, more strenuous activity such as descending a flight of stairs frequently will increase the severity of the discomfort. The symptoms of nonspecific abdominal pain are precipitated and exacerbated by problems in the individual's environment. They may also be part of a long-term psychiatric illness.

AMELIORATING FACTORS

If the patient experiences relief after eating or taking antacids, *peptic ulcer* or *peptic esophagitis* is the probable cause of pain. The pain of *gastritis*, although worsened by ingestion of food and alcoholic beverages, may be relieved by antacids. The pain of peptic esophagitis is often lessened when the patient is in an upright posture.

Pain relieved by defecation or the passage of flatus suggests an *irritable colon* or *gas entrapment* in the large bowel, whereas pain relieved by belching suggests *gaseous distention* of the stomach or esophagus. The pain of *gastroenteritis* is occasionally relieved by vomiting or diarrhea.

ASSOCIATED SYMPTOMS

The abdominal pain seen with a truly *acute abdomen* is usually of such severity that patients overlook any associated symptoms they might have. Thus, it can be said that any additional complaint (e.g., headache) contradicts the diagnosis of acute abdomen.

The timing of vomiting in relation to the onset of abdominal pain and associated symptoms may help the physician establish a precise diagnosis. The earlier the vomiting occurs in relation to the onset of abdominal pain, the less the abdominal distention. In lower intestinal obstruction, there is less vomiting and greater distention. Vomiting that precedes the onset of pain reduces the probability of an acute abdomen. Vomiting that begins after the onset of pain is more consistent with the diagnosis of an acute abdomen and frequently is seen in patients with *appendicitis.* The absence of vomiting does not preclude the diagnosis of an acute abdomen.

If vomiting occurs soon after the onset of pain and the vomitus is light in color, the vomitus probably consists of digestive juices and bile; this suggests *gastritis, cholecystitis,* or *obstruction.*

Jaundice, dark urine, and light to acholic stools may be seen in patients with abdominal pain due to *cholecystitis.* These symptoms suggest an obstructive etiology of the jaundice, and complete biliary obstruction should be suspected. **A history of occasional silver-colored stools alternating with normal or light-colored stools is virtually pathognomonic of *carcinoma of the ampulla of Vater.*** The production of silver-colored stools is a result of upper gastrointestinal blood from the ampullary carcinoma mixing with acholic stools.

Examination of vomitus from patients with acute abdominal obstruction may provide a clue to the location of the obstruction. Undigested food in the vomitus suggests that the obstruction is proximal to the stomach; this may be due to *achalasia* or *peptic esophagitis.* Occasionally, undigested food may be seen in vomitus from patients with *pyloric obstruction.* This diagnosis is most likely if the vomiting persists and does not contain bile.

Brown vomitus with a fecal odor suggests mechanical or paralytic *bowel obstruction.* The more proximal the obstruction, the more frequent the vomiting.

Constipation with small, dry stools—sometimes alternating with diarrhea or mucus in the stool—is frequently seen in patients experiencing increasing stress, and suggests an *irritable colon.*

PHYSICAL FINDINGS

Physical examination of the abdomen in patients presenting with abdominal pain should include inspection, auscultation, palpation, and percussion as well as rectal and pelvic examinations. The physical examination should begin with inspection of the abdomen, with the physician standing at the foot of the patient's bed. This part of the examination often can provide major clues to the diagnosis because it allows one to note distention, abnormal pulsations, and abdominal movement with respiration. The second part of the examination should always consist of auscultation; it is preferable for the physician to listen to bowel sounds before beginning a manual investigation. When palpating the abdomen and vaginal area, the physician should be particularly attentive to lymph node enlargements or hernias and to the quality of femoral pulses.

Specific physical findings in appendicitis, cholecystitis, diverticulitis, and bowel perforation or infarction vary with the disease. If peritonitis is present, however, certain physical findings are common, regardless of disease. The pain of peritonitis is severe, generalized, continuous, and of acute or gradual onset. There is usually abdominal tenderness with guarding, stabbing pain with gentle coughing, and pain to percussion. Abdominal rigidity occasionally is present. There is decreased movement of the abdominal wall with respiration. If rebound pain is present, it usually is found over the area of primary disease. Patients with peritonitis often are in shock, have fever or chills, and present with decreased or absent bowel sounds. The patient usually lies relatively motionless, as movement aggravates the pain. Depending on the severity of the peritonitis and the prior cardiovascular status of the patient, hypotension, tachycardia, pallor, and sweating may also be present. Younger, healthier patients are relatively resistant to hypotension but easily develop tachycardia. In contrast, elderly patients with a decreased cardiovascular reserve more readily become hypotensive. The presence of cardiac disease may impair the development of tachycardia.

APPENDICITIS. In acute appendicitis there almost always is tenderness over the inflamed appendix. There often is involuntary guarding as well as rebound tenderness over McBurney's point. Classically, there is a disproportionate rise in the pulse rate with respect to the degree of fever.

CHOLECYSTITIS. Guarding in the right upper quadrant and tenderness to palpation and percussion suggest cholecystitis. When gallbladder disease is suspected in patients with right upper quadrant pain, the examiner should begin palpation very gently in other parts of the abdomen and end gently over the gallbladder. The goal of this careful palpation is detection of an enlarged (hydrops) gallbladder. An enlarged gallbladder may not be detected by deep palpation or percussion, as such aggressive examination may result in involuntary guarding, which prevents detection of the enlarged gallbladder. In all patients with abdominal pain, the physician should begin palpation away from the painful area and gradually move toward palpation over the most painful spot.

PEPTIC ULCER. In patients with symptoms of peptic ulcer disease, there may be no abnormal physical findings except pain to gentle percussion over the midepigastrium or duodenal sweep. When peritonitis develops in patients with peptic ulcer disease, it is secondary to perforation of the involved viscus. If the viscus perforates anteriorly, extreme rigidity of the abdominal wall results. If the viscus penetrates posteriorly, back pain is a major symptom, and the symptoms of peritonitis are minimal. In the early stages of a penetrating or perforated peptic ulcer, bowel sounds may be increased or normal, but as the condition progresses, bowel sounds become diminished or absent.

INTESTINAL OBSTRUCTION. Auscultation of the abdomen may help the physician diagnose obstruction. Classically, rushes of high-pitched, tinkling peristalsis are heard. These rushes often are associated with recurring crampy, colicky pain. The physician must listen for a succussion splash in all patients complaining of vomiting. This examination requires the examiner to place the stethoscope over the stomach and to shake the abdomen gently. A succussion splash may be heard over a stomach that is dilated or distended with air and fluid. This finding is normal in infants and in adults immediately after eating. By 30 minutes after eating, the sound should not be heard unless there is an obstruction with an air-fluid level. Impaired gastric emptying occurs most commonly in patients with *pyloric obstruction* (congenital or acquired); it also occurs in patients with gastric tumors or gastric atony. Atonic gastric dilatation is most commonly seen in postoperative patients and in patients who have severe hyperkalemia or diabetic ketoacidosis.

There is a classic triad of physical findings in patients with acute intestinal obstruction: (1) sudden onset of colicky abdominal pain, (2) vomiting, and (3) obstipation. Bowel sounds are generally hyperactive and high-pitched and occur in rushes; if perforation or peritonitis occurs, the bowel sounds become reduced. When the obstruction is in the large intestine, there may be abdominal distention and general or local distention of the intestine. With *volvulus* there may be gross distention of the entire abdomen; this occurs early in the disease.

SALPINGITIS. The physical findings of salpingitis include unilateral or bilateral tenderness to palpation in the lower abdomen and increased bowel sounds. Involuntary guarding and rigidity are rare findings. Pelvic examination often elicits pain, particularly with lateral movement of the cervix and adnexal palpation. There is frequently a purulent cervical discharge.

IRRITABLE COLON. Although most patients with an irritable colon have no significant physical findings (the diagnosis is made by careful history), a tender ascending or descending colon may be palpable.

ACUTE DIVERTICULITIS. The classic triad for acute diverticulitis is (1) abdominal tenderness, (2) a palpable mass in the left lower quadrant, and (3) fever. The mass or tenderness occasionally may be detected only by rectal examination. Diarrhea and rectal bleeding are uncommon, and bowel sounds are usually decreased.

URETEROLITHIASIS. Tenderness to percussion in the costovertebral angle and ileus may be the only physical finding in patients with ureterolithiasis. This diagnosis usually is confirmed by the presence of hematuria.

DIAGNOSTIC STUDIES

Although plain or flat abdominal radiographs frequently are ordered in patients with acute abdominal pain, they are diagnostic in less than 50 per cent of cases. If an acute surgical abdomen is suspected and the diagnosis is unknown or dubious, the physician should obtain an electrocardiogram as well as chest and abdominal radiographs and should perform studies of complete blood count (CBC) with differential, electrolytes, urea nitrogen, serum amylase (if pancreatitis is suspected), and urine and stool.

Rarely, laparotomy is necessary in patients with recurrent abdominal pain if the diagnosis is not apparent. In one series of 27 laparotomies for unexplained abdominal pain, carcinoma was found in 50 per cent of patients. Laparoscopy and peritoneal cytology are helpful when surgical intervention is being considered. In patients over 50 years of age presenting with *recurrent nonspecific acute abdominal pain,* the following laboratory tests should be done to detect cancer: (1) examination of stools for occult blood (this test should be done in all patients over 50 years regardless of the presence of abdominal pain); (2) sigmoidoscopy and, if necessary, colonoscopy; and (3) barium enema.

Specific laboratory tests should be ordered when certain diagnoses are suspected: *appendicitis*—CBC with differential; *cholecystitis*—CBC with differential; isotopic and ultrasonographic scanning; *peptic ulcer*—upper GI radiographs; *perforated peptic ulcer*—radiographs to reveal free air; *acute intestinal obstruction*—abdominal radiographs; *ureterolithiasis*—intravenous pyelography; microscopic urinalysis; *pancreatitis*—serum amylase. Abdominal computed tomography (CT scans) and abdominal ultrasonography are often helpful, especially when gallbladder, pancreatic, or pelvic disease is suspected. CT scans provide information concerning the bowel wall, mesentery, and intraperitoneal and retroperitoneal structures and are useful in surgical decision making.

LESS COMMON DIAGNOSTIC CONSIDERATIONS

Abdominal pain may be due to pneumonia, particularly of a lower lobe. Abdominal pain and vomiting may be the presenting symptoms in diabetes. Right upper quadrant pain can be due to congestive heart failure resulting from stretching of Glisson's capsule. Right upper quadrant pain, jaundice, and anorexia may be the presenting symptoms of hepatitis.

Amebiasis can mimic appendicitis or diverticulitis or both. Abdominal or flank pain or both, when associated with nausea and vomiting, may be the presenting symptoms of a hydronephrosis.

An acute abdomen in a young black patient classically suggests the possibility of sickle cell crisis. Severe abdominal wall tenderness can result from a spider bite. Rarely, diffuse abdominal pain can be secondary to marked gaseous distention.

Severe pain in the back or flank, or vague, poorly localized abdominal pain may be the first presenting symptom in patients with carcinoma of the pancreas. If abdominal pain is associated with thrombophlebitis (in the absence of trauma), migratory thrombophlebitis, or the development of diabetes, carcinoma of the pancreas should be suspected. Carcinoma of the head of the pancreas usually presents with jaundice or abdominal pain early in the course of the illness.

Abdominal pain that may be associated with vomiting and that occurs in the middle of the menstrual cycle is called "mittelschmerz." It represents pain associated with physiologic rupture of an ovarian follicle.

If a child or woman of childbearing age suddenly develops severe, generalized abdominal pain, often associated with syncope or persistent dizziness, ectopic pregnancy must be considered. This is more common in younger women, in those of low parity, and in those with a history of prior pelvic sepsis or infertility. Physical findings include acute abdominal pain with guarding and rigidity, especially in the lower abdomen. Extreme tenderness to cervical manipulation has been reported in 85 per cent of patients with an ectopic pregnancy. Laparoscopy, human chorionic gonadotropin, and ultrasonography may help the physician establish the diagnosis.

Vascular causes of abdominal pain include mesenteric thrombosis and acute mesenteric occlusion by embolism or torsion. The latter may have no associated signs or symptoms—only severe abdominal pain with bloody stools occurring later. Aortic aneurysm may cause constant low back pain, which may worsen with recumbency; dissection is character-

DIFFERENTIAL DIAGNOSIS OF ABDOMINAL PAIN IN ADULTS

CAUSE	NATURE OF PATIENT	NATURE OF PAIN	LOCATION OF PAIN	ASSOCIATED SYMPTOMS	PRECIPITATING OR AGGRAVATING FACTORS	AMELIORATING FACTORS	PHYSICAL FINDINGS	DIAGNOSTIC STUDIES
Gastroenteritis	Any age	Crampy	Diffuse	Nausea, vomiting, diarrhea, fever	Food	Occasional relief with vomiting or diarrhea	Hyperactive peristalsis	
Gastritis	Especially alcoholics	Constant, burning	Epigastric	Hemorrhage, nausea, vomiting, diarrhea, fever	Alcohol, NSAIDs, salicylates, food (occasionally)			
Appendicitis	Any age: peak age 10–20 yr.; M>F	Colicky, progressing to constant	Early in epigastrium or periumbilicus; RLQ later	Vomiting (after the pain has started), constipation, fever	Pain worse with movement and coughing	Lying still	RLQ involuntary guarding; rebound to RLQ	CBC with differential
Cholecystitis and/or cholelithiasis	Adults; F>M	Colicky, progressing to constant	RUQ radiates to inferior angle of right scapula	Nausea, vomiting, dark urine, light stool, jaundice	Fatty foods, drugs, birth control pill, cholestyramine		Tenderness to palpation or percussion in RUQ	Liver function tests, CBC, amylase, ultrasonography, isotopic gallbladder scan
Diverticulitis	More common in elderly	Intermittent cramping	LLQ	Constipation, diarrhea			Palpable mass in LLQ	
Pancreatitis	More common in alcoholics and patients with cholelithiasis	Steady, mild to severe	LUQ and epigastric; radiates to back	Nausea, vomiting, prostration, diaphoresis	Lying supine	Leaning forward	Abdominal distention, decreased bowel sounds, diffuse rebound	Amylase, ultrasonography

Condition	Patient population	Character/onset	Location	Associated symptoms	Aggravating/relieving factors	Physical findings	Diagnostic tests
Intestinal obstruction	Elderly and those with prior abdominal surgery	Colicky, sudden onset		Vomiting, obstipation		Hyperactive peristalsis in small bowel obstruction	Abdominal radiographs
Intestinal perforation (peritonitis)	F>M; elderly	Sudden onset, severe; Sudden or gradual onset	Diffuse	Guarding, rebound	Pain worse with movement or coughing; Lying still	Decreased bowel sounds, guarding, diffuse rebound	Abdominal radiographs, peritoneal lavage
Salpingitis	Menstruating females	Cramplike	RLQ and/or LLQ, non-radiating	Chandelier tenderness of cervix	Pain worse while descending stairs; worse around time of menstruation	Adnexa and cervix tender to manipulation	Ultrasonography, CT scan, human chorionic gonadotropin to r/o ectopic pregnancy
Ectopic pregnancy	Fertile female with history of menstrual irregularity	Sudden onset, persistent pain	Lower quadrant	Tender adnexal mass (vaginal bleeding)			Human chorionic gonadotropin
Peptic ulcer (with perforation)	M>F; 30–50 yr	Gnawing, burning; Sudden onset	Epigastric radiating to sides, back or right shoulder		Empty stomach, stress, alcohol; Food, alkali	Epigastric tenderness to palpation or percussion	Endoscopy; radiography
Mesenteric adenitis	Children and adolescents; after respiratory infection	Constant	RLQ	Vomiting, rebound, constipation, diarrhea, fever			CBC with differential

Table continued on following page

DIFFERENTIAL DIAGNOSIS OF ABDOMINAL PAIN IN ADULTS *Continued*

CAUSE	NATURE OF PATIENT	NATURE OF PAIN	LOCATION OF PAIN	ASSOCIATED SYMPTOMS	PRECIPITATING OR AGGRAVATING FACTORS	AMELIORATING FACTORS	PHYSICAL FINDINGS	DIAGNOSTIC STUDIES
Ureterolithiasis		Colicky, occasionally progresses to constant; severe; sudden onset	Lower abdomen; flank radiating to groin	Nausea, vomiting, abdominal distention, chills, fever			CVA tenderness, hematuria	Urinalysis, IVP, ultrasonography
Dissection or rupture of aortic aneurysm	Elderly; hypertensive; 40–70 yr	Unbearable, sudden onset	Chest or abdomen; may radiate to back and legs	Shock			Shock, decrease or difference in femoral pulses	Radiography, Ultrasonography, CT scan
Reflux (peptic) esophagitis		Burning, gnawing	Midepigastrium; occasionally radiating to jaw		Recumbency	Antacids		Upper GI radiographs, endoscopy
Irritable colon	More common in young women	Crampy, recurrent	Most common in LLQ	Mucus in stools		Pain occasionally relieved by defecation	Colon tender to palpation	
Incarcerated hernia	More common in elderly	Constant	RLQ or LLQ		Coughing and straining		Hernia or mass	Upper GI radiographs
Mesenteric infarction	Elderly	May be severe	Diffuse	Tachycardia, hypotension			Decreased bowel sounds, blood in stools	Abdominal radiographs

ized by severe, excruciating pain. Other uncommon conditions simulating an acute abdomen are reviewed by Purcell (1989).

Selected References

Burnett, L. S.: Gynecologic causes of the acute abdomen. Surg. Clin. North Am. *68*:385–398, 1988.

Cope, Z.: Cope's Early Diagnosis of the Acute Abdomen. New York, Oxford University Press, 1987.

Diehl, A. K., Sugarek, N. J., and Todd, K. H.: Clinical evaluation of gallstone disease: usefulness of symptoms and signs in clinical diagnosis. Am. J. Med. *89*:29–34, 1990.

De Dombal, F. T.: Picking the best tests in acute abdominal pain. J. R. Coll. Physicians Lond. *13*:203–208, 1979.

Paterson-Brown, S., and Vipond, M. N.: Modern aids to clinical decision making in the acute abdomen. Br. J. Surg. *77(1)*:13–18, 1990.

Phillips, S. L., and Burns, G. P.: Acute abdominal disease in the aged. Med. Clin. North Am. *72*:1213–1224, 1988.

Purcell, T. B.: Nonsurgical and Extraperitoneal Causes of Abdominal Pain. Emerg. Med. Clin. North Am. *7*:721–740, 1989.

Saegesser, F.: The acute abdomen part 1: differential diagnosis. Clin. Gastroenterol. *10*:123–144, 1981.

Staniland, J. R., Ditchburn, J., and De Dombal, F. T.: Clinical presentation of acute abdomen: study of 600 patients. Br. Med. J. *3*:393–398, 1972.

Trnka, Y., and Warfield, C. A.: Chronic abdominal pain. Hosp. Pract. *19*:201–209, 1984.

Wilson, D. H.: The acute abdomen in the accident and emergency department. Practitioner *222*:480–485, 1975.

Chapter *2*

Abdominal Pain in Children

Since chronic abdominal pain is rare in children, the main emphasis of this chapter will be the differential diagnosis of acute and recurrent abdominal pain. Because abdominal pain has many causes, a detailed history and a very careful physical examination are necessary. A small number of selected laboratory studies may also be required. Accurate diagnosis is essential because abdominal pain may be a manifestation of a surgical emergency; these cases must be identified promptly. Whenever there is significant concern about the presence of a surgical condition, the patient should be hospitalized to permit serial abdominal examinations and laboratory studies.

Gastroenteritis is the most common cause of acute abdominal pain in children. *Constipation,* another common cause of abdominal pain, may be acute but is more often recurrent. Other common nonsurgical causes of acute abdominal pain include *mesenteric adenitis, nonspecific abdominal pain, urinary tract infection, sickle cell disease, poisoning,* and *diabetes. Recurrent abdominal pain* is defined as three discrete episodes of abdominal pain occurring over 3 or more months. It is quite common over the age of 5 years and often has a psychosomatic cause.

The most common surgical causes of acute abdominal pain are *appendicitis, hernia strangulation,* and *intussusception.*

NATURE OF PATIENT

Presentation and causes of abdominal pain vary according to three age groups: (1) children under 5 years, (2) patients between 5 and 12, years, and (3) adolescents. The cause of abdominal pain in very young children is difficult to determine unless abdominal tenderness, guarding,

19

doubling up, or vomiting is present. Physical examination is particularly important in this age group. *Intussusception* is likely when signs of intestinal obstruction are found in infants (peak incidence, 6 months). A lead point such as Meckel's diverticulum seldom is found. *Appendicitis* is uncommon in infants and children up to the age of 5 years, but it is the most common condition causing abdominal pain that requires surgery in this age-group. Because appendicitis seldom is considered, the diagnosis is often missed or delayed. Perforation is, therefore, more common, and a disproportionately high percentage of deaths due to appendicitis occur in children under 5 years of age. *Poisonings,* most common in children aged 1 to 4 years, are another frequent cause of abdominal pain.

In children between 5 and 12 years, the major dilemma involves *recurrent abdominal pain,* which can be a symptom of either psychosomatic or organic disease; it is usually due to psychological factors. Among children with recurrent abdominal pain, there is a high incidence of behavioral and personality disorders. These patients tend to be "highstrung" perfectionists and are often apprehensive. In this group, many patients have histories of colic and feeding problems in infancy, and there is a high incidence of stressful family and school situations. Unexplained episodes of recurrent abdominal pain occur in 10 per cent of school-aged children, but an organic cause is found in less than 10 per cent of these cases.

Inflammatory bowel disease frequently begins during adolescence and can be a cause of acute or recurrent abdominal pain. Growth failure in adolescents with abdominal pain is an important clue to this diagnosis, although it may also indicate *gluten-sensitive enteropathy. Sickle cell crises* occur almost exclusively in blacks, although they occur occasionally in people of Mediterranean descent. *Acute appendicitis* is most common in children aged 5 to 15 years, with a peak incidence occurring between 10 and 15 years.

NATURE OF PAIN

The timing of the first occurrence of abdominal pain in children may help to identify *psychological stress* as the cause. For example, abdominal pain that develops at a time of school problems, the birth of a sibling, or family discord suggests a psychological cause.

In addition to observing the severity, duration, and location of abdominal pain, the examiner must note whether the onset is gradual or sudden. A gradual onset of cramping pain often suggests an intestinal cause, such as *appendicitis,* whereas a sudden onset of noncramping constant pain suggests *torsion* of a viscus, *intussusception,* or *perforation.* The pain of *appendicitis* classically precedes the development of vomiting and anorexia, begins gradually as a crampy epigastric or periumbilical pain, and progresses to a constant pain in the right lower quadrant. In young children, this pain may be mild or discontinuous or both. Because of atypical presentations and decreased incidence in young children, this diagnosis is often missed. The pain of *mesenteric adenitis* often mimics appendicitis, although a child with the former condition is not quite as sick and is not necessarily anorexic. Mesenteric adenitis usually occurs after a viral or bacterial infection. The associated pain may be colicky in younger children and severe and episodic in older children. **There is tenderness and guarding when the pain is present, and usually no guarding when the pain is absent.** This is in contrast to appendicitis, in which the guarding persists despite the absence of pain. Guarding and abdominal tenderness are the symptoms most frequently associated with a surgical diagnosis.

Cramping, diffuse abdominal pain that follows or coincides with the onset of diarrhea, nausea, or vomiting suggests *gastroenteritis*. Cramping pain occurring primarily after meals is often due to *constipation*. This diagnosis should be accepted only when an enema yields a large amount of feces and relieves pain. Sudden onset of severe, crampy, spasmodic pain that causes an infant to scream and draw up his legs should suggest *intussusception*. This spasmodic pain often recurs at 15- to 30-minute intervals, and the child may be normal, lethargic, or sleeping between attacks.

When abdominal pain is severe and colicky and radiates to the groin or flank, *urolithiasis* should be considered. Hematuria may confirm this diagnosis. Hematuria may also be noted when an inflamed retrocecal appendix overlies the ureter. Abdominal pain associated with tenderness to percussion in the costovertebral angle region may indicate *pyelonephritis*.

The abdominal pain of *diabetic acidosis* often is generalized, and ketosis is usually present. The abdominal pain of a *sickle cell crisis* is severe, and there is usually an associated ileus. This diagnosis should be considered in all black children with severe abdominal pain. Certainly, every black child in whom the diagnosis of appendicitis is considered should have a sickle cell test before surgery. When appendicitis is suspected in patients with a positive sickle cell test, an appendectomy should not be performed until there is a clear lack of response to medical therapy for sickle cell crisis or there are progressive manifestations of sepsis. Recurrent abdominal pain suggests *sickle cell disease, inflammatory bowel disease, cystic fibrosis*, and *constipation*.

LOCATION OF PAIN

The pain of *gastroenteritis* is poorly localized, whereas the pain of constipation is usually located in the right lower quadrant. The presumed mechanism of right lower quadrant pain in *constipation* involves gaseous distention of the cecum. **Increasing localized tenderness in the right lower quadrant associated with rebound to the right lower quadrant is the single most helpful finding favoring the diagnosis of appendicitis.** Subsequent to this localization of pain in the right lower quadrant, paralytic ileus may develop. Classic findings often occur with the appendix in its usual location, but atypical symptomatology may result from an unusually located inflamed appendix. It is critical for the physician to perform a rectal examination because pain in the right upper quadrant may be due to a retrocecal appendicitis.

ASSOCIATED SYMPTOMS

A detailed evaluation of associated symptoms often helps establish the diagnosis. Some generally applicable rules concerning the differential diagnosis of acute abdominal pain are as follows:

1. When significant diarrhea is associated with abdominal pain, a surgical lesion is rare.

2. When abdominal distention—particularly with acidosis—is associated with abdominal pain, a surgical emergency is more likely.

3. When vomiting precedes abdominal pain, an extra-abdominal cause is suggested; when abdominal pain precedes vomiting, an abdominal cause is likely.

When abdominal pain is diffuse and no localizing physical signs are found, associated diarrhea, nausea, or vomiting suggests *gastroenteritis*. A preceding upper respiratory infection (e.g., pharyngitis, tonsillitis, or otitis media), a high fever, nausea or vomiting, and a good appetite suggest *mesenteric adenitis*.

Abdominal pain without systemic signs (e.g., fever or leukocytosis) or localized abdominal findings, especially when there is intense stress at home or school, suggests a *psychosomatic cause*. Some children with such findings also have nausea, vomiting, headaches, and diarrhea. Their pain is poorly localized, and there are no peritoneal signs.

A history of polyuria, polydipsia, weight loss, or diabetes in the patient or the family suggests that the abdominal pain may be caused by *diabetic ketoacidosis*.

Growth failure, particularly during adolescence, is an important clue suggesting *inflammatory bowel disease* or a *gluten-sensitive enteropathy*. Weight loss and anemia are other signs of organic disease.

PHYSICAL FINDINGS

For excellent reviews of special techniques useful in pediatric abdominal examination, one should refer to the articles by Jones (1979) and Gryskiewicz and Huseby (1980). Physical examination should include general observation of the child as well as inspection of the abdomen for distention, masses, or abnormal pulsations. The abdomen should then be auscultated prior to palpation or percussion. Diffuse and generalized hyperperistalsis suggests *gastroenteritis*, whereas rushes of high-pitched peristalsis associated with crampy pains suggest an *obstructive process.*

Patients with *appendicitis* have tenderness over the inflamed appendix. Peritoneal inflammation, present in 97 per cent of children with acute appendicitis, usually results in muscle guarding and rebound tenderness. Other signs of peritonitis include shallow breathing, absent peristalsis, low-grade fever with a disproportionate rise in the pulse rate, and leukocytosis (which may be absent during the first 24 hours). The child may lie quite still or move cautiously and often prefers to lie on his side with the right thigh flexed. With a retrocecal appendix, the child may limp and demonstrate a positive psoas or obturator sign, although these signs are difficult to elicit in very young children. The following features of acute appendicitis have been described as peculiar to children:

1. Surgery should be performed within 24 hours of symptom onset; otherwise, perforation is likely.

2. The pain may be mild and discontinuous.

3. The pain may be atypically located when the appendix is not located in the right iliac area.

Both *mesenteric adenitis* and *nonspecific acute abdominal pain* can mimic appendicitis. It is very difficult for the physician to distinguish mesenteric adenitis from acute appendicitis by physical examination alone. **The value of serial abdominal examinations and serial laboratory tests, often performed in the hospital, cannot be overemphasized, particularly when the diagnosis is unclear.** With early inflammatory processes, there may be sufficient irritation to make the abdomen diffusely tender, but not enough to produce peritoneal irritation. In these instances, there may be no muscle guarding or rebound tenderness. In mesenteric adenitis, the white blood cell count is usually not elevated, the temperature may be high (even higher than in acute appendicitis), and there is often a history or physical findings of a previous viral or bacterial respiratory infection. Mesenteric adenitis may also follow viral gastroenteritis. In these cases, crampy, diffuse abdominal pain with nausea, vomiting, or diarrhea gradually changes to constant right lower quadrant pain.

One long-term study of patients with *recurrent abdominal pain* revealed organic causes in only 2 per cent, a finding that is not encouraging to the physician who is considering the possibility of early appendicitis. If there is a history of similar pain episodes and if the current episode subsides over 24 hours, the diagnosis of recurrent nonspecific abdominal pain is more likely. Until the diagnosis is clear, active serial observations are essential. Continued pain, tachycardia, anorexia, diarrhea, pain on movement, and especially rebound tenderness all warn that the pain is not nonspecific and that surgical intervention must be seriously considered. When the temperature, blood count, sedimentation rate, urinalysis, and stool examination for occult blood and ova and parasites are normal, recurrent nonspecific abdominal pain is most likely.

A bulge in the inguinal area or the presence of an undescended testicle suggests an *inguinal hernia*. A lump may be palpated either rectally or abdominally in infants with *intussusception*. When intussusception is ileocecal (most common), a lump may be palpated in the right upper quadrant or the epigastrium. Rectal examination classically reveals bloody mucus on the examining finger. The "currant jelly" stool of dark altered blood per rectum is a late sign of intussusception. A barium enema performed carefully not only may reveal the intussusception but also may alleviate it.

Palpation of fecal material in the colon and tenderness over the course of the colon suggest pain due to *obstipation*. A firm inspissated stool may be palpated rectally. This diagnosis is confirmed if an enema yields a large amount of stool and relieves the pain. Occasionally, an enlarged kidney is detected by palpation, suggesting hydronephrosis as the cause of abdominal pain.

Physical findings associated with abdominal pain due to *diabetic ketoacidosis* include Kussmaul's respirations, diffuse abdominal pain, and sweet, fruity breath. The presence of Kussmaul's respirations and the absence of shallow respiration, usually seen with peritonitis, also suggest diabetic ketoacidosis.

DIAGNOSTIC STUDIES

Many indications for diagnostic studies were reviewed earlier in this chapter. Studies useful in the differential diagnosis of abdominal pain include complete blood count with differential, erythrocyte sedimentation rate, abdominal radiographs, stool examination for occult blood, urinalysis, and urine culture and sensitivity. **Every child should have a blood sugar test and urinalysis prior to abdominal surgery. All black patients should have a sickle cell prep.** Frequent serial tests may be necessary with acute pain. In cases of recurrent abdominal pain, the tests should be repeated, but less frequently. **When recurrent abdominal pain is the chief complaint, when there are no additional symptoms that suggest organic disease, and when a thorough history and physical examination are negative, only simple**

diagnostic studies should be performed. In special instances, gastrointestinal barium studies, cholecystography, ultrasonography, intravenous pyelography, computed tomography, endoscopy, proctoscopy, and small bowel biopsy may be helpful.

LESS COMMON DIAGNOSTIC CONSIDERATIONS

Congenital intestinal obstruction, Hirschsprung's disease, duodenal atresia, midgut volvulus, and necrotizing enterocolitis may occur in the neonate. Abdominal distention, food refusal, and vomiting are commonly present in all these conditions. Likewise, radiographs are usually diagnostic. Neonates with Hirschsprung's disease fail to pass meconium. Many with duodenal atresia or midgut volvulus demonstrate visible gastric peristalsis.

A twisted ovarian cyst should be considered in cases of acute lower abdominal pain in girls. A mass ordinarily is palpable, but a thorough rectal examination may be difficult unless it is performed with the patient under general anesthesia. Ultrasonography may help detect an ovarian cyst. A history of mittelschmerz also suggests that the pain may be due to an ovarian cyst. In older girls, salpingitis and pelvic inflammatory disease must be considered whenever a fever is observed in association with lower abdominal pain. The fever is usually higher than that observed with appendicitis, and a vaginal discharge is usually present. If a Gram stain of the vaginal secretion reveals gonococci, the diagnosis is clear.

Complete or incomplete intestinal obstruction resulting from adhesions should be considered as a cause of abdominal pain in any patient with an abdominal scar. This pain is usually cramping and commonly accompanied by bilious vomiting. Physical examination may reveal abdominal distention, and distended loops of bowel occasionally may be identified clinically or radiographically. In the early phase, high-pitched tinkling bowel sounds may occur in rushes. If the obstruction continues, peristalsis becomes lower in pitch and less frequent.

Peptic ulceration and occasional perforation may develop in children experiencing major stress as the result of serious physical trauma (e.g., burns or severe head injuries). Unfortunately, diagnosis is frequently delayed because of the severity of the other associated problems. Peptic ulceration and perforation should be considered whenever there are abdominal symptoms in children who have suffered major stress. Upright or decubitus radiographs may demonstrate free air in the peritoneal cavity.

Gallstones are rare in children and are most likely to occur in those with hemolytic anemias. Abdominal pain may be the presenting complaint in children with lower lobe pneumonias. Children with migraine

DIFFERENTIAL DIAGNOSIS OF ABDOMINAL PAIN IN CHILDREN

CONDITION	NATURE OF PATIENT	NATURE OF PAIN	LOCATION OF PAIN	ASSOCIATED SYMPTOMS	PHYSICAL FINDINGS	DIAGNOSTIC STUDIES
Gastroenteritis	All ages	Crampy	Diffuse	Diarrhea Vomiting	Hyperperistalsis Low-grade fever	
Intussusception	Under 5 yr; peak incidence at 6 mo	Severe, crampy			Rushes of high-pitched peristalsis "Currant jelly" stools Walnut-size mass, palpated abdominally or rectally	Barium enema
Constipation	Any age; peak incidence at 5–12 yr	Recurrent, crampy (especially after meals)	Often RLQ		Feces in rectum Feces may be palpable in colon	Enema yields large amount of feces and relieves pain
Psychosomatic cause	Frequently 5–12 yr High-strung, perfectionist History of colic	Recurrent (3 or more episodes)		Psychological stress	Absence of systemic signs	Laboratory studies and radiographs within normal limits

Condition					
Appendicitis	Uncommon in young children Peak incidence 5–15 yr	Atypical in children Precedes anorexia and vomiting Worse with movement	Begins gradually in epigastrium or periumbilical area and progresses to a constant RLQ pain	Poor appetite	Serial examinations useful Fever Guarding persists when pain is not present Rebound in RLQ Decreased peristalsis	Leukocytosis Abdominal radiographs
Mesenteric adenitis	As in appendicitis	As in appendicitis	RLQ	Symptoms of recent URI Good appetite	No guarding when pain is not present Fever Similar to appendicitis	CBC with differential Lymphocytosis
Inflammatory bowel disease	Adolescence			Diarrhea	Growth failure Diffuse abdominal tenderness, often without rebound	Upper and lower GI radiographs Elevated ESR
Inguinal hernia			Lower quadrant	Undescended testicle Abdominal distention	Bulge in inguinal area	

headaches also may complain of abdominal pain. Lactose intolerance can cause recurrent abdominal pain in children and should be considered if the onset of pain coincides with heavy lactose ingestion. Before invasive procedures are performed or a psychogenic origin is assumed, a lactose-restricted diet should be attempted. Blunt, nonpenetrating abdominal trauma can cause rupture of the spleen, liver, intestines, or kidneys and result in abdominal pain. Crohn's disease should be considered in adolescents who have abdominal pain associated with weight loss, anemia, rectal bleeding, diarrhea, or passage of mucus per rectum. Acute pancreatitis, although rare in children, can be caused by trauma, viral infection (especially mumps), prolonged steroid therapy, or obstruction of the common bile duct due to a stone or an inflammatory process. Patients with this condition usually have marked nausea, vomiting, low-grade fever, and severe, constant upper abdominal pain radiating to the back. Allergies to foods and drugs occasionally cause abdominal pain. Lead poisoning should be suspected if there are paroxysms of diffuse abdominal pain alternating with constipation. A history of pica may or may not be obtained from the parents or patient.

Selected References

Galler, J. R., Neustein, S., and Walker, W. A.: Clinical aspects of recurrent abdominal pain in children. Adv. Pediatr. 27:31–53, 1980.

Gryskiewicz, J. M., and Huseby, T. L.: The pediatric abdominal examination. Postgrad. Med. 67:126–138, 1980.

Jones, P. F.: The acute abdomen in infancy and childhood. Practitioner 222:473–478, 1979.

Lake, A. M.: Acute abdominal pain in childhood—finding the cause. Postgrad. Med. 65:119–127, 1979.

Lebenthal, E. B.: Recurrent abdominal pain in childhood. Am. J. Dis. Child. 134:347–348, 1980.

Reynolds, S. L., and Jaffe, D. M.: Children with abdominal pain: evaluation in the pediatric emergency room. Pediatr. Emerg. Care 6:8–12, 1990.

Shrand, H.: Problems in family practice—acute abdominal pain in children. J. Fam. Pract. 2:131–134, 1975.

Stevenson, R. J.: Abdominal pain unrelated to trauma. Surg. Clin. North Am. 65:1181–1215, 1985.

Chapter 3

Backache

NATURE OF PATIENT

Backaches in children are relatively uncommon. **In young children, backache represents serious disease more often than in adults, although the most common cause of backache in children is lumbosacral strain.** This type of sprain usually results from participation in sports. A sprained back occasionally is caused by *trauma* (e.g., injuries suffered during a motor vehicle accident or during participation in gymnastics). Because low back pain may represent serious illness in children, a thorough history and physical examination should be performed. *Infection* should be a strong diagnostic consideration, especially in suspected intravenous drug users. *Spondylolisthesis* and *spondylolysis* occur more commonly in teenagers than in younger patients. In these patients, pain usually develops after strenuous athletic activity, and the cause can best be detected with appropriate radiographs.

Regardless of cause, backache is most common in patients between 20 and 50 years of age. It is more common in people who do heavy manual labor, such as industrial workers and farmers. In young adults who complain of persistent backache, *nonbacterial inflammatory disease,* such as *Reiter's syndrome* and *ankylosing spondylitis,* should be considered. It is particularly important for the examiner to ask these patients about other inflammatory changes that may be associated with Reiter's syndrome (e.g., iritis, pharyngitis, urethritis, and arthritis). Even if the patient has spondylolisthesis, it is important for the physician to rule out inflammatory causes of backache. *Postural backaches* are more common in multigravida patients and in individuals who are obese or otherwise in poor physical condition. *Herniated discs* occur in young adults but are relatively uncommon.

The number of backaches caused by *disc disease* increases as age increases from 25 to 50 years. Disc syndromes are more common in men, particularly older ones. In older patients, backache is a common symptom but not a common chief complaint. When it is the chief complaint in patients over 50 years of age, serious illness such as *cauda equina syndrome* must be considered, although the most common cause is *osteoarthritis of the lumbosacral spine*. It has been said that everyone eventually develops some degenerative joint disease in the low back, but as a rule, clinical problems arise only when this degeneration reaches a moderate degree. It is then usually preceded by some traumatic incident, possibly minor, that precipitates the onset of symptoms. **In patients over 50 years who present with backache without significant history of prior backaches, serious conditions such as cancer and multiple myeloma must be considered.**

NATURE OF SYMPTOMS

To determine the cause of backache, the physician must consider important historical factors such as age, location of pain, possible radiation of pain, effects of motion of back or leg, and previous trauma (Table 3–1).

The pain of *acute lumbosacral strain* is characterized by a sudden onset often related to turning, lifting, twisting, or unusual physical activity. It is usually well localized at the lumbosacral region.

The pain of a *musculoskeletal strain* and a *postural backache* is often described as dull and persistent and associated with stiffness. Patients have difficulty locating a precise point of maximum pain. After trauma, this pain may have an immediate or delayed onset. Patients may state that they felt something "give way." The pain typically radiates across the lower back and occasionally into the buttocks, but rarely into the lower extremity.

The low back pain of *degenerative lumbosacral arthritis* has a gradual onset, is not usually precipitated by physical activity, and is usually associated with a history of morning stiffness. Many patients with this condition complain that their lumbosacral motion is limited by pain and stiffness that is often worse in the morning but that improves an hour or so after arising. Radiation of pain to the knee, calf, or lower leg is uncommon.

Many patients with *herniated disc syndrome* have a history of previous, less severe episodes. The pain usually has a sudden onset and often radiates into the buttock, down the posterolateral aspect of the leg, and sometimes to the foot. The pain of a disc syndrome has been compared with a toothache—sharp, lancinating, radiating pain that may be associated with paresthesias and muscle weakness (caused by nerve root pressure). Remitting pain usually indicates a posterolateral disc protrusion, but an intermittent backache also can be caused by a disc that does not produce significant root irritation. More than 90 per cent

TABLE 3–1. Differential Features of Common Causes of Pelvic Girdle Pain

Cause	Site of Pain	Aggravating and Relieving Factors	Physical Findings	Other Findings
Degenerative disc disease with facet impingement	Buttock, posterior thigh	Worse with spinal extension; relieved by rest in fetal position	Restricted spinal movement, tender spinal segment	Radiographs abnormal
Degenerative disc disease with nuclear prolapse	Buttock, posterior thigh	Worse with spinal extension; relieved by rest in fetal position	Restricted spinal movement, tender spinal segment, nerve root dysfunction	Radiographs abnormal; prolapse shown on film
Sacroiliitis	Buttock, posterior thigh	Worse at rest; relieved with activity	Often associated restriction of spinal movement	Radiographs abnormal
Osteoarthritis of hip	Groin, occasionally buttock or knee	Worse with activity; relieved with rest	Restricted hip movement	Radiographs abnormal
Meralgia paresthetica	Lateral thigh paresthesia	Worse at night	Tenderness just below anterior superior iliac spine	Relieved by local infiltration of anesthetic and steroids
Trochanteric bursitis	Lateral thigh	Worse at night and with activity	Tenderness over greater trochanter	Relieved by local infiltration of anesthetic and steroids

(From Little, H.: Trochanteric bursitis. Can. Med. J. 120:456–458, 1979.)

of lumbar disc herniations occur at L4–L5 or L5–S1. If root irritation is present, neurologic findings (sensory loss, motor weakness, or hyporeflexia) are diagnostic. There also may be tenderness to palpation in the sciatic notch.

The qualitative characteristics of low back pain can be of considerable practical diagnostic importance. Variable, diffuse, and intense sensations of pressure often occur in patients without demonstrable organic disease. When the pain is described consistently and specifically, it is easier for the physician to demonstrate organic disease. If pain is related to posture, trauma, or overly strenuous activities; if it is episodic and intermittent; if it is aggravated by action; and if it is relieved by rest and recumbency, inflammatory disease (e.g., ankylosing spondylitis) and infectious processes (e.g., tuberculosis) are not likely.

Back pain in *sacroiliac syndromes* tends to be localized over the posterior superior iliac spine. In *sacroiliitis* (an inflammatory arthritis of the sacroiliac joints), the pain may alternate from side to side, although it is usually felt in the low back and buttocks, and may radiate into the posterior thigh.

Occasionally, low back pain may be a manifestation of the *irritable bowel syndrome*. In these cases, there often is associated midback pain, abdominal pain, and a history characteristic of an irritable colon. This pain does not radiate into the leg. The low back pain from *prostatitis* is usually a vague ache that is not affected by movement or coughing and is not associated with muscle spasm or limited mobility.

Rarely, the acute pain of *renal colic* presents with excruciating pain in the back rather than in the flank or groin. In these cases, there is a gradual shift in the location of pain to the flank with radiation into the groin. With renal colic, the straight leg–raising test usually is negative, and the urinalysis generally shows hematuria.

Some patients with *depression* may experience chronic low back pain. It is often described as diffuse, accompanied by a sensation of severe pressure. When somatic pain is a manifestation of depression, the severity of the pain varies with the mental state: Pain increases with anxiety and depression and often decreases with extreme fear. If an elderly patient describes a burning or aching back pain—particularly if the pain is described as superficial and unilateral—*herpes zoster* should be suspected, since this pain often precedes the herpetic skin lesions.

ASSOCIATED SYMPTOMS

With *osteoarthritis of the lumbar spine,* patients often have pain in other joints. Patients with *herniated disc syndrome* usually have neurologic symptoms such as sciatica, paresthesias, dysesthesias, hypoesthesias, anesthesias, paresis, sphincter problems, and impotence. **Pres-**

sure on the unmyelinated fibers may cause cauda equina syndrome, a rare surgical emergency whose signs include central back pain associated with weakness of the leg muscles, impotence, urinary frequency, urinary retention (sometimes with overflow), incontinence, saddle anesthesia, and loss of sphincter tone.

Low back pain that is associated with vaginal discharge suggests a *gynecologic* cause. In men, back pain associated with burning on urination, difficulty in urination, or fever suggests *prostatitis*. If herpes zoster is associated with back pain, underlying *cancer* should be strongly considered.

PRECIPITATING AND AGGRAVATING FACTORS

Acute lumbosacral strain usually is precipitated by lifting, twisting, unusual physical activity or position, or trauma. Many patients are older and overweight and have not been physically active. When acute lumbosacral strain occurs in athletes, it may be due to poor equipment, inadequate coaching, insufficient warm-up or conditioning, or any body position that unnecessarily exaggerates lordosis. Acute lumbosacral strain in adolescent athletes may be precipitated or aggravated during periods of rapid growth, since the soft tissues, ligaments, and musculotendinous units do not keep up with bone growth. Patients with acute lumbosacral strain experience pain with motion but not with coughing and straining. *Postural backaches* worsen as the day progresses.

In patients with *herniated disc syndrome,* pain can be precipitated by trauma or certain types of movement (particularly twisting in the bent back position, as when starting a lawn mower or outboard engine). Aging also facilitates the development of this syndrome; herniation of the nucleus pulposus is the result of degenerative changes that occur with aging of the disc. The pain of a disc syndrome may be exacerbated by coughing, laughing, straining at stool, sneezing, sitting, and lateral bending; in acute cases it may be aggravated by almost any activity that results in the movement of the lower back, particularly hyperextension. The pain caused by *degenerative lumbosacral arthritis* also may be increased by lateral bending and extension of the lumbar spine. Backaches that worsen during or just after menstruation suggest a *gynecologic* cause.

AMELIORATING FACTORS

Many patients with an *acute lumbosacral strain* state that lying prone and motionless relieves the pain. Most acute back pain, which is relieved by rest, is of mechanical origin. This can be a significant point in differential diagnosis if the malingerer, neurotic, or patient with strong secondary gain can be ruled out. Many patients with low back pain due to *osteoarthritis* state that their pain diminishes when they lie on the floor or on a firm mattress. Likewise, some patients with disc syndrome are relieved by lying down. This variable, therefore, is not a truly helpful factor in the differential diagnosis of low back pain. What is helpful is that some patients with *disc syndrome* inform the physician that they feel better when walking or lying on their sides with their knees flexed (fetal position). This latter finding strongly suggests that the pain is due to disc disease. If disc pain is unrelieved after 10 to 14 days of conservative nonoperative procedures (including rest), surgery may be required.

The back discomfort due to *irritable colon* may be relieved by defecation.

PHYSICAL FINDINGS

The following is an outline for a satisfactory examination of a patient presenting with low back pain. History should include a general medical, personal, sociologic, occupational, and sexual history. Special attention should be paid to previous backaches and factors that precipitate, aggravate, or ameliorate the pain, as well as to a history of trauma or heavy physical activity. **Physical examination should include a rectal and a pelvic evaluation, especially in patients over the age of 40 years and in those without a history or physical findings characteristic of the common causes of backache.** Particular attention should be paid to observations made during examination of the breast, prostate, thyroid, lymph nodes, and peripheral pulses. Any evidence of systemic inflammatory disease such as iritis, urethritis, or arthritis should be noted. Examination of the spine should include determination of range of motion anteriorly, posteriorly, and laterally.

Examination of the back also should include observation of the patient in the anatomic position, determination of range of motion of both the trunk and lumbar spine, cervical flexion with and without trunk flexion, and gait. With the patient sitting, knee and ankle reflexes should be checked, as should extension of each leg. The examiner also should determine the strength of dorsiflexion of toes and ankles, sensation to touch and pinprick in the lower extremity, and integrity of proprioception (Figs. 3–1 to 3–3) while the patient is in this position.

With the patient supine, five tests should be performed: straight leg–raising, Lasègue's compression (Fig. 3–4), bow string, knee compression, and pelvic pressure. The range of motion of hip joints must be established, and painful areas of extremities must be palpated. With the

Figure 3–1. Dermatomes of skin. (Reprinted with permission from *Medical Trial Technique Quarterly* [pp. 456–466, 1980 Annual], edited by Fred Lane, J. D., published by Callaghan & Co., 3201 Old Glenview Rd., Wilmette, IL 60091.)

	Lumbar				Sacral		
	2	3	4	5	1	2	3
Quadriceps Femoris		█	█				
Tibialis Anterior			█	█			
Extensor Digitorum Longus				█			
Extensor Hallucis Longus				█	█		
Tibialis Posterior			█	█	█		
Long Flexor of Toes				█	█	█	
Gastrocnemius & Soleus					█	█	
Hamstrings				█	█	█	
Gluteus Maximus				█	█	█	

Figure 3–2. Nerve supply of various muscles (the main nerve roots are shaded). (Reprinted with permission from *Medical Trial Technique Quarterly* [pp. 456–466, 1980 Annual], edited by Fred Lane, J. D., published by Callaghan & Co., 3201 Old Glenview Rd., Wilmette, IL 60091.)

Cremasteric
L1

Knee
(Patellar) L3, 4

Ankle (Tendo-Achilles)
S1, 2

Figure 3–3. Root origin of reflexes. (Reprinted with permission from *Medical Trial Technique Quarterly* [pp. 456–466, 1980 Annual], edited by Fred Lane, J. D., published by Callaghan & Co., 3201 Old Glenview Rd., Wilmette, IL 60091.)

Figure 3–4. Sciatic nerve stretch test. The examiner uses the Lasègue test to invoke pain down the leg by raising the limb with knee extended. If this fails to induce pain, compression of the posterior tibial nerve in the lateral popliteal space is painful if there is nerve root involvement, or pain may be provoked by sharp dorsiflexion of the foot (Bragard test). (From Jacobs, B.: American Family Physician Monograph, Oct. 1978, p. 13.)

patient prone, the spine should be palpated, as should the sacroiliac joints; the hips should be hyperextended and the knees flexed.

Physical findings in patients with *acute lumbosacral strain* usually are limited to the lower back, which demonstrates some limitation of motion. There may be local swelling and tenderness to palpation as well as spasm of the paraspinal muscles. The neurologic examination is negative, unlike in cases of herniated disc, with which there often are associated spasm of the hamstring muscles and neurologic findings in the lower leg. During palpation over the sciatic notch, there may be pain or tenderness with some radiation to the knee or upper calf, but sensory and motor examination is intact. Often there is an increase in the lumbar lordotic curve; this lumbar curve may change very little with bending. There frequently is limited range of motion of the lower back, particularly anteriorly and posteriorly, but not as much laterally. Although a straight leg–raising test may cause back pain, it does not induce pain with a sciatic distribution.

When *osteoarthritis* causes low back pain, there may be symmetrical restriction of movement, unlike in cases of *herniated disc,* which usually causes asymmetrical limitation of motion. There may be tenderness to palpation in the lumbosacral region or at L4, L5, or S1.

When low back pain results from a *disc syndrome,* the physical findings often are markedly different from those of a *lumbosacral strain* or *osteoarthritis.* Instead of increasing the lumbar lordotic curve, a disc syndrome usually reverses the lumbar curve, often with forward or lateral tilt or both. As with osteoarthritis and lumbosacral strain, there is limitation of spinal movement with a disc syndrome. The distinguishing features are the production of sciatic pain after hyperextension or lateral tilt and diminished or absent knee jerks in patients with disc syndrome. As with the other causes of low back pain, there may be spasm of the paraspinal muscles and tenderness to palpation in the sciatic notch.

Restricted straight leg–raising implies root irritation, and is suggestive, but not diagnostic, of a herniated disc. Positive crossed, straight leg–raising usually indicates a massive or central herniated disc or a mass lesion. The location of pain elicited by straight leg–raising often suggests the area of nerve root irritation. Pain in the back or lumbosacral region suggests a higher lesion than pain in the calf or along the distribution of the sciatic nerve. Another clue to a ruptured disc may be asymmetrical hamstring tightness.

Most patients with sciatic nerve root irritation, regardless of its cause, experience pain in the calf with straight leg–raising. They usually demonstrate a positive Lasègue sign as well.

Only seldom is a surgical emergency present in patients with herniated disc syndrome. **There are three basic factors that influence the outcome of pressure on a nerve root: the amount of pressure** on the nerve root, the duration of pressure, and the amount of myelin surrounding the nerve axon. Mild pressure with local edema and inflammation causes nerve root irritation with some pain and paresthesias. Stretching the root aggravates the pain, as is the case with a positive straight leg–raising or a Lasègue sign. With increased pressure there is impaired conduction, motor weakness, reflex diminution, and some sensory loss in addition to pain. Severe pressure produces marked motor paralysis, loss of reflexes, and anesthesia. Mild to moderate pressure for short periods of time is tolerated fairly well by myelinated fibers. Prolonged pressure, however, is poorly tolerated, particularly by minimally myelinated nerves. *If paralysis following compression of myelinated fibers persists for 24 hours, it may be irreversible.* Myelin protects nerves from compression; the central parasympathetic nerve fibers to sphincters, however, are unmyelinated. **Therefore, loss of sphincter tone or urinary retention is a surgical emergency. If pressure on these unmyelinated fibers is not relieved immediately, permanent damage may ensue.**

DIAGNOSTIC STUDIES

In patients with osteoarthritis or a mechanical cause of their low back pain, the erythrocyte sedimentation rate (ESR) and alkaline phosphatase level are within normal limits. The ESR is elevated in *multiple myeloma, infectious spinal disease,* and *ankylosing spondylitis.* The alkaline phosphatase level is elevated in patients with *Paget's disease.*

Plain radiography seldom is indicated in otherwise healthy patients, aged 20 to 50, who present with acute low back pain. Radiographic examination is normal or may show increased lumbar lordosis in patients with an acute lumbosacral or low back strain. When osteoarthritis causes low back pain, radiography frequently shows narrowing of the lumbar spaces with spurring and often sclerosis of the vertebrae. Radiography may assist in the diagnosis of compression fractures, cancer, Paget's disease, and multiple myeloma. Computed tomography scans (with or without contrast media) are helpful in locating herniated discs and spinal tumors.

LESS COMMON DIAGNOSTIC CONSIDERATIONS

Although most backaches are due to lumbosacral strain, disc disease, osteoarthritis, or postural backache, there are innumerable less common causes. Backaches can result from disease of almost any system, and have been classified as viscerogenic, vascular, neurogenic, psychogenic, spondylogenic, genitourinary, musculoskeletal, and secondary to metastatic or primary tumors of bone or soft tissue. They also may be due to functional-mechanical derangement in the musculoskeletal system, resulting from poor posture or obesity. Back pain in children is a rare complaint, and may have a serious, organic cause. In older patients in whom back pain is a major complaint, particularly if it is the first attack, it is necessary for the physician to consider serious diseases such as metabolic disorders (osteoporosis, osteomalacia, chondrocalcinosis, and Paget's disease), cancer, compression fractures, and infections.

Ankylosing spondylitis most often occurs in young to middle-aged males. It has an insidious onset and lasts at least 3 months. Classically, it is associated with marked morning stiffness. In contrast to more common causes of backache, ankylosing spondylitis is associated with a significantly elevated ESR and, rarely, with fever. There may be a family history of the same illness. Other joints may be involved, and the pain is frequently worse at night. The human leukocyte antigen (HLA) B27 test seldom is positive. Fifty per cent of patients with ankylosing spondylitis develop transient arthritis of larger peripheral joints; sometimes they develop conjunctivitis or urethritis.

Vertebral fractures (compression fractures) may occur with severe trauma or, more commonly, osteoporosis of the vertebrae in elderly patients. In these patients, vertebral fractures may occur following minor trauma. They also can occur after prolonged immobilization or steroid use. The back pain usually is at the level of the fracture and radiates locally across the back and around the trunk, but seldom into the lower extremities. Vertebral fractures occur more frequently in the middle and lower dorsal spine. Radiography is useful in confirming the diagnosis.

Infectious diseases of the spine, more common in children and intravenous drug users, also cause backaches. Many patients with such infections have an elevated ESR and may be febrile. An infectious cause of backache should be considered in cachectic individuals or patients undergoing prolonged steroid or immunosuppressive therapy. Uncommon causes of disc space infection include actinomycosis, tuberculosis, brucellosis, and fungal infections.

Neoplastic disease can cause backache, particularly in the elderly. Although primary neoplasms are rare, myeloma and metastatic disease are more common. In a patient with a known cancer, the onset of back pain should suggest spinal metastases. Metastatic carcinoma is more common in older patients, and should be particularly suspected if they have a history of cancer. There often is an insidious onset of a waist-level or midback pain that becomes progressively more severe and more persistent. The pain usually is unrelieved by lying down and frequently worsens at night. Unexplained weight loss with severe back pain aggravated by rest should suggest metastatic carcinoma in the spine. Multiple myeloma can cause severe, unremitting backaches; these are present at rest and may worsen with recumbency. This diagnosis can be confirmed

DIFFERENTIAL DIAGNOSIS OF BACKACHE

CONDITION	NATURE OF PATIENT	NATURE OF SYMPTOMS	ASSOCIATED SYMPTOMS	PRECIPITATING AND AGGRAVATING FACTORS	AMELIORATING FACTORS	PHYSICAL FINDINGS	DIAGNOSTIC STUDIES
Acute lumbosacral strain	*Adults (20–50):* especially those who do strenuous work *Children:* often due to trauma or sports	*Sudden onset* Pain usually localized to the lumbosacral region		Precipitated by lifting, twisting, unusual physical activity Aggravated by motion but not by coughing or straining	Lying prone and motionless	**Neurologic examination negative** Paraspinal muscle spasm and pain Straight leg-raising causes back but not leg pain Limitation of motion of lumbosacral spine region anteriorly and posteriorly Increased lumbar lordosis	Radiographs show increased lumbar lordosis

Condition	Age/Risk group	History	Associated features	Aggravating factors	Relieving factors	Examination	Radiograph
Postural backache (low back strain)	Obese, physically unfit adults	Vague low back pain Difficult to locate point of maximum pain Occasional radiation into buttocks		Worsens as day progresses		**Neurologic examination negative** Limitation of motion anteriorly and posteriorly Increased lumbar lordosis Straight leg–raising causes back pain, not leg pain	
Degenerative lumbosacral arthritis	>50 yr	Gradual onset, not precipitated by physical activity Lumbosacral spine motion limited Pain worse in morning Pain radiation into leg is uncommon	Often arthritis in other joints	Aggravated by lateral bending and extension of lumbar spine	Lying on back on floor Better 2 hr after arising	Symmetric restriction of movement **Neurologic examination negative**	Radiograph shows disc space narrowing and spurring

Table continued on following page

DIFFERENTIAL DIAGNOSIS OF BACKACHE Continued

CONDITION	NATURE OF PATIENT	NATURE OF SYMPTOMS	ASSOCIATED SYMPTOMS	PRECIPITAT-ING AND AG-GRAVATING FACTORS	AMELIO-RATING FACTORS	PHYSICAL FINDINGS	DIAGNOSTIC STUDIES
Lumbar disc disease	More common in males age 40 or older Rare in children	Sudden onset, previous less severe episodes Pain often radiates down posterolateral aspect of leg Buttock pain or paresthesia pain can be lancinating or like a severe toothache	Hypesthesia Dysesthesia Weakness of some leg muscles	Coughing Sneezing Hyperextension of lumbar spine	Lying on side with knees flexed	Neurologic signs in lower leg Asymmetrical limitation of motion Hamstring spasm Tender to palpation in sciatic notch Reversal of lumbar lordotic curve Forward or lateral tilt Pain of sciatic distribution after hyperextension or lateral tilt Restricted straight leg-raising	CT scan of spine MRI

Gynecologic disorders			Vaginal discharge	Worse around menstruation or ovulation	Lying supine with knees flexed	Abnormal pelvic examination	
Prostatitis	Older men	Constant low back pain	Urinary hesitancy	Change in sexual frequency		Prostate tender to palpation No limitation of motion of back No muscle spasm	WBCs in prostatic secretion
Irritable colon	Young women Stressed individuals	Pain occurs in midback	Mucus in stools Abdominal pain	Stress	Defecation	Colon tender to palpation	
Depression	Adults	Severity of pain varies with mental state Diffuse, pressurelike pain	Early morning wakefulness Fatigue Constipation Anorexia	"Loss"		Depressed affect	
Neoplasm (usually backache caused by metastases)	History of cancer, especially of breast and prostate First episode of backache occurs after age 50	Gradual onset of pain	Weight loss	May be worse lying down		Rectal, pelvic, or breast examination may reveal primary tumor	Radiograph and CT scan of spine MRI
Herpes zoster	Elderly	Burning superficial pain	Herpetic lesions appear after onset of pain			Herpetic vesicles	

with radiography of the spine, pelvis, and skull; elevated ESR; and abnormal serum protein electrophoretic patterns.

The back pain of *acute pancreatitis* is invariably associated with marked gastrointestinal symptoms. Chronic low-grade pancreatitis, however, may cause vague back pain without noticeable abdominal symptoms. Patients with posterior penetrating ulcers may present with pain in the high midback as their chief complaint. This pain usually is not in the lumbar area and occasionally is relieved by antacids. Frequently, there is tenderness to epigastric palpation. Pain can be referred to the back from the urinary tract, uterus, prostate, and retroperitoneal structures.

Spinal stenosis can cause central low back pain that may radiate into one or both legs. The pain has the character of intermittent claudication: the patient is forced to rest after walking one or two blocks. An important diagnostic feature is that the pain also is relieved by flexion of the spine. It may occur at night, and the patient may find relief by walking, especially in a stooped position.

Spondylolisthesis and spondylolysis occur infrequently in the general population but are common causes of back pain in growing individuals. These conditions are caused by repetitive flexion and extension forces, particularly in congenitally predisposed individuals. They are more common in gymnasts and in football linemen. The pain is severe, worse with activity, and relieved by rest. Diagnosis is confirmed by appropriate radiographic studies.

Selected References

Bernard, T. N., Jr., and Kirkaldy-Willis, W. H.: Recognizing specific characteristics of nonspecific low back pain. Clin. Orthop. *217*:266–280, 1987.

Bunnell, W. P.: Back pain in children. Orthop. Clin. North Am. *13*:587–604, 1982.

Clancy, W. G.: Low back pain in athletes. Am. J. Sports Med. *7(6)*:361–369, 1979.

Deyo, R. A.: Early diagnostic evaluation of low back pain. J. Gen. Intern. Med. *1*:328–338, 1986.

Grabias, S. L., and Markin, H. J.: Pain in the lower back. Bull. Rheum. Dis. *30(8)*:1040–1045, 1979, 1980.

Gunn, C. C., and Milbrandt, W. E.: Early and subtle signs in low-back pain. Spine *3(3)*:267–281, 1978.

Hoppenfeld, S.: Back pain. Pediatr. Clin. North Am. *24(4)*:881–887, 1977.

Kaushal, S. P.: The aching back—the history and physical examination. Med. Trial Tech. Q. *26(4)*:456–466, 1980.

Kirkaldy-Willis, W. H.: Five common back disorders: how to diagnose and treat them. Geriatrics *33*:32–41, 1978.

Quinet, R. J., and Hadler, N. M.: Diagnosis and treatment of backache. Semin. Arthritis Rheum. *8(4)*:261–287, 1979.

Svara, C. J., and Hadler, N. M.: Back pain. Clin. Geriatr. Med. *4*:395–410, 1988.

Belching, Bloating, and Flatulence

In this chapter, *belching* is defined as the eructation of gas through the mouth; *bloating* is gaseous abdominal distention; and *flatulence* is the passage of intestinal gas per rectum.

BELCHING

Belching is not a symptom of organic disease. There is only one cause of belching, which is swallowing of air (*aerophagia*). Air is swallowed or, more accurately, sucked into the stomach and released in the form of a belch. Air-swallowing may occur with eating or drinking; more air is swallowed with liquids than with solids. Aerophagia also occurs as a conscious or, more often, as an unconscious nervous habit unassociated with food ingestion. It also can be associated with mouth-breathing, gum-chewing, orthodontic appliances, and ill-fitting dentures. Chronic, repetitive, "unintentional" belching usually is caused by repetitive inhalation of air and regurgitation of it from the stomach or esophagus in the form of a belch. Some patients who demonstrate these findings consciously or unconsciously relax the upper esophageal sphincter during inspiration.

NATURE OF PATIENT

Excessive belchers tend to be nervous, anxious, and tense. Belching often is normal in infants, although excessive belching may be the result of excessive air-swallowing during feeding. If there is an inadequate seal of the infant's lips around the real or artificial nipple, air may be ingested during nursing. This may be exaggerated if, during feeding, the child is held in a position that is too horizontal.

In some instances, patients with gastric or biliary disorders develop a habit of trying to relieve abdominal discomfort by swallowing (sometimes unconsciously) air and belching it up again; they believe that this provides some relief of their abdominal discomfort.

If associated pathology can be confidently ruled out, patients must be reassured that nothing serious is wrong. It may help to describe how a patient with a laryngectomy can be trained to swallow air; accordingly, a patient with a belching problem can be untrained. Simply instructing some patients not to belch when they feel the urge to do so may gradually stop their habit of swallowing air and belching it back. The use of antifoaming agents has not been shown to be particularly helpful. Rather, patients should be instructed to avoid chewing gum, eating quickly, smoking, and drinking carbonated beverages.

ASSOCIATED SYMPTOMS

The most common associated symptom is abdominal distention, representing gas in the stomach. Most swallowed air that is not belched up is reabsorbed in the small intestine. Usually, intestinal gas is derived by fermentation of intestinal contents. Some patients who swallow large amounts of air may experience or perceive abdominal discomfort until they belch. An urge to belch accompanied by chest pain on belching is a rare finding that may indicate an inferior wall myocardial infarction.

PRECIPITATING AND AGGRAVATING FACTORS

The most common precipitating factor is air-swallowing and subsequent relaxation of the esophageal sphincter to produce a belch. Nervous concern about belching can initiate a vicious cycle of unconscious air-swallowing and more belching. For some individuals, a supine position prevents swallowed gastric air from escaping into the esophagus, and an upright position facilitates belching. *Emotional stress* increases the likelihood of air-swallowing.

DIAGNOSTIC STUDIES

Although belching is invariably caused by swallowing air, this does not rule out coexisting unrelated pathology. If other symptoms warrant it, cholecystography, upper GI studies, and chest radiography should be considered.

LESS COMMON DIAGNOSTIC CONSIDERATIONS

Rarely, there is oral eructation of intestinal gas. In these instances, the odor is offensive, resembling that of methane or hydrogen sulfide. This suggests fermentation in stagnating gastric contents secondary to pyloric obstruction from ulcer, tumor, or previous vagotomy.

BLOATING AND FLATULENCE

Bloating and flatulence are two common complaints reported to physicians. The problem has been recognized since the time of Hippocrates, who taught that "passing gas is necessary to well-being." In the days of early Rome, it was noted that "all Roman citizens shall be allowed to pass gas whenever necessary." Because swallowed air is reabsorbed in the small bowel, most of the gas in the distal small bowel and colon is produced within the bowel by fermentation. In most instances, flatulence is not of any clinical significance, but because various pathologic conditions may be associated with it, their presence should be investigated if the flatulence is excessive.

Flatulence is usually caused by excessive production of gas in an otherwise normal individual or increased discomfort from normal amounts of abdominal gas in healthy individuals. If bloating and flatulence have persisted for several years without the development of signs of serious organic pathology (e.g., weight loss, ascites, or jaundice), the patient can be reassured that the flatulence is not of great clinical significance. It must always be remembered, however, that some patients with *gallbladder disease, colon carcinoma, diverticulitis,* and *diverticulosis* may present with a chief complaint of abdominal discomfort, bloating, and occasionally flatulence. Patients with colon carcinoma may present with vague abdominal discomfort or distention.

NATURE OF PATIENT

Flatulence is particularly common in infants up to age 3 months. This is referred to as "3-month colic" and is due to immature nervous control of the gut, which permits gas to become trapped in bowel loops. *Malabsorption* may lead to excessive fermentation of unabsorbed nutrients; this may produce an increase in flatulence. This can occur in patients with pancreatic insufficiency, pancreatic carcinoma, biliary disease, celiac disease, or bacterial overgrowth in the small intestine. A patient, particularly of African or Mediterranean descent, complaining of excess bloating or flatulence may have malabsorption and subsequent fermentation due to an *inherited lactose intolerance.* This diagnosis is confirmed if diarrhea develops or if the bloating or flatulence is exacerbated after ingestion of a lactose load (found in milk, ice cream, or other dairy products). Flatulence also may be seen in patients with *diverticulitis* or *diverticulosis*.

NATURE OF SYMPTOMS

Most gas that passes from the rectum has an unpleasant, foul odor. The gases that cause this odor are produced by intestinal bacteria. Because of their odor, these gases are detectable in minute quantity.

ASSOCIATED SYMPTOMS

Flatulence, of no clinical significance, may be associated with abdominal distention, bloating, borborygmi, abdominal discomfort, and cramping pain. When flatulence or bloating occurs, moderate abdominal pain may be associated, even in the absence of organic disease. Patients may be unable to obtain relief by passing flatus. In some individuals, this is due to disordered motility of the gut; it cannot propel the gas forward through the bowel. This is not due to an increased volume of gas, but to the patient's inability to propel the gut gas forward. Some individuals have an exaggerated pain response to bowel distention despite a normal volume of intestinal gas. *Diverticulitis* should be suspected if flatulence is accompanied by lower abdominal pain, constipation, or diarrhea. *Giardiasis* should be suspected as the cause of flatulence, particularly if it is accompanied by foul-smelling, watery, or semisolid stools or abdominal distention.

PRECIPITATING AND AGGRAVATING FACTORS

The symptoms of bloating and flatulence are exacerbated by the ingestion of unabsorbable carbohydrates; these provide a substrate for the intestinal bacterial production of carbon dioxide and hydrogen. Constipation may also aggravate the symptoms of abdominal distention. This can be explained by the increased smooth muscle spasm in the colon around the gas bubbles. **Although constipation may aggravate abdominal bloating, diarrhea usually does not relieve such distention.**

Many patients with *gas entrapment syndromes* experience a worsening of the pain when bending over to tie their shoes or when wearing a tight garment. Occasionally, this pain is exacerbated by flexion of the leg on the abdomen.

AMELIORATING FACTORS

Factors that may be associated with decreasing symptoms are diets low in undigestable carbohydrates or in lactose, failure of the patient to recline after meals, exercise, and ingestion of buttermilk or broad-spectrum antibiotics. Passage of flatus often relieves the sensation of abdominal bloating, at least temporarily. Any abdominal pain syndrome that is markedly relieved by passage of flatus should suggest gas entrapment.

PHYSICAL FINDINGS

When gas is trapped in the splenic flexure, palpation of the left upper quadrant can cause abdominal pain or pain in the chest ("pseudoangina"). With hepatic-flexure gas entrapment, the pain most frequently is in the right upper quadrant, and gallbladder discomfort may be simulated.

DIAGNOSTIC STUDIES

The physician should consider the following studies when appropriate: upper and lower gastrointestinal radiographic examination, proctosigmoidoscopy, cholecystography, and stool analysis for fat and occult blood. If these tests do not reveal organic disease, the patient should be reassured, and dietary modification recommended. Likewise, a diagnostic trial of a lactose load can be used to determine, presumptively, if a lactase deficiency is present. If this exacerbates bloating, flatulence, or diarrhea, the patient should avoid foods with lactose.

More complicated tests can be performed, such as D-xylose absorption, mucosal biopsy, and the analysis of flatus for the volume and composition of the various intestinal gases. Large quantities of carbon dioxide or hydrogen suggest malabsorption and fermentation of unabsorbable carbohydrates such as fruits and beans. Lactase deficiency also can lead to excessive quantities of hydrogen in the flatus. Flatulogenic foods include milk, onions, dry beans, celery, carrots, raisins, bananas, apricots, prune juice, apple juice, pretzels, bagels, wheat germ, brussel spouts, and ice cream. There is a tremendous individual variation with regard to the flatulogenic properties of these foods.

LESS COMMON DIAGNOSTIC CONSIDERATIONS

Incomplete or intermittent bowel obstruction, malabsorption syndromes, small bowel diverticula, maldigestion due to pancreatic or

DIFFERENTIAL DIAGNOSIS OF BELCHING, BLOATING, AND FLATULENCE

CONDITION	NATURE OF PATIENT	NATURE OF SYMPTOMS	ASSOCIATED SYMPTOMS	PRECIPITATING AND AGGRAVATING FACTORS	AMELIORATING FACTORS	PHYSICAL FINDINGS	DIAGNOSTIC STUDIES
Belching Aerophagia	Nursing infants Nervous, anxious, and tense children and adults	Occurs with eating or drinking Conscious or unconscious nervous habit	Abdominal distention	In infants: nursing while in a position that is too horizontal Mouth-breathing Gum-chewing Orthodontic appliances Emotional stress Ill-fitting dentures Supine position Gastric or biliary disorders	Behavior modification: Avoidance of gumchewing, eating quickly, smoking, and drinking carbonated beverages Upright position	Those of gas in stomach	
Bloating and Flatulence Excessive intestinal bacterial fermentation causing increased gas Increased awareness of normal amount of gas	Most common cause at any age, especially in elderly adults	Flatulence Bloating	Abdominal discomfort or pain	Ingestion of nonabsorbable carbohydrates	Avoidance of all carbohydrates, particularly the nonabsorbable ones Passage of flatus		

Malabsorption	Patients with pancreatic insufficiency, pancreatic carcinoma, biliary disease, celiac disease, and bacterial overgrowth in the small intestine	Increased flatulence	Diarrhea	Nonabsorbable carbohydrates		Greasy, foul-smelling stools	Stool analysis GI radiographs
Lactase deficiency	Common in patients of African or Mediterranean descent	Bloating Excess flatulence	Diarrhea	Lactose load (i.e., from dairy products)	Avoidance of lactose Lactase supplement		Mucosal biopsy Lactose load
Giardiasis	Campers and hikers at higher risk	Increased flatulence	Abdominal distention Watery diarrhea, often foul-smelling	Drinking water infected with *Giardia*			Stool analysis for *Giardia* Duodenal aspirate for *Giardia*
Gas entrapment Splenic flexure			"Pseudoangina"	Abdominal pain worsened by bending or wearing tight garments	Passage of flatus	LUQ pain on palpation Pain worsened by flexion of left leg on abdomen	Fluoroscopy for trapped gas
Hepatic flexure			Pain resembling gallbladder discomfort		Passage of flatus	RUQ pain on palpation Pain worsened by flexion of right leg on abdomen	

biliary disease, and short bowel syndrome may cause bloating or flatulence.

Selected References

Bond, J. H., and Levitt, M. D.: Gaseousness and intestinal gas. Med. Clin. North Am. 62:155–164, 1978.

Bouchier, I. A. D.: Flatulence. The Practitioner 224:373–377, 1980.

Hightower, N. C.: Intestinal gas and gaseousness. Clin. Gastroenterol. 6:597–606, 1977.

Levitt, M. D., and Bond, J. H.: Flatulence. Annu. Rev. Med. 31:127–137, 1980.

Raskin, J. B.: Intestinal gas. Geriatrics 38(12):77–93, 1983.

Van Ness, M. M., and Cattau, E. L.: Flatulence: pathophysiology and treatment. Am. Fam. Physician 31:198–208, 1985.

Chapter 5

Breast Lumps

Over their lifetime most women will detect a lump in their breasts. Most of these lumps are benign cysts, but current studies report that 1 out of 10 women will develop carcinoma of the breast, and about 50% of these women will die of their disease. Therefore, it is crucial to be able to separate benign from malignant lesions. Benign breast disease is a continuum from entities such as fibroadenoma and cysts with atypia to cystic changes with marked atypia. Breast cancer is the second most common cancer in women, having recently been passed in frequency by lung cancer. **Breast cancer is the most common cause of death in women aged 40 to 50.** The most common breast lesions are *fibrocystic breasts, fibroadenomas, breast cancer, mastitis,* especially in lactating women, *fat necrosis,* and *gynecomastia,* which, by definition, occurs only in males. Breast lumps are common, and occur in as many as 50 per cent of premenopausal women. Most of these lumps are benign, but because breast cancer is part of the differential, this is a problem of great concern. The following definitions were offered by Grady and coworkers (1988): Breast lumps are masses in the breast noted on physical examination and may be either benign or malignant. Benign breast disease is a pathologic diagnosis and should be applied in most instances to masses that have undergone tissue sampling. It includes fibrocystic disease, fibroadenoma, and uncommon conditions such as mastitis, lipoma, traumatic fat necrosis, and galactocele. At biopsy, 90 to 95 per cent of all benign breast disease is fibrocystic disease or fibroadenoma. Fibrocystic disease is an ill-defined group of pathologic breast lesions that includes cysts, fibrosis, adenosis, duct ectasia, hyperplasia, and papilloma.

NATURE OF PATIENT

Benign breast disease is common in women under age 30. Of these women with benign breast disease, 45 per cent have fibrocystic disease, whereas about 45 per cent have fibroadenomas. After age 30, 85 per cent of those with benign breast disease have fibrocystic breasts and 10 per cent have fibroadenomas. In other words, fibroadenomas become less common with increasing age. Breast cysts are uncommon in elderly patients, but when they occur, 50 per cent of the patients are using estrogen supplements.

Users of oral contraceptives have a lower incidence of breast cancer. Factors that increase the risk for breast cancer include a mother or sister who had breast cancer, early menarche, late menopause, and nulliparity. There is twice the risk of breast cancer in patients whose mother or sister had breast cancer and three times the risk if both mother and sister had breast cancer. There also is a rare genetic type of familial breast cancer that appears to be inherited as an autosomal dominant. Other factors that increase the risk for breast cancer include age greater than 50, first pregnancy after age 35, obesity, and benign proliferative breast disease (ductal and lobular hyperplasia or atypia).

Gynecomastia is normal in the neonatal period, during puberty, and in older males. It occurs in certain familial syndromes and various pathologic states (cirrhosis and prolactinoma) and among users of many drugs. Gynecomastia in neonates is not uncommon and is probably related to the high levels of estrogen in the placental and fetal circulation. In neonatal gynecomastia, there usually is bilateral involvement, and fluid occasionally may be expressed from the nipple. Forty per cent of pubertal boys (ages 13–14) develop gynecomastia. When it is bilateral and mild, it may be diagnosed by the physician, but it is not recognized by the patient or his family unless it is marked. Unilateral gynecomastia is a more frequent patient complaint.

NATURE OF SYMPTOMS

Fibroadenoma is the most common breast lump that occurs during adolescence, but because it is asymptomatic, it usually is detected on physical examination by the patient or her physician. These lumps usually are single, unilateral, and located in the upper outer quadrant, although they may be multiple or bilateral in 25 per cent of patients. Fibroadenomas do not vary in size with the menstrual cycle, while the lumps of fibrocystic breast disease often enlarge premenstrually.

ASSOCIATED SYMPTOMS

Pain in the breast (mastodynia) in young women suggests fibrocystic disease, especially if the pain is bilateral and increases premenstrually. **Pain in one breast in postmenopausal women is highly suggestive**

of a malignant process. Cyclic breast pain that increases premenstrually suggests a benign condition, especially fibrocystic breast disease. Mastodynia also may be caused by papillomas, sclerosing adenosis, duct ectasia, sporadic puerperal mastitis, breast lipomas, traumatic fat necrosis, and galactoceles. Other causes of chest wall pain include pectoral or intercostal muscle sprain, mastitis, costochondral separation or costochondritis.

If the lump is fixed to the skin, or if there is associated nipple discharge, or axillary adenopathy, cancer is probable.

Although nipple discharge—particularly a bloody one—suggests cancer, it occasionally occurs with fibrocystic disease and in males with adrenogenital syndrome.

PRECIPITATING AND AGGRAVATING FACTORS

Risk factors for breast cancer have been discussed earlier in this chapter. The pain and tenderness of fibrocystic breasts often worsens during the premenstrual period. Gynecomastia is exacerbated by several drugs, including marijuana, spironolactone, methyldopa, phenytoin, cimetidine, and digitalis. Fat necrosis may be precipitated by external trauma as well as surgical trauma.

AMELIORATING FACTORS

A reduction in cyst size and decreased pain occur in patients with fibrocystic breast disease when they become menopausal. Oral contraceptives, pregnancy, and reduction in the ingestion of methylxanthines contained in coffee, tea, cola, and chocolate also often alleviate the symptoms of fibrocystic disease.

PHYSICAL EXAMINATION

Fibroadenomas usually are unilateral and occur in the upper, outer quadrant. They usually present as a smooth, oval, occasionally irregular, 3- to 4-cm firm to elastic lump that is freely movable. Fibrocystic disease usually is bilateral, symmetrical, with multiple, tender, soft or cystic round lumps that have regular borders. They occasionally are single or unilateral. In contrast, malignant breast lumps are typically hard, irregular, fixed and associated with a nipple lesion or discharge, adenopathy, and occasionally pain.

All suspicious lesions must be biopsied to obtain histologic

DIFFERENTIAL DIAGNOSIS OF BREAST LUMPS

CONDITION	NATURE OF PATIENT	NATURE OF SYMPTOMS	ASSOCIATED SYMPTOMS	PRECIPITATING AND AGGRAVATING FACTORS	AMELIORATING FACTORS	PHYSICAL EXAMINATION	DIAGNOSTIC STUDIES
Fibroadenoma	Usually 20–40 yr old, rare in postmeno-pausal women unless taking estrogen	Usually asymp-tomatic	May enlarge, es-pecially during adolescence and pregnancy			Usually solitary; multiple or bi-lateral in 15%–25%. Firm, mo-bile, smooth, rubbery	Mammography, biopsy
Fibrocystic breasts	Frequency in-creases with age and peaks around meno-pause, then resolves	Cyclic breast pain especially around men-struation. Usu-ally bilateral	Rare nipple dis-charge that usually is not bloody	Pain and tender-ness worsen pre-menstrually	Menopause; reduc-tion in ingestion of methylxan-thines found in tea, coffee, cola and chocolate Oral contraceptives	Multiple tender breast lumps usually bilat-eral and in up-per outer quad-rants Occasionally sin-gle or unilat-eral	Mammography, ultrasonog-raphy

Cancer	Usually greater than age 40; common (1 in 10)	Usually none until late in disease	Occasional pain in one breast when patient is postmenopausal. Bloody nipple discharge, axillary adenopathy	Increased incidence if mother and/or sister had breast cancer; early menarche; late menopause; greater than age 50; nulliparous	Decreased incidence in users of oral contraceptives	Lump is hard, irregular, fixed	Mammography, biopsy
Fat necrosis	Older; more common in large pendulous breasts	Painful, tender to palpation		Trauma; surgical trauma		Firm, solitary, irregular, may be attached to skin	
Gynecomastia	Males, especially pubertal and elderly, alcoholics	Breast enlargement, unilateral or bilateral; often tender	Adrenogenital syndrome	Drugs; estrogens, oral and topical; marijuana; spironolactone, methyldopa, phenytoin, cimetidine, digitalis			

diagnosis even though mammography is negative and not all of the typical findings of cancer are present.

Gynecomastia usually is unilateral but may be bilateral. The lumps of fat necrosis usually are firm, solitary, and irregular and may be attached to the overlying skin.

DIAGNOSTIC STUDIES

Various organizations have different recommendations for mammography. Generally it is recommended that mammography be performed yearly after age 50. At least one mammogram should be done between ages 35 and 40 but more frequently in patients at greater than usual risk, such as those with a mother or sister or both with a history of breast carcinoma. Fine-needle aspiration, fine-needle biopsy, and excisional biopsy are all useful techniques for determining the histologic character of a breast lump. Biopsies are indicated in instances where the mammogram suggests cancer or a suspicious lesion is palpable on physical examination. Mammographic signs of cancer include (1) irregularity of the mass, (2) mass appears smaller on mammogram than on physical examination, (3) nipple retraction, (4) increased stromal density on sequential examinations, and (5) calcification appearing on the mammogram. Biopsy should be performed on all suspicious lesions to obtain a histologic diagnosis. Because mammograms can miss 10 to 15 per cent of lesions, biopsies should be performed on any suspicious mass that is palpable on physical examination. Ultrasound examination is helpful in differentiating cystic from solid lesions.

LESS COMMON DIAGNOSTIC CONSIDERATIONS

Less common causes of benign breast lumps include papillomas, sclerosing adenosis, duct ectasia, lobular neoplasia, and apocrine metaplasia. Solitary papillomas are the most common benign cause of nipple discharge and bleeding. They usually are unilateral and located in the subareolar region. They most commonly occur in perimenopausal women. There is no increased cancer risk. In contrast, multiple papillomas increase cancer risk fourfold and most commonly occur in premenopausal women. In instances of multiple papillomas, nipple discharge is rare. They are bilateral in 25 per cent of the cases and occur distal to the nipple.

Duct ectasia results from ductal dilatation and stasis of ductal contents with a subsequent inflammatory reaction. It often is associated with nipple discharge and, occasionally, ductal calcification. In women over age 55, nipple discharge is most often due to ectasia, athough one-third of the patients with nipple discharge have a ductal papilloma.

Mondor's disease is a superficial thrombophlebitis of the anterolateral portion of the breast and chest wall. It may occur spontaneously or secondary to injury or surgery. The skin may be retracted along the course of the thrombosed vein. Sporadic puerperal mastitis seldom occurs in lactating mothers, and may result in a breast abscess presenting as a lump. Fever, chills, and tenderness usually are associated.

Selected References

Eddy, D. M.: Screening for breast cancer. Ann. Intern. Med. *11*:389–399, 1989.

Grady, D., Hodgkins, M. L., and Goodson, W. H. III: The lumpy breast. West. J. Med. *149*:226–229, 1988.

Greydanus, D. E., Parks, D. S., and Farrell, E. G.: Breast disorders in children and adolescents. Pediatr. Clin. North Am. *36*:601–638, 1989.

Hendler, F. J.: Southwestern Internal Medicine Conference: breast disease and the internist. Am. J. Med. Sci. *293*:332–347, 1987.

Hutchins, L. F., Broadwater, R., Jr., Lang, N. P., Maners, A., Bowie, M., and Westbrook, K. C.: Breast cancer. Dis. Mon. *36*:63–125, 1990.

Leung, A. K.: Gynecomastia. Am. Fam. Physician *39*:215–222, 1989.

Scott, E. B.: Fibrocystic breast disease. Am. Fam. Physician *36*:119–126, 1987.

Winchester, D. P.: Evaluation and management of breast abnormalities. Cancer *66*:1345–1347, 1990.

Chapter 6

Chest Pain

Chest pain is one of the most common complaints of adult patients. Regardless of whether they admit it, they are usually concerned that this pain is due to some type of cardiac disease. Therefore, the physician must be thoroughly familiar with the differential diagnosis of chest pain. Although the physician must realize that it is in the patient's interest not to overlook any acute cardiac illness, it is just as essential that cardiac disease not be incorrectly diagnosed or inferred, since such misdiagnosis may cause some patients to become "iatrogenic cardiac cripples."

Common causes of chest pain include *angina pectoris; myocardial infarction;* musculoskeletal chest wall conditions, including *costochondritis, benign overuse myalgia, fibrositis,* and *referred pain; trauma; cervicodorsal arthritis; psychoneurosis; esophagitis; esophageal spasm; pleuritis;* and *mitral valve prolapse* (Table 6–1). Less common causes of chest pain include *lung tumors, gas entrapment syndromes, pulmonary hypertension, pulmonary embolus,* and *pericarditis*. Persons with biliary disease, including *cholelithiasis, cholecystitis,* and *common duct stones*, may also present with pain in the chest.

NATURE OF PATIENT

Chest pain due to coronary artery disease is least likely in young people. In children, chest pain is most likely to be due to *musculoskeletal system trauma* (e.g., myositis or costochondritis) or an *inflammatory disease* (e.g., pleurisy). When pain similar in quality to angina pectoris occurs in a child or adolescent, *peptic esophagitis, mitral valve prolapse,* or *cocaine abuse* should be suspected. Rarely, children with congenital anomalies of the coronary arteries may have ischemic pain. Although *pulmonary embolism* is uncommon in children, it should be suspected in any postoperative, immobilized, or bedridden patient. Likewise, females

61

TABLE 6–1. Noncardiac Causes of Chest Pain

Resembles Angina Slightly	Not Typical of Angina
Psychoneurosis*	Psychoneurosis*
Pulmonary hypertension*	Costochondritis
Esophagitis and esophagospasm*	Nonspecific myositis
	Radiculitis
	Cervicodorsal arthritis
	Bursitis
	Shoulder disease
	Pericarditis
	Pneumonia
	Aneurysm
	Gastrointestinal distention with gaseous entrapment*
	Peptic ulcer
	Gallbladder disease*
	Diaphragmatic or paraesophageal hernia*

*Relieved by nitroglycerin
From Seller, R. H. *In* Rakel, R. E., and Conn, H. F.: Family Practice. 2nd ed. Philadelphia, W. B. Saunders Co., 1978.

of any age are at increased risk for pulmonary embolism if they are taking oral contraceptives.

In an adult population, all causes of chest pain may occur. Some patients experience chest wall pain after *aortocoronary bypass* using internal mammary grafts. In older patients, *coronary artery disease, cervicodorsal arthritis, tumors, esophagitis,* and *pulmonary embolism* are the most common causes.

NATURE OF PAIN

Although it is important for the physician to differentiate chest pain of cardiac origin from other types of pain, it is not sufficient to establish whether or not the pain is of cardiac origin. Patients with pain of cardiac origin should receive varying forms of therapy and will have a different prognosis, depending on whether their pain was due to *angina pectoris, Prinzmetal's angina, hypertrophic cardiomyopathy, mitral valve prolapse,* or *pericarditis.* An accurate diagnosis usually can be made by a precise history. In eliciting the history of chest pain, the examiner should note five specific characteristics of the discomfort: the location of pain, the quality of pain, the duration of pain, the factors that precipitate or exacerbate the pain, and ameliorating factors.

The distinctive clinical characteristics of *angina pectoris* are that the pain is paroxysmal (lasting 30 seconds to a few minutes), dull, pressing, squeezing, or aching; it is located substernally; and it may radiate to the precordium, upper extremities, neck, or jaw. The term

anginal salute refers to the way patients hold a clenched fist ov
sternum to describe their pain. Some anginal patients experience no
chest pain, but only neck, arm, or jaw discomfort. The location of pain
in patients with angina pectoris may vary a great deal from person to
person, but it differs little with recurrent episodes in the same patient.
Thus, if the patient complains of chest pain in different locations during
separate episodes, the pain is probably not due to angina pectoris. Pain
of biliary tract or esophageal origin is likely to be substernal, whereas
the pain of pericarditis is likely to be precordial.

Patients with angina pectoris describe their pain as a tightness,
pressure, or heaviness, and, infrequently, as a burning sensation. Burning is relatively uncommon; if present, it suggests the possibility of
peptic esophagitis, the most frequent imitator of coronary artery disease.
**Rarely, if ever, is anginal pain described as knifelike, sharp, or
sticking. Although some patients describe the pain as "sharp,"
they usually mean that it is severe in intensity rather than knifelike
in quality.** The pain of *pulmonary hypertension,* which often occurs in
patients with mitral stenosis or primary pulmonary disease, may be
indistinguishable from the pain of *angina pectoris.* It is usually described
as a dull, pressing, substernal pain, precipitated by exertion, and relieved
by rest or administration of nitroglycerin. Although this pain may
radiate to either arm, it radiates more commonly to the right arm. It
must be recognized that patients with pulmonary hypertension and
coronary artery disease may experience chest pain as a result of pulmonary hypertension, coronary artery disease, or both.

Dull, achy, or burning chest pain also may be experienced by
patients with *peptic esophagitis* or *esophagospasm, pulmonary hypertension, cervicodorsal arthritis, gallbladder disease, diaphragmatic* or *para-
esophageal hernias,* and *mitral valve prolapse.* In these cases the associated exacerbating or ameliorating factors are most helpful in
establishing the diagnosis.

Sharp, sticking pains, especially if only of a few seconds duration,
are more characteristic of *psychoneurosis, costochondritis, cervicodorsal
arthritis, mitral valve prolapse, chest wall syndrome, pericarditis,* and
pleuritic processes. The location of the pain usually is not helpful in
differentiating the cause of the chest pain in these conditions, with a
few exceptions. Pain on the side of the chest, particularly if it is
exacerbated by respiration, is more likely to be pleuritic. Pain localized
to the costochondral junction or specific intercostal spaces is most likely
due to *costochondritis* or *intercostal myositis.* The pain of *chest wall
syndrome* may occur during exercise or at rest; occasionally, it is
nocturnal. The pain not uncommonly is described as "sticking," but it
may also be described as "dull" and "pressing." The most critical finding
in the diagnosis of chest wall syndrome is detection of chest wall
tenderness on physical examination. It frequently is located substernally,

at the left parasternal region, near the shoulder, and in the fourth or fifth left intercostal space (Fig. 6–1).

The presence of cervicodorsal arthritis or reflux esophagitis does not rule out the possibility that chest pain is due to coronary disease. Patients may have two conditions, each of which contributes to their chest pain. For example, a patient may have pain due to esophagitis as well as pain due to angina pectoris. Not uncommonly, when two conditions coexist the patient may be able to distinguish between the two types of chest pain. For instance, if questioned carefully, a patient may describe a dull substernal pain often induced by exercise and relieved by nitroglycerin but not antacids as well as another dull substernal pain radiating to the neck and arms that is not as thoroughly relieved by nitroglycerin but that is occasionally ameliorated by antacids. When further investigated, this type of patient may have documented coronary artery disease and reflux esophagitis.

ASSOCIATED SYMPTOMS

The pain of *mitral valve prolapse* occasionally may be indistinguishable from that observed in patients with coronary artery disease, in that it may occur with exertion and seldom can be relieved by nitroglycerin. More often the chest pain of mitral valve prolapse has features not typical of angina that should alert the physician to the fact that the pain is not of coronary origin. The chest pain of mitral valve prolapse usually occurs during rest. Although it may last for a few minutes, it also may last for several hours. It often is described as "sticking" and not substernally located. It frequently is alleviated by lying down; the

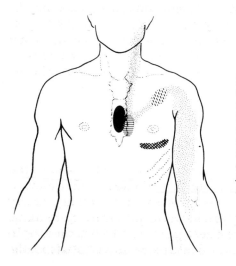

Figure 6–1. Regions of anterior chest where spontaneous pain was most commonly experienced and where tenderness could be elicited. Circumscribed areas represent primary site of pain and of tenderness; stippled areas represent radiation of pain. (From Epstein, S. E., et al.: Chest wall syndrome: a common cause of unexplained cardiac pain. J.A.M.A. *241*:2793–2797, 1979. Copyright 1979, the American Medical Association.)

pain of *angina pectoris* often is worsened by recumbency, as is the pain of *reflux esophagitis*. **If atypical chest pain is associated with arrhythmias (particularly tachyarrhythmias) and lightheadedness or syncope, mitral valve prolapse should be suspected.**

Patients with *pneumonia* or *pulmonary embolism* may have chest pain, but they usually also have fever, cough, or hemoptysis. Patients who have protracted or vigorous coughing may experience chest pain resulting from intercostal muscle or periosteal trauma. In these instances, local chest wall tenderness usually is present.

Patients with *hypertrophic cardiomyopathy* (HCM) may have typical angina pectoris, but their chest pain is not necessarily due to coronary artery disease. **In patients with HCM, the most common symptom is dyspnea, which usually precedes the development of chest pain.** In any person with angina pectoris who has coexisting or antecedent dyspnea, a careful search for HCM should be made.

Although the pain due to *esophagitis* often is similar to anginal pain, the associated symptoms are helpful in establishing the differential diagnosis. The pain of esophagitis usually is not related to exertion but is related to overeating and recumbency. The pain commonly awakens the patient at night. This symptom is rare in patients with angina pectoris unless they have angina decubitus. Patients with angina decubitus usually have congestive heart failure, and their pain often is precipitated by minimal exertion.

Cervicodorsal arthritis may produce chest pain. This pain seldom is similar to that of angina pectoris. More often it is sharp and piercing, although the pain occasionally may be described as a deep, boring, dull discomfort. The major characteristics of *root pain* are (1) pain with movement of the body, (2) pain on coughing and sneezing, and (3) pain after prolonged recumbency. The pains may occur in any part of the chest or shoulder girdle and radiate down the arms. The pains may be bilateral or unilateral. Chest pain may be precipitated by bending or hyperextension of the upper spine or neck. Usually, the pain is not related to exercise and is fleeting and thus is not truly relieved by rest.

The chest pain associated with *pericarditis* may be pleuritic or heavy and steady.

AMELIORATING FACTORS

Nitroglycerin usually relieves *angina pectoris* within 2 to 4 minutes; rest alone usually brings relief in less than 10 minutes. Unfortunately, a positive response to nitroglycerin does not confirm coronary artery disease as the cause of pain. Nitroglycerin works primarily by relaxing smooth muscle. **It also may relieve chest pain due to peptic esophagitis and esophageal spasm, biliary dyskinesia and cholelithiasis,**

gas entrapment syndrome, pulmonary hypertension, mitral valve prolapse, and, occasionally, psychoneurotic chest pain. Pain can be due to coronary artery disease and yet not be relieved by nitroglycerin. The pain may be too severe or the nitroglycerin may be outdated or administered improperly. If the symptoms suggest coronary artery disease and sublingual nitroglycerin does not provide relief, the physician should determine whether the patient is taking the medication properly. A helpful method is to take a tiny piece of paper, crumple it into the size of a nitroglycerin tablet, and have the patient place it under his tongue. The patient should be instructed to let the nitroglycerin dissolve and remain under his tongue unswallowed. He should be told to expect a warm, flushing feeling and to keep the saliva under his tongue until the pain is relieved. At this point, the patient may either swallow the saliva or expectorate it. **The Valsalva maneuver also may give prompt relief of angina pectoris, but it does not usually relieve the chest pain of obstructive HCM.** Occasionally, patients with HCM get relief of chest pain by squatting, which decreases outflow obstruction.

If antacid relieves a patient's chest pain, this strongly suggests that the discomfort is due to *reflux esophagitis.* Relief of chest pain by recumbency suggests *mitral valve prolapse,* whereas relief by squatting suggests *HCM.* Relief of chest pain by passage of flatus suggests *gas entrapment* in the hepatic or splenic flexure.

PRECIPITATING AND AGGRAVATING FACTORS

Anginal pain often is precipitated by physical exertion, emotional stress, sexual activity, exposure to cold, and, occasionally, eating (Table 6–2). *Prinzmetal's angina* occurs at rest. Chest pain due to pulmonary hypertension also is induced by exertion.

Chest pain due to *peptic esophagitis* often is precipitated by overeating and recumbency. It frequently awakens the patient at night. Chest pain due to *esophageal spasm* can be precipitated by swallowing certain substances, particularly cold liquids and anything that stimulates the production of endogenous gastrin. Thus, chest pain that follows ingestion of alcohol should suggest the possibility of esophageal spasm. Chest pain that occurs during exercise such as jogging may be due to esophageal reflux rather than angina pectoris. The former is relieved by antacids.

If the pain is exacerbated or reproduced when pressure is applied over the painful area, *costochondritis, Tietze's syndrome, rib fractures, chest wall syndrome,* and *nonspecific myositis* are more likely. Reproduction or exacerbation of pain with chest wall pressure does not usually occur in patients with ischemic cardiac pain.

Although a few patients with chest pain due to *HCM* obtain relief with nitrates, the pain of HCM usually is exacerbated and the murmur

TABLE 6–2. Diagnosis of Chest Pain

Condition	Chest Pain		Dizziness, Vertigo, Syncope	Response to		Cardiac Auscultation	Abnormal EKG		Stress EKG	Symptoms Reproduced at Bedside
	Typical	Atypical		Nitrates	Propranolol		QRS	ST–T		
Coronary heart disease	+++	+	Rare	++++	++++	–To+++	Common	Common	+++	–
Angina with normal coronary arteries	++	++	Rare	++	++	–	Occasional	Common	+++	–
Hypertrophic cardiomyopathy	+++	+	++	+	+++	–To+++ Variable	Common	Common	+++	Rare
Mitral valve prolapse	+	+++	++	+	+++	–To+++ Variable	Rare	Common	++	Rare
Hyperventilation syndrome	+Rare	++	++	–	+	–	–	Rare	+	++
Esophageal disease	+(?)	+++	–	+	–	–	–	–	–	–
Radicular syndromes	+	+++	+	+(?)	–	–	–	–	–	+++
Chest wall syndromes	–	+++	–	–	–	–	–	–	–	+++

From Levine, H. J.: Difficult problems in the diagnosis of chest pain. Am. Heart J. *100*:108–117, 1980.

is intensified by nitroglycerin. **Just as chest pain associated with dyspnea should alert the physician to the possibility of HCM, chest pain made worse by nitrates should likewise alert the physician to the possibility of HCM, as should the association of lightheadedness, dizziness, or syncope.**

PHYSICAL FINDINGS

Few physical findings are diagnostic of *angina pectoris*. A sinus tachycardia or a bradycardia may coincide with anginal pain. Signs of *congestive heart failure* in patients with chest pain suggest that the pain probably is due to myocardial ischemia. If a careful examination performed during an episode of ischemic heart pain reveals a palpable systolic bulge near the apex, paradoxical splitting of the second sound, a diastolic filling sound (S_3 or S_4), or a transient mitral regurgitant murmur, this strongly suggests that ischemic heart disease is the cause of chest pain. Likewise, *hypertension, diabetic retinopathy,* or the presence of cutaneous manifestations of atherosclerosis such as *xanthomas,* increase the probability of coronary artery disease as the cause of chest pain.

Squatting decreases outflow tract obstruction and thus diminishes the characteristic midsystolic murmur of *HCM*. The systolic murmur of HCM is increased with the patient in the upright position and during the Valsalva maneuver. Atrial and ventricular arrhythmias are common in HCM and occasionally may be the earliest manifestation. Chest wall tenderness to palpation or auscultation of a pericardial friction or a pleural friction may help in diagnosis.

Tenderness in the region of spontaneous pain, especially if the quality of pain can be reproduced by pressure on the area, strongly suggests *chest wall syndrome*. In addition to application of pressure on various areas of the chest, certain maneuvers—including horizontal flexion of the arm and the "crowing rooster" maneuver—also may cause the pain of chest wall syndrome. *Mitral valve prolapse* is suggested by auscultation of a midsystolic "click," late systolic murmur, or both. Patients may have mitral valve prolapse with absent or transient auscultatory findings.

DIAGNOSTIC STUDIES

Resting electrocardiograms may be normal in 50 per cent of patients with angiographically confirmed coronary artery disease. An ECG obtained during a bout of chest pain is more likely to be abnormal. Some studies have revealed that even during an episode of chest pain, ST segment depression occurs in only 50 per cent of patients. **An appropriately administered exercise electrocardiogram is probably the single most useful and noninvasive test in the diagnosis of coronary artery disease.**

Myocardial perfusion scanning and radionuclide cineangiography have greatly enhanced our ability to diagnose coronary artery disease using noninvasive tests. Coronary angiography should be reserved for those patients who will probably need, and who consent to have, coronary artery surgery as well as for certain other selected patients.

The electrocardiogram of *mitral valve prolapse* may show changes similar to those of coronary artery disease. If electrocardiographic changes are present, they usually include ST-segment depression and T-wave inversion or abnormalities in leads II, III, and AVF and occasionally in the precordial leads. The ST–T wave changes of mitral valve prolapse may be differentiated from those of coronary artery disease by the oral administration of 40 mg of propranolol. The ST–T wave abnormalities seen in some patients with mitral valve prolapse (and in some athletes) may diminish or disappear 1 to 2 hours after propranolol administration, whereas patients with angina pectoris are unaffected.

The electrocardiogram usually is abnormal in patients with *obstructive hypertrophic cardiomyopathy,* although a normal electrocardiogram may be obtained. The most common electrocardiographic abnormalities include those of left ventricular hypertrophy, intraventricular conduction defects, and nonspecific ST–T wave changes. The electrocardiographic findings (P wave abnormalities) most helpful in the diagnosis of HCM are those that are not generally seen in patients with coronary artery disease. These P wave abnormalities suggestive of atrial enlargement are common in patients with HCM and uncommon in patients with coronary artery disease. An ECG picture of transmural infarction (Q waves in the anteroseptal or inferior leads) also may be seen in some patients with HCM.

The echocardiogram is the preferred study for the diagnosis of both mitral valve prolapse and hypertrophic obstructive cardiomyopathy.

LESS COMMON CAUSES OF CHEST PAIN

The pain of costochondritis and costochondrodynia usually is localized to the costochondral junction. The pain may be constant or may be exacerbated by movement of the chest wall, including respiratory motion. One may confirm the diagnosis by applying pressure over the painful area, thus replicating the pain.

Gas entrapment syndromes (gas trapped in the hepatic or splenic flexure) are suggested by a history of chest pain when the patient bends over or wears a tight garment. The pain may be exacerbated by bending,

DIFFERENTIAL DIAGNOSIS OF CHEST PAIN

CONDITION	NATURE OF PATIENT	NATURE OF PAIN	ASSOCIATED SYMPTOMS	AMELIO-RATING FACTORS	PRECIP-ITATING AND AGGRAVAT-ING FAC-TORS	PHYSICAL FINDINGS	DIAGNOSTIC STUDIES
Angina pectoris	Adult	Achy, dull, tight, severe, pressing, not usually sharp or sticking Substernal		Nitroglycerin Rest Valsalva maneuver	Exertion, cold exposure, emotional stress	Sinus tachycardia, bradycardia, apical systolic bulge coincident with pain Xanthomas Signs of heart failure	Exercise EKG Coronary arteriography Radionuclide tests
Prinzmetal's angina	Adult	Achy, dull, tight, severe, pressing, not usually sharp or sticking Substernal		Nitroglycerin Rest	Often occurs at rest		EKG during attack Coronary arteriography
Esophagitis	Any age	Burning Tightness May be identical to that of angina	Water brash "Heartburn" after alcohol	Antacids	Overeating Recumbency (may awaken from sleep) Occasionally precipitated by exertion		Esophagoscopy Infusion of dilute acid into the esophagus (Bernstein test)
Esophageal spasm	Especially obese adults	May be identical in quality to angina		Occasionally relieved by nitroglycerin	Often induced by ingestion of alcohol or very cold liquids		Esophageal manometry

Condition	Age	Pain quality	Associated symptoms	Relieving factors	Aggravating factors	Physical findings	Diagnostic tests
Mitral valve prolapse	Any age	Usually not substernal Often has a sticking quality May last several hours Not typical of angina	Palpitations Arrhythmias Often occurs at rest Syncope	Beta-blockers Recumbency		Click and/or late systolic murmur	Echocardiogram Phonocardiogram
Hypertrophic cardiomyopathy	Any age	Pain may be similar to that of angina	Dyspnea Arrhythmias Lightheadedness	Beta-blockers Squatting	Pain may be aggravated by nitroglycerin	Murmur intensified by nitroglycerin and Valsalva maneuver Decreased by squatting	Echocardiogram
Intercostal myositis	Any age	May be sticking in quality			May intensify with inspiration	Localized tenderness to palpation No pleural friction	
Cervicodorsal arthritis	Adult	May be sharp or sticking Duration only a few seconds			May be precipitated by certain movements (e.g., neck exercises and twisting) Not related to stress		Radiographs of cervicodorsal spine

Table continued on following page

DIFFERENTIAL DIAGNOSIS OF CHEST PAIN *Continued*

CONDITION	NATURE OF PATIENT	NATURE OF PAIN	ASSOCIATED SYMPTOMS	AMELIORATING FACTORS	PRECIPITATING AND AGGRAVATING FACTORS	PHYSICAL FINDINGS	DIAGNOSTIC STUDIES
Chest wall syndrome	Adult	Often sharp and sticking Fleeting			May be aggravated by recumbency and certain positions	Local tenderness to palpation "Crowing rooster" maneuver may precipitate pain	
Pericarditis	Any age	Sharp or dull Protracted duration	Fever Recent viral infection			Pericardial friction	EKG Echocardiogram CBC
Myocardial infarction	Adult	Severe Crushing Precordial Protracted duration	Sweating Fatigue Nausea	Not relieved by nitroglycerin			EKG Enzymes Radionuclide studies
Gas entrapment syndrome	Any age Often obese	Dull, achy	Flatulence	Passage of flatus Nitroglycerin	Aggravated by bending and tight garments	Flexing thigh and palpation of colon may elicit pain	Gas in hepatic or splenic flexure on radiographs

flexing the thigh on the chest, or palpation of the colon. The pain may be relieved by passage of flatus or by ingestion of sublingual nitroglycerin.

The pain of pulmonary hypertension may be indistinguishable from that due to angina pectoris and other causes of exercise-induced chest wall pain. It also can be relieved by sublingual nitroglycerin. It should be suspected in patients with mitral stenosis or other causes of pulmonary hypertension, pulmonary disease, an accentuated pulmonary second sound, or electrocardiographic signs of right atrial disease (peaked P waves) or right ventricular overload. The pain of a pulmonary embolus in the acute phase may be due to pulmonary hypertension. Subsequently, the pain is related to pulmonary infarction with associated pleurisy. The pain usually is not related to exercise, and tends to become more constant (often with a pleuritic component) in the later stages.

Pericarditis should be suspected in the presence of continual chest pain associated with diffuse electrocardiographic changes. This pain tends to be aggravated by changes in position. A pericardial friction rub confirms the diagnosis.

Lung and mediastinal tumors often present with chest pain, which tends to be constant, especially in the later stages. **Whenever the diagnosis of chest pain is not clear, particularly in adult patients, one should obtain a chest radiograph to detect any tumors that may be present.**

Selected References

Diehl, A. M.: Chest pain in children: tip-offs to cause. Postgrad. Med. 73(6):335–337, 340–342, 1983.

Editorial: Diagnosis of chest pain. Lancet 1:129–130, 1977.

Epstein, S. E., Gerber, L. H., and Borer, J. S.: Chest wall syndrome—a common cause of unexplained cardiac pain. J.A.M.A. 241:2793–2797, 1979.

Fam, A. G.: Approach to musculoskeletal chest wall pain. Prim. Care 15:767–782,1988.

Hecht, H. S., et al.: Reproducibility of equilibrium radionuclide ventriculography in patients with coronary artery disease: response of left ventricular ejection fraction and regional wall motion to supine bicycle exercise. Am. Heart J. 104:567–584, 1982.

Levine, H. J.: Difficult problems in the diagnosis of chest pain. Am. Heart J. 100:108–117, 1980.

Schroeder, J. S., Lamb, I. H., and Hu, M.: The prehospital course of patients with chest pain. Analysis of the prodromal, symptomatic, decision-making, transportation and emergency room periods. Am. J. Med. 64:742–748, 1978.

Selbst, S. M.: Chest pain in children. Am. Fam. Physician 41:179–186, 1990.

Zoob, M.: Differentiating the causes of chest pain. Geriatrics 33:95–101, 1978.

Chapter 7

Colds, Flu, and Stuffy Nose

It might appear that the differential diagnosis of colds, flu, and stuffy nose is unimportant, as most of these conditions have no specific cures. However, because upper respiratory infections are the most common affliction of adults and children, the sheer case volume requires the physician to be particularly expert in the diagnosis and symptomatic treatment of these conditions.

Many different *viruses* are responsible for causing colds, upper respiratory infections, and flu. It is important that the physician be able to differentiate these viral infections from *allergic rhinitis* (both perennial and seasonal), *chronic rhinitis,* and the common complications of these viral infections, which include *sinusitis, otitis media, bronchitis,* and *pneumonia.* These last four complications usually are secondary to superimposed bacterial infections, which will respond to appropriate antibiotic therapy. The constitutional complaints often associated with upper respiratory infection also may represent the prodrome of other viral infections, such as *infectious mononucleosis, measles,* and *mumps.*

NATURE OF PATIENT

Children commonly experience severer constitutional symptoms with upper respiratory infections or colds than do adults. After a *common cold,* adults with a history of bronchitis, allergies, asthma, heavy cigarette smoking, or immune incompetence and children with a history of recurrent bronchitis, allergies, or cystic fibrosis develop lower respiratory tract infections more frequently than other people. *Influenza* tends to be milder in neonates and children; severity increases with the age of the patient. Many elderly patients develop a superimposed *bacterial pneu-*

monia. More than 70 per cent of deaths recorded during known influenza epidemics have occurred in patients over age 65. Other high-risk groups include patients with acquired immunodeficiency syndrome (AIDS), chronic cardiorespiratory disease, chronic renal disease, diabetes, and third trimester pregnancies. *Rhinitis medicamentosa* should be suspected in patients who frequently use nasal drops, sprays, or inhalers. It is most important for the physician to be alert for the development of complications of common upper respiratory infections. *Sinusitis* is more likely to occur in a patient with a history of recurrent sinusitis; *otitis media* is more common in young children; *bronchitis* is more common in smokers and those with underlying *pulmonary disease*; and *pneumonia* is more common in older and diabetic patients.

NATURE OF SYMPTOMS

Symptoms of common *viral upper respiratory infections* are well known. These symptoms largely depend on the particular infective viral agent, the patient's age, and the underlying medical conditions. The incubation period is 1 to 3 days. Usually, there is a profuse nasal discharge and congestion with complaints of stuffy nose, sneezing, postnasal drip, cough, and sore throat. Patients may complain of headache, fever, malaise, and hoarseness. They also may note pharyngeal exudates, oropharyngeal vesicles, and lymphadenopathy. In children, there may be vomiting, diarrhea, abdominal pain, and wheezing. Although an upper respiratory infection is the most frequent cause of nasal airway obstruction, less common causes must be considered, including polyps, foreign body, herpes simplex, furuncle (folliculitis of nasal vibrissae), and less common infections. In neonates, unilateral nasal obstruction may be caused by a congenital abnormality (e.g., choanal atresia). In a child with unilateral nasal obstruction as the presenting symptom, the physician should consider the possibility of a foreign body.

Although the symptoms of influenza and common upper respiratory infection may be similar, *influenza viral infections* often can be differentiated from the symptoms of a common cold by the sudden onset of typical signs of flu: shivering, chills, malaise, insomnia, marked aching of the limb and back muscles, dry cough, retrosternal pain, and loss of appetite. Patient with *type A influenza* may not have coryza.

In addition to acute stuffy nose, chronic stuffy nose is a common complaint. *Chronic rhinitis* is most frequently due to allergy (both seasonal and perennial), *nonallergic rhinitis with eosinophilia* (NARES), drugs (topical and systemic), and *vasomotor rhinitis*. Chronic rhinitis is characterized by nasal congestion, postnasal drip, rhinorrhea, sneezing, and nasal itchiness. It is difficult to determine the specific cause on the basis of the symptoms alone.

Nasal sprays, antihypertensive drugs, hormones, and psychotropic agents often cause chronic nasal congestion. The more frequent offenders are reserpine, methyldopa, prazosin, beta blockers, estrogens, oral contraceptives, thioridazine, chlordiazepoxide, amitriptyline, and perphenazine. Aspirin can cause nasal stuffiness, rhinorrhea, asthma, and nasal polyposis.

It is particularly important for the physician to recognize *allergic* and *chronic rhinitis* as causes of nasal stuffiness. There are two types of allergic rhinitis: *perennial* and *seasonal*. Patients who have perennial rhinitis usually complain of nasal airway blockage with a persistent watery mucoid drainage. Their nasal turbinates are pale and boggy. Patients who have seasonal rhinitis usually complain of sneezing, itching eyes, lacrimation, and a watery discharge from the nose. They usually have a seasonal variation in their symptoms. The perennial group does not.

Chronic, or idiopathic, rhinitis is not known to have a specific cause. Most patients with this condition have persistent engorgement of the nasal turbinates, which leads to nasal obstruction and a profuse watery rhinorrhea. Their symptoms are exacerbated by allergy, stress, hormonal changes (e.g., those associated with menstruation and menopause), marked temperature variations, and chemical irritants. These patients often complain of persistent nasal obstruction that may alternate from side to side. Sneezing is not as common as it is in allergic rhinitis.

When symptoms of a cold and cough persist longer than the patient's fever, the upper respiratory infection may have subsided, and the persistent symptoms may be due to a sinusitis of bacterial origin.

AMELIORATING FACTORS

Ameliorating factors are not particularly helpful in differential diagnosis.

PHYSICAL FINDINGS

The physical examination is most helpful in the detection of complications such as otitis media, sinusitis, pneumonia, and other bacterial infections. The physician should suspect something more serious than a simple upper respiratory infection if the temperature is greater than 102° F. If there is severe sore throat, exudative pharyngitis, earache, severe head or neck pain, or wheezing, it is particularly important for the physician to exclude complications such as *streptococcal pharyngitis, otitis media, sinusitis, meningitis,* and *bacterial pneumonia,* since these conditions respond well to appropriate antibiotic therapy.

DIFFERENTIAL DIAGNOSIS OF COLDS, FLU, AND STUFFY NOSE

CONDITION	NATURE OF PATIENT	NATURE OF SYMPTOMS	COMPLICATIONS	PRECIP- ITATING AND AGGRAVAT- ING FACTORS	PHYSICAL FINDINGS	DIAGNOSTIC STUDIES
Common cold/ viral upper respiratory tract infec- tions	Anyone	Constitutional symptoms worse in chil- dren Incubation period 1–3 days Profuse nasal drainage Nasal congestion Sneezing Postnasal drip Cough Sore throat Headache Fever (<102° F) Hoarseness General malaise	Lower RTI,* espe- cially in adults with history of bronchi- tis, allergies, asthma, heavy ciga- rette smoking, im- munoincompetence Sinusitis, especially in patients with history of recurrent sinusitis Bronchitis in smokers and patients with pulmonary disease Pneumonia in elderly and diabetics Nasal airway obstruc- tion Streptococcal pharyn- gitis Meningitis		Mucopurulent na- sal discharge Nasopharyngeal mucosal infec- tion and swell- ing Temperature usu- ally <102° F Pharyngeal exu- dates less fre- quent than with bacterial infec- tions Lymphadenopathy	Throat culture (to rule out strepto- coccal infection and pharyngitis) Monospot (to rule out infectious mononucleosis)
	Children	Vomiting Diarrhea Abdominal pain Wheezing	Lower RTI in children with history of re- current bronchitis, allergies, cystic fi- brosis Otitis media		Fever, may be >102° F Wheezing when bronchiolitis is associated	

*RTI = respiratory tract infection.

	History	Symptoms	Precipitating Factors	Physical Findings	Diagnostic Evaluation
Allergic rhinitis Perennial	Onset before age 20 Family history of allergic disease	Nasal airway blockage Persistent watery nasal discharge No seasonal variation		Pale/boggy nasal turbinates Watery nasal discharge	Nasal smear shows eosinophils
Seasonal		Sneezing Itchy eyes Lacrimation Watery nasal discharge Seasonal variation	Allergens such as dust, pollen, spores	Pale/boggy nasal turbinates	
Chronic (idiopathic) rhinitis		Persistent nasal obstruction May alternate sides Profuse watery rhinorrhea Sneezing not common	Allergy Stress Hormonal changes Marked temperature changes Chemical irritants	Swollen nasal turbinates	
Sinusitis	Prior history of sinusitis	Often recurrent pain over sinuses Early: unilateral dull Later: bilateral severe	Coughing Sneezing Percussion of involved sinuses		Sinus radiographs Transillumination of sinuses
Maxillary		May present as toothache		Pain with percussion of teeth	

Table continued on following page

DIFFERENTIAL DIAGNOSIS OF COLDS, FLU, AND STUFFY NOSE *Continued*

CONDITION	NATURE OF PATIENT	NATURE OF SYMPTOMS	COMPLICATIONS	PRECIPITATING AND AGGRAVATING FACTORS	PHYSICAL FINDINGS	DIAGNOSTIC STUDIES
Ethmoid		Retro-orbital pain Mucopurulent nasal discharge (may be bloody)	Visual loss Cavernous sinus thrombosis Brain abscess	Coughing and sneezing may cause retro-orbital pain	Chemosis Proptosis Extraocular muscle palsy Orbital fixation	
Rhinitis medicamentosa	Frequent users of nasal drops, sprays, or inhalants Hypertensive patients taking certain antihypertensive drugs	Nasal congestion Nasal stuffiness		Nasal medications Reserpine Beta blockers Clonidine Hydralazine Methyldopa Prazosin Estrogens Oral contraceptives Chlordiazepoxide Amitriptyline	Mucosa injected	No eosinophils on nasal smear

Patients with acute *sinusitis* often have pain over the involved sinuses that usually is unilateral and dull in the early stages but that may become bilateral and more severe later. Coughing, sneezing, and percussion over the involved sinuses often exacerbate the pain. Percussion of the teeth may produce pain when the maxillary sinuses are infected. In fact, some people may present with a toothache as an early manifestation of sinusitis. Patients with ethmoid sinusitis often experience retro-orbital pain on coughing or sneezing. They also may demonstrate chemosis, proptosis, extraocular muscle palsy, or orbital fixation. A mucopurulent nasal discharge, with or without blood, frequently is present. Examination should include not only palpation and percussion over the sinuses but also careful observation of the pharynx, cranial nerves, eyes (including evaluation of visual acuity), ears, nose, and mouth. Visual loss, cavernous sinus thrombosis, and brain abscesses are serious sequelae to be avoided. When correctly performed, transillumination may be helpful in the diagnosis of frontal and maxillary sinusitis.

DIAGNOSTIC STUDIES

Throat cultures may be useful in cases of streptococcal pharyngitis. The Monospot test is helpful in the diagnosis of infectious mononucleosis. Nasal smears allow one to detect eosinophils in allergic rhinitis. Sinus radiographs help one detect sinusitis. Computed tomography permits one to visualize intracranial lesions.

LESS COMMON DIAGNOSTIC CONSIDERATIONS

Frequent respiratory infections should alert the physician to the possibility of an anatomic abnormality, immunoincompetence, or mucoviscidosis. Less common causes of nasal blockage include nasal polyps, tumors, foreign body, collagen vascular disorders, and congenital malformations in neonates.

Selected References

Beare, A. S.: Upper respiratory infections. Practitioner 227:953–961, 1983.
Busse, W. W.: Chronic rhinitis—a systemic approach to diagnosis and treatment. Postgrad. Med. 73:325–335, 1983.
Middleton E.: Chronic rhinitis in adults. J. Allergy Clin. Immunol. 81:971–975, 1988.
Newman, R. K., and Johnson, J. T.: Nasal airway obstruction—approach to diagnosis and management. Postgrad. Med. 68:184–191, 1980.
Reed, S. E.: The common cold. Practitioner 223:753–757, 1979.

Solomon, W. R.: Newer approaches to the diagnosis of rhinitis. Ear Nose Throat 65:42–46, 1986.
Stevenson, J.: Influenza. Practitioner 223:759–763, 1979.
Stott, N. C. H.: Management and outcome of winter upper respiratory tract infections in children aged 0–9 years. Br. Med. J. 6:29–31, 1979.

Chapter 8

Constipation

Constipation is common in Western society. The frequency with which physicians diagnose constipation depends on both the patient's and the physician's definition of the problem. One bowel movement each day is what most patients consider normal. Many physicians, however, may accept two to three hard and dry stools a week as normal if this is usual and customary for the individual. Some experts in the field believe that anyone who strains to defecate or who does not effortlessly pass at least one soft stool daily is constipated. By this definition, constipation is very common.

Constipation may also be defined as a change in the person's normal bowel pattern to less frequent or more difficult defecation. In this chapter, constipation is defined as straining with bowel movements or bowel movements that occur less than five times per week. Constipation has been attributed to the deficiency of dietary fiber in the customary Western diet. Dietary fiber has been replaced by excessive ingestion of refined carbohydrates.

Constipation usually is not due to a serious disease. In most instances, it can be corrected by decreasing the amount of refined carbohydrates and increasing the amount of fiber ingested. It is particularly important for the examiner to ask whether the constipation is of recent onset and constitutes a change in previous bowel habits, as such findings may indicate serious disease.

The most common causes of constipation are *laxative habit, diets high in refined carbohydrates and low in fiber, change in daily habits or environment, drug-induced, irritable bowel syndrome,* and *painful defecation due to a local anorectal problem.* Less common causes include *bowel tumors, fecal impaction, pregnancy,* and *metabolic disorders* (e.g., *hypothyroidism, diabetes,* and *hypercalcemia*). The common causes of constipation can be divided into three categories: simple, disordered motility, and secondary constipation. *Simple constipation* usually results from a diet that contains excessive refined carbohydrates and is deficient in fiber. It may be influenced by environmental factors such as uncomfortable lavatories, suppression of the urge to defecate, and travel. *Disordered motility,* the next most common category, is seen with idiopathic slow transit (most common in the elderly), idiopathic megacolon and megarectum (more common in children), irritable bowel syndrome, and uncomplicated diverticular disease. *Secondary constipation,* the third common form of constipation, can be a response to drugs (e.g., codeine, morphine, analgesics, phenytoin, calcium channel blockers, aluminum-containing antacids, antiparkinsonian drugs, cough mixtures, and antidepressants), chronic laxation, prolonged immobilization, and organic disease of the anus, rectum, or colon (anal fissures, strictures, and carcinoma).

NATURE OF PATIENT

Constipation is uncommon in neonates; if it occurs, it is usually due to *anal fissures* or *feeding problems.* In children, the most common cause of constipation is a change in their daily habits or environment. The earlier in childhood constipation begins, the greater the likelihood of an organic cause.

Disorders of defecation in children are common, difficult to manage, and negatively perceived by the family. Approximately 85 to 95 per cent of constipation in children is functional. In children from 6 months to 3 years, it frequently results from some psychological cause. Early diagnosis of psychological causes of constipation in children facilitates treatment. In some cases, toilet training may have occurred recently, or constipation may have developed because the child had a condition, such as a rectal fissure, that caused painful defecation. Fearing painful defecation, the child suppresses the urge to defecate, perpetuating the production of hard, dry stools, which continue to irritate the rectal fissure.

In adults, most constipation is due to *dietary fiber deficiency* or *laxative habit.* Laxative use is more common in women than in men. Constipation is a common complaint in the elderly, although 80 to 90 per cent of patients over the age of 60 years have one or more bowel movements per day. Despite this, 50 per cent of patients over the age of 60 years use laxatives. This apparent discrepancy may be due to the fact that older people have a greater preoccupation with bowel function than do younger people. Constipation in elderly patients most often is due to inappropriate diet, decreased activity, poor dentition, use of constipating medications, and impaired motility. Constipation ranks with joint pain, dizziness, forgetfulness, depression, and bladder problems as one of the major causes of misery in older patients.

Obstipation (the regular passage of hard stools at 3- to 5-day intervals) and *fecal impaction* are most common in elderly patients. Some patients with fecal impaction will have continuous soiling (liquid passing around hard stools), which they describe as diarrhea. Elderly patients who are confined to bed, drink small amounts of fluid, or take constipating drugs are particularly vulnerable to fecal impaction. Although fecal impaction is more common in the elderly, the physician must be aware that it can occur in any patient subjected to sudden immobility, bed rest, or a marked change in diet or fluid consumption.

Tumors of the bowel are uncommon in children and young adults, but their frequency increases after age 40. **In any patient over age 40 who presents with recent constipation or marked change in bowel habit, carcinoma of the colon and rectum must be ruled out.**

NATURE OF SYMPTOMS

The most important factor in determining when constipation should be investigated for a serious cause or treated symptomatically and by dietary modification is whether the constipation is chronic or of recent onset. Patients who have long-standing constipation and those whose constipation developed with a recent depressive illness, change in diet, recent debility, or ingestion of constipating medicine can be treated symptomatically. Their clinical status should be reassessed after a few weeks of appropriate therapy. **Patients with unexplained constipation of recent onset or a sudden aggravation of existing constipation associated with abdominal pain, passing of blood or mucus, a progressive decrease in the number of movements per day, or a substantial increase in laxative requirements should be investigated even in the absence of abnormal physical findings.** These patients should have a sigmoidoscopic examination as well as a barium enema, and stools should be tested for occult blood. **It is notable that constipation occurs in less than one-third of patients with carcinoma of the colon and is less common than diarrhea in these patients.**

Ribbonlike stools suggest a motility disorder. They can also be caused by an organic narrowing of the distal colon or sigmoid. A progressive decrease in the caliber of the stools suggests an organic lesion. If the patient complains of stools that have a toothpaste-like caliber, a fecal impaction should be suspected.

Tumors of the descending colon are more common in older adults. Right-sided lesions increase in frequency as the patient grows older. One-third of colon cancers in patients older than 80 years are right-sided, and less than one-half of these patients have altered bowel habits. They usually present late with an anemia or a palpable mass on the right side of the colon.

ASSOCIATED SYMPTOMS

In children, simple constipation often is associated with abdominal distention, decreased appetite, irritability, reduced activity, and soiling. Children who are obstipated (i.e., those who pass hard, dry stools every 3 to 5 days) also may have overflow soiling. If soiling persists after the constipation or obstipation has improved, the physician should search for some *psychological disturbance*; fecal impaction is relatively rare in children. When children have abdominal distention associated with constipation, it usually is caused by improper diet or decreased motility; intestinal obstruction is a rare cause of constipation in children. When observed in children, signs of psychological disturbances (e.g., acting out, school problems, and difficulties with interpersonal relationships) should suggest that the constipation has a psychological cause.

If constipation is associated with steatorrhea and greenish-yellow stools, a *small bowel* or *pancreatic lesion* should be suspected. Constipation with early-morning rushes, hypogastric cramps, tenesmus, and passage of blood per rectum all suggest that the constipation is of colonic origin.

In adults, colicky pain, abdominal distention, anemia, decreased effectiveness of laxatives, weight loss, anorexia, and blood, pus, or mucus in the stool should suggest a *colonic tumor*. It should be remembered that weight loss, anorexia, and anemia usually are observed only in the late phases of colonic tumors. Rectal discomfort, leakage of stool, bleeding, urgency, tenesmus, diarrhea alternating with constipation, and rectal prolapse all suggest a *rectosigmoid tumor*. In contrast, abdominal distention and sudden onset of obstipation suggest a more proximal colon lesion.

Constipation—particularly if it alternates with diarrhea or is accompanied by passage of hard scybala or intermittent left- or right-sided iliac pain that occasionally radiates through to the back—is probably due to *irritable bowel syndrome*. A change in stool frequency or consistency associated with abdominal pain also suggests an irritable colon, as do abdominal distention and mucus in the stools.

Fecal incontinence (which some patients actually describe as diarrhea) should suggest a *fecal impaction*. Most patients with this condition must strain at stool, do not have normal formed stools, often have a toothpaste-like stool, and often have continuous soiling. Rectal examination usually reveals large quantities of hard feces in the rectal ampulla.

Constipation that develops after painful *hemorrhoids* suggests that the constipation is secondary to suppression of defecation because it induces pain. Patients with this condition, as well as others with local anorectal problems, often report blood in the bowel movements. When questioned, they usually recognize that the blood is on the surface of their stool, on the toilet paper, or in the toilet bowl rather than mixed in with the stool.

PRECIPITATING AND AGGRAVATING FACTORS

Patients and their family members should be questioned about stressful problems such as divorce, death of a spouse, or loss of a job. It is interesting to note that 20 per cent of children have moderate constipation when they begin to become effectively toilet-trained. Functional constipation may be precipitated by admission to the hospital, traveling, suppression of the urge to defecate, uncomfortable lavatory environment (such as a latrine), and immobilization. Reduction in laxative dose or change in brand of laxative occasionally precipitates constipation.

In elderly patients, constipation can be aggravated by limited variety in meals, decreased fluid or fiber intake, poor dentition, increased costs of fresh high-fiber foods (e.g., fruits and vegetables), impaired motility, debilitating illnesses, confinement to bed, and frequent ingestion of constipating drugs.

Certain drugs commonly cause constipation. These include antacids that contain aluminum hydroxide or calcium, anticholinergics, antiparkinsonian drugs, diuretics, tricyclic antidepressants, opiates, phenytoin, codeine (in analgesics or cough medicine), morphine-containing drugs, calcium channel blockers, iron-containing compounds, and certain antihypertensive and antiseizure drugs.

AMELIORATING FACTORS

A diet that is high in fiber (whole-grain cereals, bran or vegetable fiber) and low in refined sugar often alleviates constipation. Many patients find that weight-reduction diets that are low in carbohydrates and high in fiber relieve constipation. Increased fluid intake, particularly in patients who do not drink enough fluids or who take diuretics, often is helpful. Relief of painful anorectal problems frequently alleviates constipation. If a change in daily routine (e.g., rushing off to work or giving up the morning cigarette) has caused constipation, instructing the patient to readjust daily activities to permit bowel movements at the time of the urge to defecate often is effective.

PHYSICAL FINDINGS

A rectal examination should be performed in all patients with a significant complaint of constipation. This examination allows the phy-
Text continued on page 92

DIFFERENTIAL DIAGNOSIS OF CONSTIPATION

CONDITION	NATURE OF PATIENT	NATURE OF SYMPTOMS	ASSOCIATED SYMPTOMS	AMELIORATING FACTORS	PRECIPITATING AND AGGRAVATING FACTORS	PHYSICAL FINDINGS	DIAGNOSTIC STUDIES
Simple Constipation Low dietary fiber	Most common cause of constipation in adults	Dry, hard stools Stool frequency less than 5 times/week Straining at stool	In children: May be associated with abdominal distention	Increased dietary fiber Decreased intake of refined carbohydrates	Excessive intake of refined carbohydrates		
Functional (environmental/daily-habit changes)	Most common cause of constipation in children Common cause in adults	Vague abdominal discomfort	In children: Abdominal distention Decreased appetite Irritability Decreased activity Soiling	Resume prior habits	Toilet-training Traveling Uncomfortable lavatories Immobilization		
Disordered Motility Irritable bowel syndrome	Any age, especially young adults	Change in stool frequency and consistency Constipation alternates with diarrhea Mucus in stools	Abdominal distention Abdominal pain	Increased dietary fiber Decreased environmental stresses	Stress	Colon tender to palpation	

Obstipation/fecal impaction	Most common in elderly and in those subject to sudden immobility, bed rest, or decreased fluid consumption	Regular passage of hard stools at 3- to 5-day intervals / Possible continuous soiling that patients describe as diarrhea / Toothpaste-caliber stools / Fecal incontinence / Straining at stool			Large quantities of hard feces in rectal ampulla	
Idiopathic slow transit	Most common in elderly people	Dry, hard stools / Decreased stool frequency	Increased exercise / Increased dietary fiber / Increased fluids / Improved dentition	Decreased exercise / Decreased dietary fiber / Decreased fluid intake		
Hirschsprung's disease (aganglionic megacolon)	Rare cause of constipation in children	Present from birth / Soiling is absent			Rectum is empty	Barium enema
Secondary Constipation / Anal fissure	Affects any age	Patient suppresses painful defecation / Hard stools	Blood on surface of feces, on toilet paper, or in toilet		Anal fissure	Anoscopy

Table continued on following page

DIFFERENTIAL DIAGNOSIS OF CONSTIPATION *Continued*

CONDITION	NATURE OF PATIENT	NATURE OF SYMPTOMS	ASSOCIATED SYMPTOMS	AMELIO-RATING FACTORS	PRECIPITATING AND AGGRAVATING FACTORS	PHYSICAL FINDINGS	DIAGNOSTIC STUDIES
Secondary Constipation *Continued* Hemorrhoids	Adults	Patients suppress painful defecation	Blood on surface of feces, on toilet paper, or in toilet	Pregnancy Prior hemorrhoid problems		Hemorrhoids	Anoscopy
Drug-induced condition	Chronic laxative users Patients taking other medications Most common in elderly patients			Ingestion of: Laxatives Codeine Morphine Analgesics Aluminum-containing antacids Antiparkinsonian drugs Cough mixtures Antidepressants Iron and calcium supplements Antihypertensives Calcium channel blockers			

Bowel tumors	Uncommon in children Frequency increases after age 40	Constipation occurs in less than ⅓ of patients with colon cancer (diarrhea is more common) Early-morning rushes Decreased laxative effectiveness Blood, pus, or mucus in stool	Elderly patients with right-sided lesions may present late with anemia Weight loss, anorexia Colicky abdominal pain, distention	Possible palpable mass	Rectal examination Stool examination for occult blood Colonoscopy Barium enema
Rectosigmoid tumor		Rectal discomfort Stool leakage Urgency, tenesmus Progressive narrowing of stool caliber	Rectal bleeding Rectal prolapse		Sigmoidoscopy
Proximal colon tumors		Sudden onset Obstipation	Abdominal distention	Anemia	Colonoscopy Barium enema

sician to determine whether the rectum is full or empty, whether there is an anorectal problem (e.g., fissure or hemorrhoids), and whether there is a rectal mass; it also allows him to obtain a stool specimen that will be observed for occult blood. The physician should conduct an abdominal examination, with special attention to the colon, to detect palpable masses (fecal or otherwise) or abdominal tenderness. Normally, the colon is neither palpable nor tender. If the colon can be palpated and if it is tender—particularly over the descending or ascending regions—an irritable or spastic colon is probable. Stigmata of myxedema and abdominal distention should suggest that the constipation is secondary to hypothyroidism. Anemia, manifested by tachycardia and conjunctival pallor, should suggest a right-sided colonic lesion.

DIAGNOSTIC STUDIES

Examination of stools for occult blood, hematocrit or hemoglobin, and a sedimentation rate are appropriate, inexpensive, and noninvasive tests that the physician should use to evaluate constipation. Anoscopy, sigmoidoscopy, colonoscopy, and barium enema also are helpful.

LESS COMMON DIAGNOSTIC CONSIDERATIONS

In neonates, Hirschsprung's disease (aganglionic megacolon) is the most prevalent of the less common causes of constipation. It is important that it be diagnosed early. To differentiate between Hirschsprung's disease and chronic constipation, one should be aware that each condition is associated with characteristic symptoms. In Hirschsprung's disease, symptoms usually date from birth, soiling is absent, and the rectum is empty. In cases of chronic constipation, the onset may occur from ages 6 months to 3 years, soiling is common, and the rectum is usually full of feces. Other less common causes of constipation in children include anorectal stenosis, chronic lead poisoning, hypothyroidism, hyperparathyroidism, medication, anal fissures, allergy to cow's milk, and neurologic abnormalities such as spina bifida.

If constipation is associated with nausea, polyuria, fatigue, and, sometimes, a history of kidney stones, hypercalcemia, although uncommon, may be the cause of the constipation. Other metabolic and endocrinologic causes of constipation include diabetes, pregnancy, and hypothyroidism. Constipation may be the presenting symptom in patients with classic myxedema. Myxedematous patients frequently have an adynamic bowel with moderate abdominal distention. Adynamic bowel also occurs with senility, scleroderma, and spinal cord injuries and diseases. Idiopathic megacolon and megarectum also can produce severe constipation.

Psychiatric causes of constipation include depressive illness and anorexia nervosa. Occasionally, constipation is induced in depressed patients as the result of the anticholinergic effect of antidepressant drugs. Marked prostatic enlargement may contribute to constipation. Disease or weakness of the abdominal muscles, neurologic diseases, diverticular diseases, occult rectal prolapse, pancreatic carcinoma, and lead poisoning are all rare causes of constipation.

Selected References

Bramble, M. G., and Record, C. O.: Drug-induced gastrointestinal disease. Drugs *15:*451–463, 1978.

Castle, S. C.: Constipation—endemic in the elderly? Gerontopathophysiology, evaluation, and management. Med. Clin. North Am. *73:*1497–1509, 1989.

Nivatvongs, S., and Hooks, V. H.: Chronic constipation: important aspects of work-up and management. Postgrad. Med. *74:*313–323, 1983.

Painter, N. S.: Constipation. Practitioner *224:*387–391, 1980.

Pettei, M. J.: Chronic constipation. Pediatr. Ann. *16:*796–813, 1987.

Steinheber, F. U.: Interpretation of gastrointestinal symptoms in the elderly. Med. Clin. North Am. *60:*1141–1157, 1976.

Thompson, W. G., and Heaton, K. W.: Functional bowel disorders in apparently healthy people. Gastroenterology *79:*283–288, 1980.

Chapter 9

Cough

When evaluating patients with a cough, the physician should remember that (1) most healthy people seldom cough, and (2) the main function of coughing is airway clearance. The complaint of cough should be taken seriously, since it is one of the few ways by which abnormalities of the respiratory tree manifest themselves. Cough can be initiated by irritation of upper or lower airways. The most common causes of an acute cough are *infections* (most commonly *viral upper respiratory tract infection, bronchitis,* and *laryngitis*), *allergies* (often seasonal), and *postnasal drip*. The common causes of a chronic cough include *chronic bronchitis, postnasal drip, asthma, gastroesophageal reflux, chronic obstructive pulmonary disease (COPD), heart failure, tuberculosis, lung tumor,* and *habit*. The most common causes of recurrent cough in children are *asthma, viral bronchitis,* and *allergies*.

NATURE OF PATIENT

Viral infections are the most common cause of acute cough at all ages. This is particularly true of preschool children and even more likely if they are in close daily contact with many other children. In school-age children, *Mycoplasma pneumoniae* is quite common. Because its incubation period is long (approximately 21 days), infection spreads slowly. *Bacterial pneumonias* also cause coughing and have their highest incidence in winter months. **Recurrent viral bronchitis is most prevalent in preschool and young school-age children and is the most common cause of a persistent cough in children of all ages.** There may be a genetically determined host susceptibility to frequently recurring bronchitis. Young patients with recurrent cough often are asthmatic. Physicians should be suspicious of underlying asthma contributing to a recurrent cough when there is a family history of allergies, atopy, or asthma.

95

A chronic cough in children frequently is due to *allergic rhinitis, chronic sinusitis,* or *enlarged adenoids.* Although rare, chronic cough in very young children (under age 12 months) should suggest congenital malformations or neonatal infections, including viral and chlamydial pneumonias. Other relatively rare causes of chronic cough in young infants include recurrent aspiration of milk, saliva, or gastric contents and cystic fibrosis. A chronic cough in children between ages 1 and 5 years should suggest bronchiectasis or cystic fibrosis after the more common causes have been ruled out.

Chronic cough in adults most commonly is due to *chronic bronchitis* (especially in smokers), *asthma, environmental irritants, allergies, postnasal drip,* and *habit.* In older adults, any chronic cough without an obvious explanation should suggest *tumor* or *tuberculosis.*

NATURE OF SYMPTOMS

When the cough is of sudden onset and associated with fever or symptoms of an acute infection, a *viral* cause is most likely. In these cases, the cough is noisy, produces minimal sputum, and often is worse at night. With *bacterial* and *mycoplasmal infections,* cough often is the most prominent symptom. Its onset may occur over hours or days, and the sputum produced is usually thick and yellowish. In mycoplasmal infections, the cough may be severe and persist for 1 to 4 months, although all other signs and symptoms abate within 7 to 10 days.

The cough caused by a viral upper respiratory infection or viral bronchitis usually lasts for 7 to 10 days. If the cough persists for longer than 14 days, there may be a secondary bacterial infection. If the cough is associated with shortness of breath and bilateral wheezing, asthma is likely. The cough of asthma usually is nonproductive; if it is productive, there is a minimal amount of clear mucoid secretions.

Patients with an acute or chronic cough secondary to a *postnasal drip* may not be aware of this condition. They should be questioned about whether they are aware of swallowing mucus, frequent throat-clearing, "hawking," or a cough that is worse in the morning. Oral examination may reveal mucoid secretions in the posterior pharynx.

A nocturnal cough associated with shortness of breath should suggest *paroxysmal nocturnal dyspnea* or *congestive heart failure.* A nocturnal cough without associated dyspnea indicates an *allergic origin.* A cough that recurs in late afternoon or early evening also often is of allergic origin. This type of cough may occur in people who work in the city (where the pollen count is low) and then return in late afternoon or evening to their suburban homes (where the pollen count is higher). A seasonal incidence of cough is highly suggestive of an allergic cause.

In smokers, a chronic minimally productive cough, often worse in the morning, probably is related to the irritant effect of *inhaling tobacco smoke*. Although this is more common in cigarette smokers, it also can occur in cigar and pipe smokers who inhale.

The evaluation of all patients whose chief complaint is cough should include a complete history, with particular attention given to duration and character of the cough, smoking history, environmental and occupational experiences, antecedent allergies, asthma, sinusitis, symptoms of upper respiratory tract infections, heartburn, or shortness of breath or fainting while coughing ("tussive syncope"). *Gastroesophageal reflux* should also be considered if cough is precipitated by chocolate, caffeine, or other foods such as onions that facilitate reflux. Exercise-induced cough may also be due to reflux.

ASSOCIATED SYMPTOMS

If a runny nose, a sore throat, or generalized aches and pains are present, an *infectious* cause of the cough is most probable. The presence of fever, chills, exudative or nonexudative pharyngitis, conjunctivitis, otitis, abdominal pain, headache, or pleuritic chest pain suggests the presence of *bacteria* or *Mycoplasma*. Because a *postnasal drip* (one cause of cough) may coexist with other conditions that produce chronic cough, such as *bronchiectasis, heart failure, bronchogenic carcinoma*, and *tuberculosis*, the physician should not automatically assume that the postnasal drip is the only cause of the cough.

If sneezing, a boggy edematous nasal mucosa, conjunctivitis, tearing, itching of the roof of the mouth, or itching of the eyes is present, an *allergic* cause of an otherwise unexplained cough is most likely.

Elderly patients, whose physical activity may be restricted by arthritis or other associated disease, may not present with the usual symptom of dyspnea on exertion. The chief complaint instead may be a chronic unexplained cough that may occur only at night while the patient is recumbent or that may worsen at night. Therefore, any unexplained nocturnal cough in elderly patients should suggest congestive heart failure.

PRECIPITATING AND AGGRAVATING FACTORS

In all cases of unexplained cough (particularly in children) when exercise precipitates the cough, an asthmatic cause should be suspected, even when there is no typical wheezing. Some coughs are precipitated by exposure to very dry, superheated air. This frequently is the case in patients whose homes are heated with forced hot air. This cough may be exacerbated by sensitivity to spores in the dry, super-heated air.

Chronic debilitating conditions such as alcoholism, malnutrition, diabetes, uremia, leukemia, and antitumor therapy may facilitate the development of infections that produce coughing. Long-term *cigarette smoking*, chronic exposure to *industrial irritants*, or *chronic respiratory disease* in childhood predisposes the patient to the development of lung disease and cough.

Patients with *allergic rhinitis* and *chronic sinusitis* are predisposed to postnasal drip and its resultant cough. This cough may be worse at night, when the patient is recumbent, because more mucus drips into the throat when one is in this position. **Other coughs that are worse when the patient is in the recumbent posture or at night include those caused by allergies, paroxysmal nocturnal dyspnea, asthma, reflux esophagitis, and breathing dry, hot air.**

AMELIORATING FACTORS

In patients with allergic rhinitis, antihistamine therapy may ameliorate coughing by reducing secretions in the nose and paranasal sinuses. If smokers with chronic cough stop smoking, the cough usually abates. In one study of 200 patients, "smoker's cough" stopped in 77 per cent of patients who ceased smoking, and a marked reduction in coughing was noted in 13 per cent. Most of the 77 per cent in whom the cough disappeared lost their cough after 1 month of not smoking.

PHYSICAL FINDINGS

Special attention should be paid to examination of the ears, nose, mouth, throat (including indirect laryngoscopy), sinuses, neck, lungs, and cardiovascular system. The patient should always be asked to cough so that the cough characteristics may be heard and the sputum examined. A mucopurulent sputum suggests *infection*, although some *allergic* coughs are productive. If a large number of eosinophils are observed in a stained sputum specimen, an allergic cause is probable.

In patients with an acute cough secondary to infection, the chest examination often is normal, but the pharynx may be injected or pale, boggy, and swollen. The sinuses should be palpated, percussed, and transilluminated for evidence of *sinusitis*. When the mucosa of the nose and oropharynx has a cobblestone appearance (from chronic stimulation of submucosal lymphoid follicles), *postnasal drip* probably is causing the cough. If the lung fields are hyperresonant to percussion and auscultation reveals distant breath sounds, scattered rhonchi or wheezes, or prolonged expiration, *COPD* should be suspected.

It should be noted that cough may be the earliest symptom of *heart failure*, particularly in patients with pulmonary hypertension or mitral stenosis. Cough may occur before the usual findings of chronic congestive heart failure (rales, edema, tachycardia, gallop) are evident.

DIAGNOSTIC STUDIES

Tests used to determine the cause of cough include complete blood count, an eosinophil count, sinus and chest radiographs, and cytologic and microscopic sputum examination. Pulmonary function tests, bronchoscopy, and cardiovascular studies may help in some cases.

The chest radiograph may be negative in some patients with diffuse infiltrative lung disease. Approximately 5 per cent of patients with *sarcoidosis* have normal chest films. Likewise, patients with cough due to a tracheobronchial lesion may have a normal chest radiograph.

If an asthmatic cough is suspected and wheezing is absent, pulmonary function tests that measure response to isoproterenol should be performed. In rare instances, bronchial provocation with methacholine may be performed, but only with extreme care. If these tests are positive, asthma is the most likely cause of the cough.

A simple outpatient diagnostic test for a cough due to congestive heart failure is the administration of a potent oral diuretic for 2 to 3 days. If the patient diureses several pounds and at the same time demonstrates marked improvement of the cough, one may assume that the cough was due to pulmonary congestion secondary to heart failure.

LESS COMMON DIAGNOSTIC CONSIDERATIONS

Most people who complain of cough do not have bronchogenic carcinoma. However, 70 to 90 per cent of patients with bronchogenic carcinoma develop a cough at some time during the course of their disease. Various studies have documented that cough was the presenting symptom in 21 to 87 per cent of patients with bronchogenic carcinoma. The possibility of bronchogenic carcinoma is especially strong in chronic cigarette smokers who develop a cough that lasts for months or who demonstrate a marked change in the character of their cough. Pulmonary tumors often are characterized by change in the cough pattern, hemoptysis, chest pain, and enlarged supraclavicular nodes.

In patients with a lung abscess, cough is the dominant symptom more often than bloody sputum, pain, or dyspnea. The cough observed in patients with bronchiectasis usually is of long duration; productive of

DIFFERENTIAL DIAGNOSIS OF COUGH

CONDITION	NATURE OF PATIENT	NATURE OF SYMPTOMS	ASSOCIATED SYMPTOMS	AMELIO-RATING FACTORS	PRECIPITATING AND AGGRAVATING FACTORS	PHYSICAL FINDINGS	DIAGNOSTIC STUDIES
Acute Cough Viral upper respiratory tract infections	Most common cause of acute cough in all ages	Acute onset of noisy cough (over hours or days) Cough is worse at night and may persist for 7–10 days Sputum is thick and yellowish, but minimal amount is produced	Fever Runny nose Sore throat General aches and pains			Pharynx may be injected or pale, boggy, and swollen Coarse rhonchi	
Mycoplasma Bronchitis or pneumonia	Common cause of acute cough in school-aged children Frequent cause of persistent cough in adults	Long incubation period (about 21 days) Severe cough may persist for 1–4 months Other symptoms (fever, etc.) abate within 10 days	Same as for bacterial pneumonia but not usually as severe			Scattered rales Signs of pneumonia	Chest radiograph Cold agglutinins Complement fixation
Viral bronchitis	Recurrent infections are the most common cause of persistent cough in children who are often asthmatic	Cough may persist for 7–10 days	Fever				
Allergies	History of allergy in family	Minimally productive May be nocturnal Recurrent cough without dyspnea May have seasonal incidence	Sneezing Conjunctivitis Tearing Itching of eyes and roof of mouth Postnasal drip	Antihistamine		Boggy, edematous nasal mucosa	Stained sputum smear for eosinophils

Condition	History	Symptoms		Precipitating/Aggravating Factors	Physical Findings	Diagnostic Studies
Bacterial pneumonia		~~Noisy cough~~ ~~Incidence highest in winter~~ ~~Acute onset~~ ~~Cough is worse at night~~	~~Fever, chills~~ ~~Signs of acute infection~~ ~~Pharyngitis~~ ~~Conjunctivitis~~ ~~Otitis~~ ~~Abdominal pain~~ ~~Headache~~ ~~Pleuritic chest pain~~	Chronic debilitating conditions	Signs of pneumonia	Chest radiograph Sputum and blood cultures
Chronic or Recurrent Cough Postnasal drip	May not be aware of condition	Frequent throat-clearing and hawking Cough worse in morning		Recumbency Allergic rhinitis Chronic sinusitis	Mucoid secretions seen in posterior pharynx Palpation, percussion, and transillumination of sinuses reveal sinusitis Mucosa of nose and oropharynx has cobblestone appearance	
Asthma	May have family history of allergies, atopy, or asthma	Recurrent cough that is minimally or not productive (if productive, secretions are clear and mucoid)	Shortness of breath	Exercise May be worse during seasonal allergies	Bilateral wheezing	Pulmonary function tests Response to isoproterenol and methacholine

Table continued on following page

DIFFERENTIAL DIAGNOSIS OF COUGH *Continued*

CONDITION	NATURE OF PATIENT	NATURE OF SYMPTOMS	ASSOCIATED SYMPTOMS	AMELIORATING FACTORS	PRECIPITATING AND AGGRAVATING FACTORS	PHYSICAL FINDINGS	DIAGNOSTIC STUDIES
Chronic obstructive pulmonary disease (COPD)	Elderly patients		Shortness of breath			Lungs are hyperresonant to percussion. Auscultation reveals distant breath sounds, scattered rhonchi, wheezes, or prolonged expiration	Pulmonary function tests
Chronic bronchitis	Most common cause of chronic cough in adults (especially smokers)	May be minimally productive. Often worse in morning		Smoking		Scattered rhonchi	
Congestive heart failure	Elderly patients present differently. May have only chronic, unexplained cough	Cough often is nocturnal	Dyspnea on exertion. Paroxysmal nocturnal dyspnea	Diuresis	Recumbency. Exercise	Rales. Pitting edema. Tachycardia. Gallop	Chest radiograph. Potent diuretic for 2–3 days should improve patient's symptoms
Gastroesophageal reflux	Usually adults	Irritative, nonproductive	Heartburn, eructation	Antireflux measures, including diet, drugs, and elevating head of bed	Recumbency; ingestion of chocolate, caffeine, or alcohol; exercise	Usually none	Upper GI radiograph. Esophagoscopy. Esophageal pH monitoring

loose, moist, purulent sputum; and, occasionally, associated with hemoptysis. The cough of tuberculosis often is chronic (although it may be acute), and associated with hemoptysis, fever, night sweats, apical rales, and weight loss.

The physician should be particularly suspicious of disorders of the trachea or larynx in patients with inspiratory stridor or a dry, brassy, high-pitched, and unproductive cough. If the cough is associated with marked dyspnea, tachypnea, tachycardia, calf tenderness, prolonged immobility, atrial fibrillation, pleural friction, or hemoptysis, pulmonary embolism should be suspected.

Patients ranging in age from 3 months to 6 years may develop croup (laryngotracheobronchitis). This cough has a barking quality. Intercostal retraction with inspiration, inspiratory or expiratory wheezing, hoarseness, and difficulty with air movement all suggest this potentially critical condition. Hospitalization for intensive therapy may be necessary. In young children, the possibility of an inhaled foreign body also must be considered as the cause of coughing.

A rare, frequently written about, and usually unrecognized cause of chronic cough is impaction of cerumen, foreign body, or hair in the ear canal, which stimulates a cough through a reflex (ear-cough) mechanism. This cough is triggered by irritation of the external auditory canal or tympanic membrane.

Exposure to noxious gases, dusts, industrial pollutants, and smog can produce cough. This is particularly true in people who have underlying lung disease.

Reflux esophagitis does not usually present with cough, but patients with this condition may cough when recumbent. It should be considered in all instances of unexplained chronic cough.

Ornithosis, although rare, should be considered in patients who have a dry, hacking, unproductive cough with fever and who are in contact with fowl or pet birds. These patients often have a normal physical examination except for fever and cough. Coccidioidomycosis should be suspected if cough develops after the patient has visited an endemic area such as the San Joaquin Valley.

When complete history and thorough physical and laboratory examinations reveal no cause of cough, a subdiaphragmatic process (abscess or tumor) should be considered. If no organic cause for a chronic cough is found, a psychogenic cause may be strongly considered. In such cases, patients do not cough at night and often can stop coughing if so instructed. This cough seldom is productive. In children, it may be an attention-getting device; in adults, it may be associated with other signs of hysterical behavior.

Selected References

Brashear, R. E.: Cough: diagnostic considerations with normal chest roentgenograms. J. Fam. Pract. *15*:979–985, 1982.

Fedson, D. S., and Rusthaven, J.: Acute lower respiratory disease. Prim. Care 6:13–41, 1979.

Fitzgerald, J. M., Allen, C. J., Craven, M. A., and Newhouse, M. T.: Chronic cough and gastroesophageal reflux. Can. Med. Assoc. J. 140:520–524, 1989.

Irwin, R. S., and Demers, R. R.: Management of the patient with cough. Comp. Ther. 5:43–49, 1979.

Irwin, R. S., Rosen, M. J., and Braman, S. S.: Cough: a comprehensive review. Arch. Intern. Med. 137:1186–1191, 1977.

Loudon, R. G.: Cough: a symptom and a sign. Basics of RD. Am. Thorac. Soc. 9:1–6, 1981.

Parks, D. P., Ahrens, R. C., Humphries, C. T., and Weinberger, M. M.: Chronic cough in childhood: approach to diagnosis and treatment. J. Pediatr. 115:856–862, 1989.

Chapter 10

Diarrhea

In this chapter, *diarrhea* is defined as an increase in frequency, fluidity, or volume of bowel movements relative to the usual habit for a person. It is notable that acute diarrhea is second in frequency only to acute respiratory tract disease in American families. Diarrhea most commonly is due to *acute gastroenteritis* caused by a virus or, less commonly, by bacteria or protozoans. Other common causes of diarrhea include *irritable bowel syndrome* (also called irritable colon, mucous colitis, or functional diarrhea) and ingestion of *antibiotics, anti-inflammatory agents, magnesium-containing substances, alcohol,* and excessive (intolerable) amounts of *lactose.* Patients with *diabetes* also frequently suffer with diarrhea.

When evaluating a patient's complaint of diarrhea, the physician must question the usual frequency and pattern of bowel movement; the current pattern of bowel movements; the presence of nocturnal diarrhea; the presence of blood or mucus in the stool; travel within the United States or abroad; recent diet changes; exacerbation of diarrhea by particular foods such as dairy products; recent drug ingestion; change in nature of food intake; and any significant previous medical or surgical history.

NATURE OF PATIENT

In all age groups, *viral gastroenteritis* is the most common cause of acute diarrhea. This usually is a benign, self-limiting condition in adults; it can, however, result in severe dehydration in infants and children. In infants under age 3, *rotovirus* is responsible for about 50 per cent of wintertime, nonbacterial gastroenteritis. This winter peak is even greater in temperate climates, such as those found in the United States. *Salmonella,* as a cause of gastroenteritis, is more common in children aged 1 to 4 years. Epidemics of *Shigella* have been noted in children aged 1 to 4 years and in people living in closed environments, particularly those with substandard sanitation (e.g., prisons and custodial institutions for children and retarded people).

Giardiasis is not common in children, but infants are susceptible. Infants may be quite ill in contrast to adults, who are often asymptomatic. However, acute or subacute diarrhea with marked symptomatology also may occur in some adults with giardiasis. Reports of symptomatic giardiasis have increased, primarily among hikers and campers, who are most likely to drink *Giardia*-infected water.

Whenever diarrhea in infants less than 1 year of age corresponds to increased ingestion of dairy products, *lactose intolerance* (lactase deficiency) should be suspected. This form of diarrhea is not limited to infants and young children: It is being reported with increasing frequency in adults, particularly those of Mediterranean extraction. Although these people may not have previously demonstrated lactose intolerance, it should be remembered that lactase production normally decreases with age; in some people, this decrease is more pronounced. In these people, diarrhea seems to follow acute or chronic ingestion of large quantities of lactose, as found in milk, cheese, ice cream, and other dairy products. A transient lactase deficiency is common after infectious gastroenteritis.

Middle-aged women with chronic diarrhea are more likely to have functional diarrhea or an *irritable colon*. This condition seems to have a predilection for young women who are raising children, especially if they have the added responsibility of a job outside the home. It affects other stressed people as well. Another form of diarrhea reported to be more frequent among middle-aged women is the misuse or surreptitious use of purgatives. Patients who use laxatives surreptitiously often demonstrate other features of hysterical behavior. The addition of sodium hydroxide to the stool provides a simple test for some forms of laxative abuse. Ex-Lax, Feen-a-Mint, and Correctol contain phenolphthalein, which turns the stool red when alkali (sodium hydroxide) is added to the stool.

Diabetics with associated neurologic dysfunction also may suffer with chronic diarrhea. Some diabetics have gastric stasis and poor bowel motility. This permits bacterial overgrowth in the small bowel, which may produce an uncontrollable, explosive, postprandial diarrhea. In some instances, patients with this condition refrain from eating before leaving their homes to avoid uncontrollable diarrhea at an inconvenient time. A therapeutic trial with tetracycline may effectively stop the diarrhea by combating the bacterial overgrowth.

Although acute diarrhea usually is benign and self-limiting, the following patients are particularly prone to serious complications from acute and chronic diarrhea: neonates, elderly people, patients with sickle cell disease, and those who are immunocompromised (by underlying disease or chemotherapy). Diarrhea due to enteric infections with protozoal, fungal, bacterial, and viral pathogens is common in patients with acquired immunodeficiency syndrome.

NATURE OF SYMPTOMS

A useful approach to the differential diagnosis of diarrhea is to separate *acute diarrhea* (which has an abrupt onset, lasts for less than 1 week, and may be associated with nausea, vomiting, or fever) from *chronic diarrhea* (in which the initial episode lasts longer than 2 weeks or symptoms recur over months or years). **The acute onset of diarrhea in a previously healthy patient, without signs or symptoms of other organ system involvement, suggests an infectious cause that most commonly is viral.**

Chronic diarrhea most frequently is caused by the irritable bowel syndrome. Irritable bowel syndrome may present as chronic or intermittent diarrhea (which classically alternates with constipation) or as flare-ups of diarrhea that occur during stressful periods. A history of hard, often marblelike stools alternating with soft bowel movements, especially if associated with mucus in the toilet bowl or on the surface of the stool, also suggests *irritable bowel syndrome*. It is important to remember that although a patient suffers from a chronic irritable colon, the possibility of a superimposed case of viral gastroenteritis, salmonellosis, or giardiasis must still be considered. In such patients, a new cause of diarrhea should be sought if there is a change in the character or exacerbation of the usual diarrhea associated with their irritable colon.

Persistent diarrhea with frothy, foul-smelling stools that sometimes float suggests a *pancreatic* or *small bowel* cause. Foul-smelling, watery, explosive diarrhea with mucus often is seen in *giardiasis*. The latency period may be 1 to 3 weeks. The onset of diarrhea due to giardiasis may be acute or gradual; it may persist for several weeks or up to 6 months.

Functional diarrhea almost never occurs at night and seldom awakens the patient. It is commonly present in the morning. There may be copious amount of mucus, but there seldom is blood in the stool, except that from hemorrhoidal bleeding. If questioned, the patient may admit to noticing undigested food in the stool and rectal urgency.

ASSOCIATED SYMPTOMS

It often is diagnostically helpful for one to classify acute diarrhea into two groups: *toxin-mediated diarrhea* (small-bowel diarrhea) and *infectious diarrhea* (colonic diarrhea). Patients with a toxin-mediated diarrhea have an abrupt onset (often a few hours after eating potentially contaminated foods) of large-volume, watery diarrhea associated with variable nausea, vomiting, increased salivation, crampy abdominal pain, general malaise, but little or no fever. The onset of neurologic symptoms in association with diarrhea suggests *Clostridia toxin (botulism)*. Diarrhea of an infectious cause should be suspected if there is a history of prior good health, acute onset of diarrhea, and no signs or symptoms of involvement of systems other than the gastrointestinal tract. This type of diarrhea is due to *colonic mucosal invasion* and has also been referred to as *dysentery syndrome*. The presence of fever, vomiting, nausea, abdominal cramps, headache, general malaise, and myalgia along with a watery diarrhea suggests a *viral,* Salmonella, or Campylobacter *gastroenteritis*. Diarrhea of *colonic origin* should be suspected if fever, early-morning rushes, hypogastric cramps, tenesmus, blood in the stools, or soft stools mixed with copious mucus are associated with diarrhea. Patients with fever and symptoms of small bowel or colonic diarrhea may have *shigellosis;* this is more common in summer. Diarrhea caused by *Salmonella* may have an acute or subacute onset, or may even present as chronic diarrhea. When a patient known to have intermittent chronic diarrhea due to an irritable colon presents with an increase in diarrhea, the cause may be additional stress or an infectious diarrhea (e.g., *Salmonella*) superimposed on an irritable colon. *Campylobacter jejuni* has recently been implicated in a large number of cases of food-borne diarrhea. It is usually associated with fever, bloody diarrhea, and abdominal pain.

Blood on the surface of stools or on toilet paper suggests blood of anal origin, most often a bleeding hemorrhoid or small anal fissure, particularly if the bleeding occurs after hard stools are passed. Copious bleeding or blood mixed with the stools suggests a more serious cause, such as *ulcerative colitis*. Marked weight loss associated with persistent diarrhea and frothy, foul-smelling stools that sometimes float suggests a pancreatic or small bowel cause of *steatorrhea* and diarrhea. When acute diarrhea and severe vomiting (out of proportion to the diarrhea) begin 2 to 4 hours after eating potentially contaminated foods (especially milk products or meats), a *toxic staphylococcal gastroenteritis* should be suspected. The diagnosis is confirmed presumptively if these symptoms also developed in several other people who ate the same foods.

In addition to foul-smelling, watery, explosive mucoid stools, patients with giardiasis may have increased flatulence, nausea, and, in severe cases, anorexia and weight loss. Some patients complain of abdominal distention and occasional greasy stools.

Diarrhea associated with perianal excoriation (related to acidic stools), abdominal distention, occasional vomiting, fever, anorexia, and, in children, failure to thrive indicates *lactose intolerance*.

Muscle weakness, lassitude, and hypokalemia can be seen in all patients with protracted, copious diarrhea, but their presence should make the physician suspicious of surreptitious *laxative abuse,* particularly if other components of a hysteric personality are present.

PRECIPITATING AND AGGRAVATING FACTORS

Drug-induced diarrhea should be suspected if diarrhea develops after the administration of antibiotics or other drugs. The most commonly implicated antibiotics are ampicillin, tetracycline, lincomycin, clindamycin, and chloramphenicol. The diarrhea ranges from mild and watery with nonspecific crampy abdominal pain and low-grade fever to a severe colitis with pseudomembrane formation. *Pseudomembranous enterocolitis* is life-threatening and is of the colonic or dysentery type. It is more common if several antibiotics have been administered but classically is due to a clindamycin-permitted *Clostridium difficile* superinfection. Symptoms may begin during or after the course of antibiotic therapy. In addition to antibiotics, magnesium-containing antacids, guanethidine, methyldopa, digitalis, beta blockers, systemic anti-inflammatory agents, iron-containing compounds, laxative abuse, colchicine, quinidine, phenothiazine agents, and high doses of salicylates can cause diarrhea.

If the onset of diarrhea is temporally related to acute stress, particularly *emotional,* a functional cause is probable. In these instances, the onset of diarrhea may be gradual or acute, and the duration may be protracted.

Ingestion of *contaminated water* or *food* may occur at any time, but especially during travel abroad or camping, thus producing "traveler's diarrhea."

AMELIORATING FACTORS

The diarrhea of *lactose intolerance* abates with fasting or avoidance of foods that contain lactose. Functional diarrhea is alleviated with decreased stress.

PHYSICAL FINDINGS

Physical examination must include a careful abdominal examination and, in some instances, a rectal examination. Fever in association with acute diarrhea suggests an infectious cause. The colon may be tender to palpation in patients with irritable bowel syndrome. Stools should be examined with the naked eye for blood or mucus and microscopically for fecal leukocytes, ova, and parasites.

DIAGNOSTIC STUDIES

Studies have shown that a specific causative agent cannot be isolated in about 60 per cent of patients with acute gastroenteritis. Examination of patients with persistent, unexplained diarrhea should include colonoscopic examination with particular attention to the colonic mucosa. This frequently helps to establish the cause of diarrhea when radiographs and routine sigmoidoscopy are negative. Patients with invasive (so-called colonic) diarrhea have an erythematous colonic mucosa that may have ecchymoses, friability, excess mucus, and small ulcerations. These ulcerations must be differentiated from the ragged ulcers of *ulcerative colitis* and the discrete, punched-out ulcers that are almost pathognomonic of *amebic colitis.*

In addition to obtaining a precise history, the physician must examine the stool for fecal polymorphonuclear or mononuclear leukocytes. It is a simple test: A fleck of mucus or liquid stool is placed on a microscope slide, mixed with an equal volume of Löffler's methylene blue, and examined after 2 to 3 minutes with the "high, dry" objective. Because fecal leukocyte production is stimulated by bacteria that invade the colonic mucosa, these leukocytes are frequently seen in infections caused by *Salmonella, Shigella, Yersinia,* and invasive *Escherichia coli.* If fecal leukocytes are present, the stool should be cultured; blood should be cultured if high fever is present. Fecal leukocytes also are seen with disorders associated with colonic mucosa inflammation, such as *ulcerative colitis,* when blood and stool cultures are not remarkable.

Organisms that cause diarrhea by toxin production (*E. coli, Clostridium perfringens, Vibrio cholera,* and *Staphylococcus*) or by induction of small bowel lesions (*Giardia* and viruses) may cause a watery stool without fecal leukocytes. Amebic dysentery usually is not associated with fecal leukocytes.

Microscopic examination of the stools reveals *Giardia* cysts in 50 per cent of patients with giardiasis. If negative, a string test, jejunal biopsy, and jejunal or duodenal aspiration also may reveal *Giardia* cysts.

In patients with diarrhea caused by laxative abuse, proctoscopic examination may reveal melanosis coli, urine and stool tests may be positive for phenolphthalein, and a barium enema may show increased haustral markings.

The stool pH is less than 6.0, and the stool sugar is greater than 1 gram per cent in patients with lactose intolerance.

LESS COMMON DIAGNOSTIC CONSIDERATIONS

Less common causes of diarrhea include amebiasis, bacterial overgrowth after abdominal surgery, achlorhydria, gastric stasis (in diabetes), carcinoid syndrome, blind loop syndrome with bacterial overgrowth, inflammatory bowel disease, Crohn's disease, and ulcerative colitis.

Antidiarrheal drugs can result in obstipation. With obstipation and fecal impaction (which is more common in the elderly), there may be frequent small, loose, and watery bowel movements without much solid stool. Fecal impactions usually can be diagnosed by rectal examination. In inflammatory bowel disease there usually are frequent small stools or diarrhea with passage of blood, mucus, and occasionally pus. Patients with this disease often have rectal leakage, nocturnal diarrhea, pain, urgency, and early-morning rushes. In the acute form, patients may appear toxic and have malaise, fever, dehydration, and tachycardia. With chronic inflammatory bowel disease, there may be weight loss, anemia, joint pains, and skin lesions (e.g., erythema nodosum).

Malabsorption conditions other than lactose intolerance include adult nontropical sprue (actually a gluten sensitivity); intolerance to carbohydrates, cow's milk, or protein; and loss of absorptive surface due to bowel resection, sprue, or pancreatic insufficiency.

Pancreatic islet cell tumors and colorectal carcinoma may present initially with diarrhea. The latter is more common in middle-aged than in elderly patients. It may present with any change in bowel habits, most commonly in diarrhea alternating with constipation. Diarrhea may be the only presenting symptom, particularly if the lesion is in the cecum or ascending colon.

CHRONIC DIARRHEA IN CHILDREN

The term "chronic" normally refers to prolonged diarrhea; the specific time that must elapse to be considered chronic is a matter of controversy. Although there is some agreement that persistence for 2 weeks justifies diagnosing chronic diarrhea in adults, the prevalent feeling is that diarrhea in a child must persist for 1 or more months to be considered chronic. In addition, the child must have either lost weight or failed to gain weight during that period for the situation to be considered clinically significant.

It is particularly important for the physician to have a concept of normal stool patterns in children. Under age 4 months, breast-fed infants pass two to four stools daily that are yellow to golden and soft, and have a pH near 5.0. Formula-fed infants under age 4 months have two to three stools daily that are firm and have a pH around 7.0. From ages 4 to 12 months, most children pass one to three stools per day. These stools are darker yellow and firmer. After age 1, children's stools are formed, and resemble adult stools in odor and color.

One approach of the differential diagnosis of chronic diarrhea in children is to clarify them by type of stool: watery stools, fatty stools, or

DIFFERENTIAL DIAGNOSIS OF DIARRHEA

CONDITION	NATURE OF PATIENT	NATURE OF SYMPTOMS	ASSOCIATED SYMPTOMS	PRECIPITATING AND AGGRAVATING FACTORS	AMELIORATING FACTORS	PHYSICAL FINDINGS	DIAGNOSTIC STUDIES
Acute Diarrhea Viral or bacterial gastroenteritis	All ages	Abrupt onset lasts for <1 week No symptoms of other organ involvement Most common cause of diarrhea In adults: benign, self-limiting condition In children: may lead to severe dehydration	Nausea and vomiting Fever Crampy abdominal pain			Hyperactive peristalsis Fever	Stool culture
Rotavirus	Most common in infants under age 3	Symptoms have peak incidence in winter					
Salmonella *Shigella*	Peak incidence in children ages 1–4 years						Stool culture

Drug-induced laxatives	Mostly women	Diarrhea Muscle weakness Lassitude		Proctoscopic examination Stool sodium hydroxide test for phenolphthalein Barium enema Hypokalemia
Antibiotics	Taking antibiotics	Mild, watery diarrhea	Ampicillin Tetracycline Lincomycin Chloramphenicol Clindamycin	
Pseudomembranous enterocolitis	Taking antibiotics, especially clindamycin	Severe colitis with pseudomembrane formation Life-threatening diarrhea of colonic or dysenteric type	Use of several antibiotics Classically, clindamycin-permitted *Clostridia difficile* superinfection	
Other drugs			Iron or magnesium-containing compounds, high doses of salicylates, quinidine, anti-inflammatory agents, beta blockers, methyldopa, digitalis, phenothiazines	

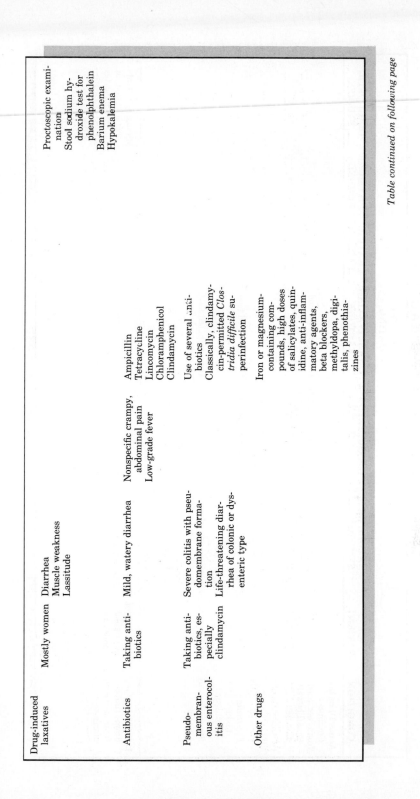

Table continued on following page

DIFFERENTIAL DIAGNOSIS OF DIARRHEA *Continued*

CONDITION	NATURE OF PATIENT	NATURE OF SYMPTOMS	ASSOCIATED SYMPTOMS	PRECIPITATING AND AGGRAVATING FACTORS	AMELIORATING FACTORS	PHYSICAL FINDINGS	DIAGNOSTIC STUDIES
Acute Diarrhea *Continued*							
Toxin-mediated (small bowel) diarrhea		Abrupt onset of large-volume, watery diarrhea	Nausea and vomiting Increased salivation Crampy abdominal pain General malaise Little or no fever	Contaminated food			
Clostridia toxin (botulism)			Neurologic symptoms	Contaminated food			
Staphylococcus toxin		Severe vomiting and diarrhea begins 2–4 hours after eating contaminated food (especially meat or dairy products)		Contaminated food			
Dysentery syndrome (infectious or colonic diarrhea)	Has history of prior good health	No symptoms other than GI involved Acute, watery diarrhea	Fever Nausea and vomiting Abdominal cramps Headache General malaise Myalgia				Microscopic stool examination for fecal leukocytes If leukocytes are present, obtain stool culture If high fever is present, obtain blood culture

Chronic Diarrhea

Condition	Predisposing	Clinical course	Symptoms	Precipitating factors		Physical findings	Diagnostic tests
Inflammatory bowel disease	In adults: / In children:	Initial episode is >2 weeks / May recur over months or years / Diarrhea must persist for >1 month	Weight loss / Bloody stools / Fever / Arthralgia / Failure to gain weight	Enteritis / Intestinal infections		Fever / Anemia	Proctoscopy / Colonoscopy / Gastrointestinal radiographs
Irritable bowel syndrome (irritable colon, mucous colitis, functional diarrhea)	Most common in young women with children and in other stressed people	Chronic or intermittent diarrhea, which classically alternates with constipation / Hard, marblelike stools alternating with soft bowel movements / Seldom occurs at night or awakens patient / Commonly present in morning / May have rectal urgency	Mucus in toilet bowl or on stool surface	Stress	Reduction in stress	Colon tender to palpation	
Lactase deficiency	Infants < age 1 year / Adults, especially those of African and Mediterranean descent	Diarrhea	Flatulence / Perianal excoriation / Abdominal distention / Vomiting / Fever / Anorexia / In children: failure to thrive	Lactose load / Infectious gastroenteritis			Lactose tolerance test / Mucosal biopsy
Diabetes	Diabetics	Uncontrolled, explosive postprandial diarrhea	Neurologic dysfunction	Meals	Antibiotics		Blood sugar / Colony count of gastric contents
Giardiasis	Severe in children / Adults may be asymptomatic / Hikers and campers at higher risk	Foul-smelling, watery, explosive diarrhea / Latency period of 1–3 weeks / Onset may be acute or gradual and may persist from a few weeks to 6 months	Mucus in stool / Increased flatulence / Nausea / Anorexia and weight loss / Greasy stools / Abdominal distention	Drinking water, infested with *Giardia lamblia*			Microscopic stool examination for *Giardia* / Duodenal aspirate for *Giardia*

bloody stools. Watery stools are most commonly seen in the following situations: (1) *persistent postenteritis* diarrhea (with or without secondary carbohydrate intolerance); (2) *intestinal infections* from viruses, bacteria *(Shigella, Salmonella, E. coli, Yersinia),* and *parasites* (particularly *Giardia*); and (3) *disaccharidase deficiency.* A *lactase deficiency* secondary to an acute gastroenteritis is much more common than a primary lactase deficiency. A sucrase-isomaltase deficiency is rare. Allergic gastroenteropathies, in which the child is allergic to cow's milk protein or soy protein, may also cause watery diarrhea in infants and children. Other, much less common causes of watery diarrhea include *Hirschsprung's disease, short bowel syndrome,* primary immune defects, and diarrhea associated with endocrine disorders.

Fatty stools suggest *cystic fibrosis, pancreatic insufficiency, celiac disease,* or *allergic gastroenteropathy.* Rarely, drugs like neomycin may induce steatorrhea.

Chronic bloody diarrhea suggests *Shigella* or *Salmonella, dysentery, inflammatory bowel disease* (including ulcerative colitis and Crohn's disease), *amebic dysentery,* or, less commonly, antibiotic-induced pseudomembranous colitis.

Selected References

Arau, T. S., Wylie, R., and Fitzgerald, J. F.: Chronic diarrhea in infants and children. Am. Fam. Physician *19*:87–94, 1979.

Bramble, M. G., and Record, C. O.: Drug-induced gastrointestinal disease. Drugs *15*:451–463, 1970.

DuPont, H. L.: Enteropathogenic organisms. New etiologic agents and concepts of disease. Med. Clin. North Am. *62*:945–960, 1978.

Kane, J. A., and Blachlow, N. R.: Infectious diarrhea. Prim. Care *6*:63–80, 1979.

Matseshe, J. W., and Phillips, S. F.: Chronic diarrhea—practical approach. Med. Clin. North Am. *62*:141–154, 1978.

Satterwhite, T. K., and DuPont, H. L.: The patient with acute diarrhea—an algorithm for diagnosis. J.A.M.A. *236(23)*:2662–2664, 1976.

Smith, P. D., and Janoff, E. N.: Infectious diarrhea in human immunodeficiency virus infection. Gastroenterol. Clin. North Am. *17*:587–598, 1988.

Chapter 11

Dizziness/ Lightheadedness and Vertigo

Most patients who complain of dizziness do not have an ear problem. A careful history is particularly important in these patients. When a patient complains of dizziness, the physician must first determine whether the patient has true vertigo or dizziness/lightheadedness. True vertigo, a hallucination of movement, is classified as objective or subjective. Objective vertigo is the illusion that one's surroundings are moving. Subjective vertigo is the feeling that, with eyes closed, one's body or head is moving or turning in space. In contrast, lightheadedness, dizziness, and giddiness represent a sensation of being about to faint, or near syncope; this is not accompanied by true syncope or a feeling of rotation or movement. Some patients describe lightheadedness as a lack of strength or a generalized weakness, and may state that they feel they would pass out if they did not lie down; this symptom usually improves rapidly with recumbency.

TRUE VERTIGO

Nature of Patient

Most vertiginous episodes in children are benign and self-limiting, except those associated with a seizure disorder. Although true vertigo is uncommon in children, they may complain of vertigo after an *upper respiratory tract infection* or an acute *viral infection* in which hearing was also disturbed. Vertigo may be secondary to an acute *viral labyrinthitis* or due to benign paroxysmal vertigo. Children with *serous otitis*

117

media usually do not complain of dizziness or vertigo but may have nondescript balance disturbances. Vertigo or headaches may develop in children several weeks after a *head injury*. Some physicians believe that when paroxysmal vertigo occurs in children with a family history of migraine, it may represent a *migraine equivalent*. Vertigo seldom is the initial symptom of a seizure; when it is, it may be followed by transitory unconsciousness or amnesia of the event.

In adults, true vertigo frequently is caused by *benign positional vertigo, Meniere's syndrome,* and *labyrinthitis*. Ototoxic and salt-retaining drugs, acoustic neuroma, and brainstem dysfunction are less common causes.

Nature of Symptoms

Although the clinical differential diagnosis of vertigo is best made on the basis of associated symptoms, physical findings, and diagnostic studies, there are some distinguishing features about the nature of vertigo. Recurrent attacks often are associated with *benign positional vertigo* and *Meniere's syndrome*. *Labyrinthitis* usually is not recurrent. The vertigo associated with *otitis media* has a gradual onset and may persist after the otitis subsides. If the vertigo has been continuous and progressive for several weeks or months, a *mass lesion* should be suspected.

Benign positional vertigo, Meniere's syndrome, and labyrinthitis have varying duration of symptoms. In positional vertigo, symptoms last from minutes to hours; in Meniere's syndrome, from hours to days; in toxic labyrinthitis or brainstem lesion, from days to weeks.

In many instances, prior episodes of vertigo may have been correctly diagnosed. However, if the previous physician did not obtain a precise history and perform an appropriate physical examination, prior episodes of vertigo may have been misdiagnosed as "nerves," "tension," or "low blood pressure." Lack of physician awareness of *benign positional vertigo* is a common cause of the misdiagnosis of dizziness in elderly people.

Associated Symptoms

Tinnitus, ear fullness, and other hearing disturbances usually are present with Meniere's syndrome, rare in labyrinthitis, and absent in benign positional vertigo. Nausea and vomiting may be present in all. If vertigo is associated with an acute onset of unilateral weakness, uncoordination, diplopia, or numbness, the vertigo is due to *brainstem disease*. In these cases, hearing usually is normal, although there are other signs of brainstem dysfunction (e.g., vertical, lateral, or rotatory nystagmus). These signs also are observed in *Meniere's syndrome* and *benign positional vertigo*. If there has been a chronic, progressive, unilateral hearing deficit with tinnitus, facial numbness, or weakness, an *acoustic neuroma* should be suspected. Café au lait spots or neurofibromatosis also may be observed in patients with acoustic neuromas.

Precipitating and Aggravating Factors

By definition, positional changes such as head-turning precipitate or aggravate benign positional vertigo; this usually is not so in Meniere's syndrome. The latter is thought to have its onset around *menstruation* as well as during times of excessive *emotional stress. Ototoxic drugs* (e.g., ethacrynic acid, aminoglycosides, and, rarely, furosemide) also may cause vertigo. Recurrent vertigo may be present when salt-retaining drugs (e.g., steroids or phenylbutazone) are ingested.

An acute onset of isolated vertigo suggests a viral infection or *lesion of the middle or inner ear;* repeated vertigo episodes associated with nausea and vomiting of many years' duration suggest *Meniere's syndrome* or *benign positional vertigo.*

Ameliorating Factors

During attacks of benign positional vertigo, patients may be comfortable when they are still. Vertigo persists in patients with Meniere's syndrome, otitis, labyrinthitis, and acoustic neuroma even if they do not move.

Physical Findings

The symptoms caused by benign positional vertigo can be replicated with caloric stimulation, Barany testing, or certain postural maneuvers. Nystagmus occurs in benign positional vertigo, Meniere's syndrome, and labyrinthitis. Vertical nystagmus occurs only with central causes of nystagmus, and its presence excludes the aforementioned (labyrinthine) causes of vertigo.

The typical lateral nystagmus of benign positional vertigo occurs within a few seconds after the patient assumes a provocative posture or performs a provocative maneuver. The nystagmus abates after a few seconds and also fatigues (does not occur) with serial repetition of the maneuver.

There is no latency or fatigue when the nystagmus is caused by a central lesion.

Diagnostic Studies

For detailed discussions of the use of diagnostic studies, the reader is referred to the articles listed in the references at the end of this chapter, particularly those by Drachman and Hart (1972), Singleton (1978), and Lehrer and Poole (1987).

Less Common Diagnostic Considerations

Less common otologic causes of vertigo include tumors of the middle and inner ear, cholesteatoma, and impacted cerumen. Less common neurologic causes of vertigo include cerebellopontine angle tumors, brainstem tumors, multiple sclerosis, and vertebrobasilar insufficiency (more common in elderly patients). Vertigo may be a migraine equivalent.

LIGHTHEADEDNESS/DIZZINESS AND GIDDINESS

Many patients describe these symptoms as a sensation of generalized, nonspecific weakness or as the feeling that they are going to faint without actually fainting. Patients may feel that this symptom abates when they recline. The most common causes of lightheadedness include *psychological problems, circulatory problems* (sometimes related to *hypotensive drugs), arrhythmias,* and *hyperventilation.*

Nature of Patient

When this symptom occurs in children, especially in those who are at or near puberty, a *psychological cause* (e.g., stressful home or school environments) should be suspected. Syncope and orthostatic lightheadedness occasionally occur during the adolescent growth spurt. Although much less common in children than in adults, *hyperventilation syndrome* may produce symptoms of lightheadedness.

When episodes of dizziness are associated with syncope or palpitations, the patient (child or adult) may be suffering from sick sinus syndrome. Some children and adults experience symptoms of lightheadedness during the rapid tachycardia of *Wolff-Parkinson-White (WPW) syndrome.* If the child is old enough, he should be asked whether he is aware of any rapid or irregular heartbeat during the episode of lightheadedness.

Patients may complain of lightheadedness or unsteadiness due to *drug ingestion.* Antihypertensive agents of all types, particularly the more potent drugs, can produce orthostatic hypotension, the most common cause of recurrent dizziness and falls in elderly people. Phenytoin and psychotropic agents can produce feelings of unsteadiness. Ototoxic drugs (e.g., gentamicin, streptomycin, neomycin, quinine, and salicylates in high doses) may cause lightheadedness without true vertigo.

An initial onset of lightheadedness in elderly patients suggests a *cardiovascular disturbance* or *cerebrovascular insufficiency;* vascular insufficiency secondary to cervical arthritis is less common. Postural dizziness related to *unstable vasomotor reflexes* is more common in elderly people but can be seen at any age. When a patient who frequently visits the doctor complains of transient lightheadedness and no specific cause can be found after a reasonably complete history and physical, the lightheadedness probably is of psychogenic origin. When a patient who rarely sees a doctor complains of lightheadedness, a more thorough history and physical should be done so that a specific cause can be ascertained. In this case, psychogenic cause should be a diagnosis of exclusion. When lightheadedness occurs in a patient with a significant psychiatric disorder, *hyperventilation syndrome* or a *reaction to psychotropic agents* should be considered.

Nature of Symptoms

Psychogenic dizziness may be recurrent but often is persistent. Drug-induced giddiness also is persistent. Orthostatic hypotension, reactive hypoglycemia, and arrhythmias cause recurrent episodes of lightheadedness. Psychogenic dizziness and that due to hypoglycemia are not particularly related to position.

Associated Symptoms

There often are many "functional" complaints in patients with *psychogenic dizziness*. If circumoral or digital paresthesias are present, the dizziness probably is due to hyperventilation. An irregular or rapid heartbeat suggests an *arrhythmia* as the cause of the lightheadedness. Nervousness and sweating indicate *hypoglycemia*.

Precipitating and Aggravating Factors

If giddiness occurs while the patient is standing, *orthostatic hypotension* should be suspected. This most commonly is induced by anti-hypertensive drugs, vasodilators used for angina, and tricyclic antidepressants. Some patients who have significant systolic pressure reduction, especially elderly people, experience lightheadedness when they assume the erect posture, despite systolic levels of greater than 120 mm Hg, particularly if the blood pressure has been reduced rapidly with antihypertensive agents. Orthostatic hypotension also may be secondary to severe diabetic or alcoholic neuropathy.

If dizziness has a temporal periodicity (mid to late morning, mid to late afternoon, or approximately 2 to 4 hours after eating), *reactive hypoglycemia* should be suspected. The dizziness can be due either to the hypoglycemia itself or to hypoglycemia-induced paroxysmal tachycardia. Dizziness on arising in the morning should suggest orthostatic hypotension or hypoglycemia, particularly if the patient is receiving a long-acting insulin.

If transient episodes of lightheadedness (without syncope) have been occurring for many years, and a reasonably complete history and physical examination do not suggest a specific cause, the patient should be reassured that he probably has no serious illness. In such a case, the symptom may be a manifestation of tension, and the patient should be instructed to record associated signs and symptoms as well as precipitating factors until his next visit.

Ameliorating Factors

If lightheadedness abates with recumbency, *orthostatic hypotension* should be suspected. If recurrent lightheadedness and dizziness abate when the patient is on vacation or removed from stressful situations, a *psychogenic cause* should be suspected. If ingestion of carbohydrates or rebreathing in a paper bag alleviates the symptom, hypoglycemia or hyperventilation should be considered, respectively.

Physical Findings

There usually are no abnormal physical findings with psychogenic dizziness. Occasionally, the patient can replicate the symptoms of hyperventilation syndrome (dizziness, circumoral numbness) by hyperventilating voluntarily. Patients with reactive hypoglycemia may manifest excessive sweating and tachycardia. Intermittent tachycardia or bradycardia may be observed in patients with WPW syndrome or sick sinus syndrome, respectively. Orthostatic hypotension may be secondary to drugs but also may be secondary to a diabetic or alcoholic neuropathy.

Less Common Diagnostic Considerations

Less common diagnostic considerations include cardiac arrhythmias such as bradyarrhythmias, paroxysmal atrial fibrillation, complete heart block, paroxysmal atrial tachycardia, and WPW syndrome (especially in younger patients). Older patients with subclavian steal syndrome feel lightheaded after movement of their arms. These people may have a decreased left carotid pulse, a bruit, or a decreased blood pressure in the left arm. Some patients with hemodynamically significant aortic stenosis or idiopathic hypertrophic obstructive myocardiopathy may experience lightheadedness primarily after exertion.

DIFFERENTIAL DIAGNOSIS OF DIZZINESS/LIGHTHEADEDNESS AND VERTIGO

CONDITION	NATURE OF PATIENT	NATURE OF SYMPTOMS	ASSOCIATED SYMPTOMS	AMELIORAT-ING FACTORS	PRECIPITAT-ING AND AGGRAVAT-ING FACTORS	PHYSICAL FINDINGS	DIAGNOSTIC STUDIES
True Vertigo Benign positional vertigo	Adults Uncommon in children	Recurrent over many years **Not** associated with tinnitus or hearing loss Episodes are of short duration (minutes to hours)	Nausea and vomiting No neurologic defect	Some relief if patient is motionless	Positional changes (e.g., head-turning)	Nystagmus and vertigo occur a few seconds after assumption of a provocative posture Lateral or rotatory nystagmus	Symptoms can be replicated by caloric stimulation, Barany testing, or certain postural maneuvers Electronystagmography
Otitis media	More common in children	Persistent vertigo	Earache		Upper respiratory infection	Those of otitis media (acute or chronic)	Audiometric testing Tympanogram
Meniere's syndrome	Adults	Sudden onset of vertigo Not precipitated by sudden movement Recurrent Duration hours to days	Tinnitus Hearing loss Ear fullness Nausea and vomiting		Menstruation Emotional stress	Lateral or rotatory nystagmus No nystagmus between attacks Hearing deficit	Audiometric testing
Labyrinthitis (peripheral vestibulopathy)	Any age	Sudden onset of vertigo Lasts hours to days	Rarely associated with tinnitus Nausea and vomiting Hearing loss possible		May be precipitated by viral infection		Caloric and postural maneuvers Electronystagmography

Table continued on following page

DIFFERENTIAL DIAGNOSIS OF DIZZINESS/LIGHTHEADEDNESS AND VERTIGO *Continued*

CONDITION	NATURE OF PATIENT	NATURE OF SYMPTOMS	ASSOCIATED SYMPTOMS	AMELIORATING FACTORS	PRECIPITATING AND AGGRAVATING FACTORS	PHYSICAL FINDINGS	DIAGNOSTIC STUDIES
True Vertigo *Continued* Acoustic neuroma	Adults	Gradual onset Persistent vertigo	Chronic, progressive unilateral hearing deficit Tinnitus Facial numbness Weakness Café au lait spots			May be café au lait spots Hearing loss Other neurologic problems	CT scan
Drugs: ototoxic		Persists days to weeks		Stop drug	Ethacrynic acid Aminoglycosides Furosemide Steroids Phenylbutazone		
salt-retaining		Vertigo recurs when patient is taking drugs					
Brainstem dysfunction (vertebrobasilar insufficiency or tumors)	Elderly	Acute onset of vertigo Normal hearing Recurrent Progressive with mass lesions	Blurred vision Diplopia Slurred speech Paresthesia Uncoordination Usually no nausea and vomiting			Vertical, lateral, or rotatory nystagmus	Electroencephalogram
Dizziness/Lightheadedness Psychogenic	Most common cause of dizziness in children	Recurrent Often persistent Without relation to posture	Many "functional" complaints	Stress reduction	Emotional stress		

Condition							
Hyperventilation syndrome	More common in adults Anxious	Recurrent	Circumoral or digital paresthesias	Rebreathing in paper bag	Emotional stress	Hyperventilation is not observed often Symptoms may be replicated by having patient hyperventilate voluntarily	
Reactive hypoglycemia		Recurrent Dizziness has temporal periodicity Onset is 2–4 hours after meals	Hypoglycemia-induced paroxysmal tachycardia Trembling Sweating	Temporary relief from carbohydrates Avoidance of excessive carbohydrate ingestion	Carbohydrate ingestion	Sweating Tachycardia	5-hour glucose tolerance test
Orthostatic hypotension	Elderly Hypertensives Diabetics	Recurrent Giddiness on standing	Occasional syncope	Recumbency	Erect posture Antihypertensive medication	Orthostatic hypotension	
Drugs		Persistent lightheadedness or unsteadiness without true vertigo		Phenytoin Psychotropic drugs Ototoxic drugs			
Sick sinus syndrome	Adults Rare in children	Recurrent dizziness	Syncope Palpitations			Irregular pulse May be normal Bradycardia	Electrocardiogram Holter monitor His bundle study
Wolff-Parkinson-White syndrome		Recurrent	Palpitations			May be normal between attacks	Electrocardiogram Holter monitor His bundle studies

Selected References

Donaldson, J. A.: Differential diagnosis of vertigo. AFP Family Practice Annual, 1982, pp. 5–17.

Drachman, D. A., and Hart, C. W.: An approach to the dizzy patient. Neurology 22:323–334, 1972.

Gantz, B. J.: Differential diagnosis and management of the dizzy patient. Prim. Care 9(2):413–427, 1982.

Hinchcliffe, R.: Outpatient problems—dizziness. Br. J. Hosp. Med. 20:202–203, 1978.

Hybels, R. L.: History-taking in dizziness: the most important diagnostic item. Postgrad. Med. 75(3):41–46, 1984.

Jongkees, L. B. W.: The dizzy, the giddy, and the vertiginous. ORL J. Otorhinolaryngol. Relat. Spec. 40:293–302, 1978.

Lehrer, J. F., and Poole, D. C.: Diagnosis and management of vertigo. Compr. Ther. 13:31–40, 1987.

Singleton, G. T.: Dizziness: an approach to its evaluation. J. Fla. Med. Assoc. 65:712–716, 1978.

Smith, J. D.: Evaluating vertigo. Emerg. Med. 12:45–51, 1980.

Towler, H. M. A.: Dizziness and vertigo. Br. Med. J. 288:1739–1743, 1984.

Venna, N.: Dizziness, falling, and fainting: differential diagnosis in the aged. Geriatrics 41:30–36, 39, 42, 1986.

Chapter 12

Earache

Otalgia usually is a sign of an acute or chronic infection of the external auditory canal or mastoid or of an acute infection of the middle ear. These infections can easily be identified with careful examination. **If otologic examination fails to show the source of the pain, referred pain should be considered.** Because the ear is innervated partially by sensory branches of the vagus nerve (Arnold's nerve), glossopharyngeal nerve (Jacobson's nerve), trigeminal nerve (auriculo-temporal nerve), as well as the facial nerve and branches of C2 and C3, pathologic conditions including infection and malignant disease of the upper aerodigestive tract (carcinoma of the larynx, hypopharynx, oropharynx, and base of the tongue) and odontogenic disease also can cause otalgia (Fig. 12–1).

Most earaches are caused by an *acute infection of the middle ear or of the external ear canal.* Usually a careful examination will reveal the cause promptly; occasionally, the differential diagnosis is more difficult. Other common causes of ear pain include *acute serous otitis media, acute otitic barotrauma, mastoiditis, traumatic perforation of the tympanic membrane, foreign bodies,* and *referred pain* (as with temporomandibular joint dysfunction and impacted third molars).

NATURE OF PATIENT

Otitis externa is more frequent in adults, particularly elderly diabetics. This infectious process also is more common in patients who suffer from seborrheic dermatitis or psoriasis of the scalp. "Swimmer's ear" is common in people who swim frequently, but also occurs in those who clean their ears with cotton swabs, paper clips, towel tips, and so forth.

Otitis media is more common in children, particularly those younger than age 8 years. Various studies suggest that 20 per cent of all children

Figure 12–1. Nerve supply to the ear. (From Beddoe, G. M.: Am. Fam. Phys. *11*:108, 1975.)

have at least three episodes of otitis media in their first year of life and that two-thirds of all children have at least one episode before age 2 years. After upper respiratory infection and tonsillopharyngitis, otitis media is the third leading reason for pediatric office visits. Premature children on respirators are at higher risk, as are those with cleft palate and Down syndrome.

Serous otitis also is more common in children. It usually is not associated with severe pain, except when an acute infection results in an acute otitis media. Serous otitis media often is asymptomatic but frequently is detected on routine audiometric testing of schoolchildren, as it is the most common cause of hearing deficiencies in children.

Local causes of ear pain predominate in children, whereas the incidence of referred pain increases with age. One study showed that 60 per cent of patients referred to an ear, nose, and throat clinic suffered from referred pain to their ears. The mean age among this group was 36 years. In 80 per cent of the patients, the ear pain was caused by *cervical spine lesions, temporomandibular joint dysfunction,* or *dental pathology. Impacted third molars* are more common in women between ages 15 and 25 years and are not an uncommon source of referred ear pain. In the elderly, *malignant lesions* of the oropharynx and larynx can cause referred otalgia. It should be noted, however, that referred pain to the ear does not rule out a local painful process. *Barotrauma* should be considered in patients who have recently traveled by air and in scuba-diving enthusiasts. Pain from direct trauma can result from a blast or a slap on the ear and in ear pickers.

NATURE OF SYMPTOMS

Otitis externa is easily differentiated from otitis media in that patients with otitis externa find movement or pressure on the pinna extremely painful. In addition, they may have tender swelling of the outer ear canal. **Bilateral pain in the ears is more suggestive of otitis externa.** Bilateral pain is unlikely in otitis media and virtually rules out a referred source of the pain. The pain of otitis media has been described as a deep-seated, severe pain that often prevents the patient from sleeping. Children who are too young to talk may present with irritability, restlessness, fever, poor feeding, or rubbing of the affected ear. In addition, there frequently is a history of a recent upper respiratory infection.

Serous otitis is painless unless the ear is infected. It usually is not associated with a severe earache, but there may be some intermittent discomfort. Patients may state that they hear crackling or gurgling sounds. Severe pain in, and especially behind, the ear is experienced in patients with *acute mastoiditis*. People with this condition have exquisite tenderness on pressing over the mastoid process.

The pain of *barotrauma* may be severe and persistent, and a superimposed otitis media occasionally develops. The pain most frequently is experienced during descent in an airplane, especially if the patient has a concurrent upper respiratory infection with eustachian tube dysfunction. The pain may be excruciating.

Patients with *impacted cerumen* also may complain of severe pain in the ear, or they may have only a vague sensation of discomfort that is sometimes associated with impaired hearing. On questioning, the patients may admit to a long-standing problem with cerumen accumulation in their ears, with exacerbation leading to visits to the physician.

The pain of *temporomandibular joint dysfunction* usually is intermittent and often is worse in the morning if associated with night grinding. The pain also may occur toward the end of the day, especially if it is secondary to tension-induced bruxism. For further discussion of temporomandibular joint dysfunction, see chapters on facial pain and headache.

ASSOCIATED SYMPTOMS

The usual sequence of symptoms in *otitis media* is a blocked feeling in the ear, pain, fever, discharge if the tympanic membrane perforates, and some relief of pain and fever with perforation. Patients with *serous otitis* usually are well and afebrile. They frequently present with impaired hearing as their only complaint, although they also may complain of a feeling of fullness in the ear, popping or crackling sounds, or tinnitus. Symptoms commonly associated with *temporomandibular joint dysfunction* include vertigo, tinnitus, headache, and a jaw click. The pain may be worse in the morning if the patient is a night grinder.

PRECIPITATING AND AGGRAVATING FACTORS

Otitic barotrauma is aggravated by upper respiratory infections, hay fever, middle ear effusion, or stuffy nose. It often is precipitated by an increase in atmospheric pressure, as occurs with descent in an airplane. *Acute otitis media* often precedes acute mastoiditis by 10 to 14 days. Pain in the ear that is referred from the second and third spinal nerve may be worse with flexion of the neck. Otalgia exacerbated by swallowing suggests *Eagle's syndrome,* an elongated styloid process.

AMELIORATING FACTORS

Barotrauma may be alleviated somewhat by chewing, Valsalva maneuver, and nasal decongestants. *Temporomandibular pain* may be eased by a dental bite appliance.

PHYSICAL FINDINGS AND DIAGNOSTIC TESTS

The physical findings of otitis externa, otitis media, and serous otitis are well known (see references) and will not be described here. It should be emphasized that the physician must perform an accurate, complete examination of the eardrum to rule out otitis media. If an adequate view is obstructed owing to wax accumulation or secondary external ear canal infection, otitis media cannot be ruled out; it can only be excluded if the entire drum is normal and there is no conductive hearing loss. In serous otitis, a serous or glutinous fluid accumulates in the middle ear space.

The drum may look abnormal because of the effusion, or it may be injected with noticeable radial vessels. Occasionally, it is retracted and shows decreased mobility on pneumo-otoscopy (Fig. 12–2). Impedance tympanometry (Fig. 12–3) helps one to confirm the diagnosis.

When the patient complains of ear pain, has a fever and noticeable swelling behind the ear, or experiences tenderness to palpation over the mastoid process, *acute mastoiditis* is probable. The tympanic membrane often is red, bulging, and immobile because of an associated otitis media. It should be suspected whenever there is a continuous discharge from the middle ear for more than 10 days. Radiographs help one establish the diagnosis.

Whenever a patient complains of pain in the ear and examination of the ear canal and drum is normal, referred pain is most probable. One of the common causes of referred pain to the ear is *temporomandibular joint dysfunction.* This may be either acute, resulting from opening the mouth extremely wide, or chronic, resulting from malocclusion or arthritis of the temporomandibular joint which occurs more frequently in patients with *rheumatoid arthritis.* Malocclusion or enlarged masseter muscles caused by bruxism may be apparent on physical examination. In addition, there often is tenderness to palpation over the temporomandibular joint. Occasionally, the examiner may hear

Speculum

Middle ear

Lens cap

Airtight interface

Tympanic membrane

Eustachian tube

Rubber tubing gasket

Pneumatic tubing

Figure 12–2. Pneumatic otoscopy. (From Schwartz, R. H.: New concepts in otitis media. Am. Fam. Phys. *19(5)*:91–98, 1979.)

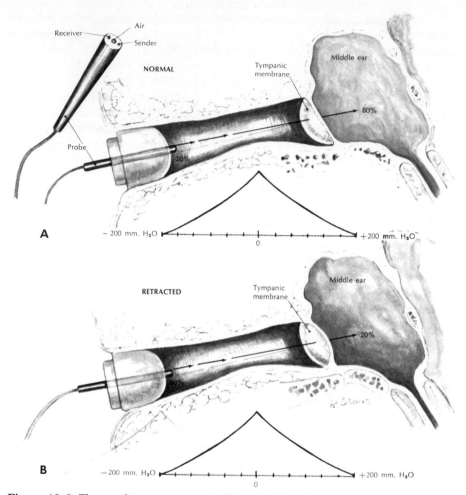

Figure 12–3. Theory of tympanometry. *A,* Normal. A low-frequency (220 Hz) probe tone is emitted from a tiny aperture in the probe tip of the instrument and is directed to the tympanic membrane. When the tympanic membrane is stiffened by positive or negative pressure, a greater amount of sound energy is reflected off the membrane and directed back down the ear canal. A small microphone housed in the probe assembly reads the amount of reflected sound energy. When the tympanic membrane is in a neutral position, the pressure in the middle ear is equal to that of atmospheric pressure and is thus in its most mobile position. Here, most of the sound energy from the probe tone is absorbed by the tympanic membrane into the middle ear and the least amount is reflected back down the ear canal. *B,* Retracted. The retracted tympanic membrane reflects negative pressure in the middle ear relative to atmospheric pressure. The most compliant position of the membrane (peak of tympanogram) is found when artificially induced negative pressure is introduced from the manometer of the instrument (see blue peak at -200 mm, H_2O). Thus, the pressure point at which the peak of the tympanogram occurs represents an indirect measure of middle ear pressure. Note that greater sound energy is reflected off the tympanic membrane until the pressure introduced down the ear canal is equal to the pressure in the middle ear (in this case, -200 mm, H_2O). (From Schwartz, R. H.: New concepts in otitis media. Am. Fam. Phys. *19(5)*:91–98, 1979.)

DIFFERENTIAL DIAGNOSIS OF EARACHE

CONDITION	NATURE OF PATIENT	NATURE OF SYMPTOMS	ASSOCIATED SYMPTOMS	PRECIPITATING AND AGGRAVATING FACTORS	PHYSICAL FINDINGS AND DIAGNOSTIC STUDIES
Otitis media	Children, especially <8 years	Pain is unilateral, deep, and severe	Irritability Restlessness Fever Poor feeding Ear feels full	Upper respiratory infection	Tympanic membrane inflamed and bulging Decreased light reflex
Serous otitis media	Children Some adults	Not usually painful Unilateral	Decreased hearing Crackling and gurgling sounds		Fluid behind tympanic membrane Tympanic membrane shows decreased mobility Decreased conductive hearing Impedance tympanometry
Otitis externa	Adults Diabetics Patients with seborrhea Ear pickers Swimmers	Often bilateral			Pain on manipulation of pinna

Table continued on following page

DIFFERENTIAL DIAGNOSIS OF EARACHE *Continued*

CONDITION	NATURE OF PATIENT	NATURE OF SYMPTOMS	ASSOCIATED SYMPTOMS	PRECIPITATING AND AGGRAVATING FACTORS	PHYSICAL FINDINGS AND DIAGNOSTIC STUDIES
Otitic barotrauma		Pain may be severe	Upper respiratory infection, nasal stuffiness	Worse on airplane descent	
Mastoiditis		Pain in and behind ear	Fever Drainage from middle ear for more than 10 days	Otitis media 10–14 days previously	Exquisite pain with pressure on mastoid process Swelling behind ear Radiograph of mastoid
Foreign body Cerumen	Children Adults	Pain or vague discomfort	May impair hearing Recurrent problem		Foreign body or cerumen in ear
Referred otalgia as with temporomandibular joint dysfunction, dental problems, and tumors	Adults (increases with age)	Rarely bilateral Temporomandibular joint dysfunction is intermittent and often worse in morning	Resemble those of temporomandibular joint dysfunction: vertigo, tinnitus, jaw click Pain referred from infected tooth may be worse with hot or cold foods	Temporomandibular joint arthritis Malocclusion or bruxism Impacted molar	Normal ear examination

clicking or palpate crepitus over the temporomandibular joint. Patients with *impacted third molars* may have trismus and pain when pressure is applied above and behind the angle of the mandible. The diagnosis can be confirmed by dental radiographs.

LESS COMMON DIAGNOSTIC CONSIDERATIONS

Pain in the ear can be caused by infections such as impetigo, insect bites, chondrodermatitis chronicus helicis (an exquisitely tender nodule of the helix seen in older adults), perichondritis of the pinna, or gouty tophi (which usually are not painful). Rarely, tumors of the middle ear and meatus can produce nonremitting pain. In herpes zoster oticus (Ramsay Hunt syndrome), there is severe pain in one ear for several days, after which vesicles appear on the auricle or in the meatus. These vesicles also may appear on the tympanic membrane and occasionally on the palate. Concurrent with the vesicles there usually is a complete lower motor neuron lesion of the seventh cranial nerve associated with pyrexia, constitutional disturbances, deafness, tinnitus, vertigo, and nystagmus.

If otalgia develops in a child within 2 weeks of orthodontic treatment and otologic examination is normal, *temporomandibular joint dysfunction* should be considered, especially if otalgia recurs after orthodontic therapy. Pain referred to the ear can occur from lesions of the fifth cranial nerve, dental caries, abscesses of lower molars, trigeminal neuralgia, sinusitis, and parotid pathology. Ear pain can be referred from the ninth and tenth cranial nerves with lesions of the vallecula, posterior third of the tongue, tonsils, larynx, migraine, glossopharyngeal neuralgia, and carotidynia (persistent sore throat with normal pharynx, ear pain aggravated by swallowing, and a tenderness over the carotid bulb).

Selected References

Clark, J. L.: Otalgia: identifying the source. Postgrad. Med. *70(4)*:99–103, 1981.
Ingvarsson, L.: Acute otalgia in children: findings and diagnosis. Acta Paediatr. Scand. *71(5)*:705–710, 1982.
Fletcher, M. M.: The Painful Ear. Resident Staff Physician, pp. 45–51, July 1980.
Ludman, H.: Pain in the ear. Br. Med. J. *281*:1538–1541, 1980.
Schwartz, R. H.: New concepts in otitis media. Am. Fam. Physician *19(5)*:91–98, 1979.
Thaller, S. R., and DeSilva, A.: Otalgia with a normal ear. Am. Fam. Physician *36*:129–136, 1987.
Thaller, S. R., and Thaller, J. L.: Head and neck symptoms. Postgrad. Med. *87*:75–77, 80, 83–86, 1990.

Chapter 13

Facial Pain

Because the practitioner usually can differentiate headache from other causes of facial pain, the differential diagnosis of headache is discussed in Chapter 16. Commonly, by the time a patient consults a physician for facial pain, he already has visited a dentist several times. This illustrates the diagnostic difficulty.

The common causes of facial pain are diseases of local structures such as *dental disease, eye disease* (glaucoma), *nose* or *sinus disease* (sinusitis), and *temporomandibular joint (TMJ) dysfunction*; vascular pain such as *migraine* and *temporal arteritis;* neurologic pain such as *trigeminal neuralgia* and *sphenopalatine ganglion neuralgia;* referred pain, rarely from *angina pectoris* and occasionally due to *muscle contraction headaches;* and psychogenic pain, as seen with *atypical facial pain, hysteria,* and *depression.* Because pain is a symptom and cannot be seen or easily measured, the evaluation and diagnosis must depend on the patient's description; therefore, details that the clinician elicits are important. A patient's reaction to pain can be seen and may indicate the severity of the pain. In cases of chronic pain, the initial symptoms may have been psychologically based, further complicating the diagnostic process. Despite the fact that depressed, anxious, or neurotic people may seek help for organic causes of facial pain more frequently than other people, chronic or recurrent episodes of facial pain can lead to depression and anxiety.

NATURE OF PATIENT

Trigeminal neuralgia is more common in patients over age 50. If facial pain occurs in a younger patient (less than age 40), trigeminal neuralgia is less likely, and other conditions that can mimic tic douloureux should be considered. These include *multiple sclerosis, acoustic neuroma,* and *trigeminal neuroma,* especially if the upper division (pain in the forehead or eye) is involved or if the symptoms are unilateral. Likewise, *glaucoma* is more common in the elderly; it affects 2 per cent of those over age 40. It is more common in people who are farsighted than in those who are nearsighted.

Atypical facial pain is most common in women between ages 30 and 50; 60 per cent of these patients have a similar family history. It tends to occur in people who present with a history of high stress, drug addiction, low self-esteem, impotence or frigidity, marital or family conflicts, or prior episodes of anxiety or depression. The typical patient is an edentulous, haggard-looking, middle-aged woman. She may have a history of concomitant psychiatric illness as well.

Facial pain from sinusitis can occur at any age but is less common in children and teenagers. *TMJ dysfunction* is more common after age 40, but it can accompany severe malocclusion or mandibular trauma at any age. There appears to be a higher incidence of TMJ dysfunction in patients with rheumatoid arthritis.

NATURE OF SYMPTOMS

Dental pain is often severe, throbbing, and poorly localized. Excruciating, lancinating, stabbing, paroxysmal pain is characteristic of the *trigeminal, sphenopalatine,* and *glossopharyngeal* neuralgias. The pain of *glaucoma* is described as dull and frontally located. The pain of *acute narrow-angle glaucoma,* however, can cause severe pain of abrupt onset.

Pain is relatively uncommon in patients with chronic or subacute sinusitis; it commonly is seen with episodes of *acute sinusitis* (which may be superimposed on subacute sinusitis). Sinusitis pain usually is dull and relatively constant; occasionally, it may be described as throbbing. This pain usually is located over the affected sinus or behind the orbit. With sphenoid sinusitis, however, pain may present at the vertex of the head and radiate to the neck and orbit. Sinusitis pain usually is unilateral but can be bilateral.

The neuralgia pains usually have a sudden onset. A typical attack may consist of two to three stabbing pains over a 1-minute period. Episodes may become more frequent with time, and there may be several attacks in a single day wih spontaneous remission for weeks or months. Although the pain may be recurrent, it usually is paroxysmal and instantaneous. Although the actual pain may last only a few seconds and then disappear, some patients experience a gradual transition from lancinating pain to a vague ache or burning. Trigeminal neuralgia pains usually occur during the day, whereas glossopharyngeal pains often develop at night. Over time, the episodes of trigeminal neuralgia may become more frequent and occur one or more times daily. These pains seldom awaken patients from their sleep.

The pain of *glaucoma* may be worse in dark rooms. It usually is gradual in onset, although the pain of acute narrow-angle glaucoma can begin suddenly and present as a dramatic emergency. The pain of sinusitis usually develops gradually and can last for days to weeks if not adequately treated.

Most causes of facial pain (including trigeminal neuralgia, sinusitis, glaucoma, and TMJ dysfunction) present with unilateral pain; occasionally, all can be bilateral or alternating. The pain of *trigeminal neuralgia* is located over the course of one of the three divisions of the fifth cranial nerve. It usually is unilateral but can be bilateral in 5 to 10 per cent of patients. These bilateral attacks tend to be more common in certain families and possibly more common in women. Trigeminal neuralgia most commonly occurs along the distribution of the second (maxillary branch) or third (mandibular branch) division and seldom over the first division (ophthalmic branch). Most patients report that the pain is on the surface in contrast to being deep inside the head, which is more common with sphenopalatine ganglion neuralgia. **Both the lancinating nature of neuralgia pain and the fact that it tends to be remittent and possibly associated with trigger areas distinguish it from the more chronic pain of sinus infection, dental abscesses, and glaucoma.** The anatomic distribution of the pain helps differentiate neuralgia from *atypical facial pain*, which is not confined to an anatomic distribution of any cranial or cervical nerve. In cases of atypical facial pain, the entire side of the head as well as the face, neck, or throat may be involved.

The pain of *subacute glaucoma* usually causes frontal headaches, whereas the pain of *acute glaucoma* often is described as pain in the eye or just behind the eye radiating to the head, ears, or teeth. The pain of *sinusitis* corresponds in location to the sinus involved. Patients with maxillary sinusitis usually complain of pain over the cheek or under the eye; the pain of frontal sinusitis is above the eyes or in the forehead; the pain of ethmoid sinusitis is most often supraorbital and may occasionally radiate to the vertex of the head. Sphenoid and ethmoid sinusitis seldom occur as isolated phenomena; they usually are associated with other forms of sinusitis.

Pain of *temporomandibular arthritis* or *TMJ dysfunction* normally is located in the TMJ area, although it may be referred to the ear or temples, thus simulating the pain of a tension headache. **Any time a patient complains of pain in the ear and physical examination of the ear is negative, the physician should palpate over the TMJ, question the patient for other signs and symptoms of TMJ dysfunction, and consider other causes of referred otalgia.** The pain of TMJ dysfunction may radiate to either the teeth or the ear.

ASSOCIATED SYMPTOMS

Involuntary facial contractions may occur with the severe pain of *trigeminal neuralgia*. Results of suffering from a chronic painful syndrome include sleeplessness, weight loss, anxiety, depression, and, rarely, a suicidal tendency. Patients with *sinusitis* often have—or recently have had—symptoms of an upper respiratory infection. Patients with *atypical facial pain* commonly are depressed and emotional, and they have a large affectual component to their illness. Patients with cluster headaches *(Horton's cephalalgia)* may have ipsilateral lacrimation or rhinorrhea.

When patients see halos or rainbows around lights, have temporary obscuring of vision, and experience pain in and around the eye, *glaucoma* should be suspected. Occasionally, these patients also will complain of nausea and vomiting. This latter finding sometimes leads to the erroneous diagnosis of migraine headaches. The associated symptoms of *TMJ dysfunction* include clicking, popping, crepitation, tinnitus, vertigo (rarely), pain in the ear, jaw clenching, bruxism, neckache, and headache. Patients may report that it is difficult for them to open their mouths widely because this action elicits the aforementioned symptoms.

PRECIPITATING AND AGGRAVATING FACTORS

Dental pain may increase with ingestion of hot, sweet, or acidic foods. *Neuralgia* pains often are induced by touching of trigger points or by temperature extremes. *Sphenopalatine neuralgia* may be precipitated by sinusitis or a postnasal drip. Coughing and sneezing may exacerbate sinus pain. Erect posture may worsen pain that is due to *maxillary sinusitis,* whereas recumbency exacerbates *frontal sinus* pain. Darkness and drugs, which cause pupillary dilatation, often precipitate the pain of *glaucoma. TMJ pain* may be aggravated by bruxism and by opening the mouth widely. Mastication and temperature extremes may exacerbate dental pain.

AMELIORATING FACTORS

Sinus pain often is relieved by postural changes: Some sinuses drain better when the patient is erect, whereas others drain more effectively when the patient is recumbent. Because frontal sinuses drain better when the patient is erect, the pain of *frontal sinusitis* lessens as the day progresses. In contrast, the pain of *maxillary sinusitis* improves with recumbency, as the maxillary sinuses drain better when the patient is in this position.

Effective relief of pain with carbamazepine (Tegretol) suggests that the pain is due to *neuralgia*. Phenytoin also will relieve neuralgic pain, but it seldom is effective in patients wih migraine headaches. Patients with *atypical facial pain* rarely obtain relief from anything other than psychotherapy or antidepressants. The pain of TMJ dysfunction occasionally is relieved by tranquilizers, anti-inflammatory agents, and muscle relaxants. Depending on what is causing the TMJ pain, bite plates or correction of a malocclusion may be helpful. One should note that correction of the malocclusion may correct the malalignment of the TMJ but not necessarily correct arthritic changes that have occurred in the joint, either primarily or secondarily to the malocclusion. Therefore, even extensive dental work does not always completely relieve TMJ pain.

PHYSICAL FINDINGS

The physician must conduct a meticulous examination of eyes, ears, nose, nasopharynx, mouth, and hypopharynx to determine the source of facial pain. The physical examination usually is normal in patients with atypical facial pain and the various neuralgias. Rarely, patients with trigeminal neuralgia may have a sensory deficit over the division involved and, possibly, pupillary inequality. If the trigeminal neuralgia is atypical or bilateral or occurs in patients under age 50 years, the physical examination should focus particularly on findings that could be caused by a basilar artery aneurysm, multiple sclerosis, or cerebellar dysfunction. Patients who have suffered with long-standing undiagnosed *neuralgia* may be partially or completely toothless; extractions may have been performed to relieve pain thought to be of dental origin.

The physical findings of *glaucoma* include increased intraocular pressure, as determined by tonometry, dilated pupil, and conjunctival injection. In the early stages of simple glaucoma, the patient usually does not notice any pain, obscuring of vision, halos, or visual field cuts. Patients with subacute glaucoma may have their vision temporarily obscured and see halos or rainbows around lights. Patients with acute glaucoma may have marked conjunctival injection; acute glaucoma, therefore, is part of the differential diagnosis of the patient with a "red eye." In patients with acute glaucoma, other physical findings include edema of the eyelids, a hazy and "steamy" cornea, decreased corneal sensation, an injected discolored iris, and a pupil that is mildly dilated and occasionally vertically oval. The intraocular tension is raised, and the eye is hard to the touch and tender to gentle palpation. Acute glaucoma can be differentiated from iritis (which may be painful) and conjunctivitis by the appearance of the cornea and the pupil. In conjunctivitis and iritis, the cornea is clear and sensitive (Table 13–1). In

TABLE 13–1. Summary of the Points of Distinction Between Conjunctivitis, Iritis, and Acute Glaucoma

Condition	Conjunctivitis	Iritis	Acute Glaucoma
Conjunctiva	Conjunctival vessels bright red and injected; movable over subjacent sclera; injection most marked away from corneoscleral margin; color fades on pressure	Ciliary vessels injected, deep red or bluish-red; most marked at corneoscleral margin; color does not fade on pressure	Both conjunctival and ciliary vessels injected
Cornea	Clear, sensitive	Clear, sensitive	Steamy, hazy, insensitive
Anterior chamber	Clear; normal depth	Aqueous turbid; anterior chamber slightly shallow	Very shallow
Iris	Normal color	Injected, swollen, adherent to lens, and muddy-colored	Injected
Pupil	Black, active	May be filled with exudate Small, fixed	Dilated, fixed, oval
Intraocular tension	Normal	Normal	Raised

From Hart, F. D. (Ed.): French's Index of Differential Diagnosis. 10th ed. © 1973, The Williams & Wilkins Co., Baltimore

142

conjunctivitis the pupil is active, whereas in iritis it is small and fixed. In both conjunctivitis and iritis, intraocular tension is normal.

Patients with *acute sinusitis* have ipsilateral nasal fullness and pain over the affected sinus that is exacerbated by palpation or percussion. Transillumination over the affected sinus is impaired. Patients may complain of toothaches or tenderness on percussion of the upper teeth because the roots of these teeth are close to the floor of the maxillary sinus. Because maxillary sinusitis is very common, it occasionally is misdiagnosed as hay fever or chronic allergic rhinitis, and vice versa.

There are fewer physical findings and symptoms associated with *subacute* or *chronic sinusitis*. Patients with subacute sinusitis may complain of headache, postnasal drip, or purulent discharge from the nose or posterior pharynx when the sinus ostea permit drainage in this subacute phase. Patients with chronic sinusitis may have a mucopurulent discharge that is unresponsive to medical management. They may complain of vague ear pain or hearing loss that is secondary to a serous otitis. Often they have a sore throat secondary to a postnasal drip.

Patients with *TMJ dysfunction* may experience pain with palpation of the joint when they open and close the mouth. The masseter muscles may be prominent in patients who grind their teeth. Auscultation over the joint may reveal a clicking sound with opening and closing of the mouth.

DIAGNOSTIC STUDIES

All patients with *unexplained* facial pain should be evaluated with dental, sinus, and skull radiographs or CT scans, tonometry, studies of erythrocyte sedimentation rate, and a very thorough examination of the nose, nasopharynx, larynx, oropharynx, and hypopharynx.

The radiograph in *chronic sinusitis* may be negative or show haziness of the sinus cavity or thickening of the sinus mucosa. Likewise, in *acute sinusitis,* radiographs can be negative in the very early stage and become positive later. In other words, positive radiographic findings are confirmatory, although negative findings do not absolutely rule out the presence of acute or chronic sinusitis. Nasal endoscopy and modified CT scan of the sinuses may be abnormal and explain facial pain despite normal radiographs. The absence of radiographic changes significantly decreases the likelihood of chronic recurrent sinusitis. Radiographic findings of *TMJ dysfunction* include the loss of the TMJ space, thinning or loss of lamina over the condylar head or glenoid fossa, flattening of the condylar head, and spur formation. Routine mandibular radiographs may be negative, but tomographic studies may show arthritic changes in the TMJ.

LESS COMMON DIAGNOSTIC CONSIDERATIONS

Vague facial pain, neuralgia and headache, or aching or sharp stabbing pain on swallowing, head movement, yawning, or coughing suggest the possibility of *Eagle's syndrome*. This syndrome may be related to an elongated styloid process that is present in 4 per cent of the population. Only 4 per cent of those with elongated styloid process have symptoms. The diagnosis may be confirmed radiographically.

Symptoms of burning, constant, and persistent pain that affects the upper division or any other division of the trigeminal nerve that begins after a recognized bout of herpes may be a postherpetic neuralgia. This is most common in older patients who, after a bout of trigeminal neuralgia, continue to have local neuralgic pain with intermittent exacerbations.

Pain that usually occurs at night (in contrast to trigeminal neuralgia, which usually occurs during the day) should suggest the possibility of a glossopharyngeal neuralgia. Patients (usually older) describe the pain as stabbing, jolting, burning, or continuous. The pain may last seconds to minutes, and attacks tend to occur in clusters, lasting from days to months. The pain often is localized to the posterior half of the tongue, the tonsils, and the pharynx, although it may radiate to the ear, the neck, and the jaw. This diagnosis should be suspected when the pain begins at night or if it is triggered by swallowing, talking, yawning, or eating spicy, salty, or bitter foods. Its incidence is quite rare compared with that of trigeminal neuralgia.

When a patient complains of constant unilateral burning or aching in the region of the mandible, maxilla, or frontotemporal area, and if the pain is described as "deep" instead of "on the surface," the problem may be sphenopalatine neuralgia (Sluder's syndrome). It can be differentiated from trigeminal and glossopharyngeal neuralgia in that it usually is a constant pain. It will last hours to days, and there may be inflamed nasal mucosa ipsilaterally. It often develops in patients who have sinusitis or postnasal drip. A diagnosis often may be made by anesthetization of the sphenopalatine ganglion. Cocaine or other topical anesthetics can be used on the tip of a nasal swab that is inserted straight back through the nares after the nasal mucosa is shrunk.

The presentation and differential diagnosis of temporal arteritis are described in Chapter 16. If a patient complains of dull, aching pain in the lower jaw (either unilaterally or bilaterally) that occurs with physical exertion, it may be atypical referred anginal pain. The diagnosis is confirmed if the jaw pain is relieved by administration of sublingual nitroglycerin. Pain that is located in the nasal cavity, in the ethmoid region, or deep in the midface and that is not due to one of the more common causes of facial pain should suggest the possibility of nasal neoplasm, particularly if the patient is elderly.

DIFFERENTIAL DIAGNOSIS OF FACIAL PAIN

CONDITION	NATURE OF PATIENT	NATURE OF PAIN	ASSOCIATED SYMPTOMS	PRECIPITATING AND AGGRAVATING FACTORS	AMELIORATING FACTORS	PHYSICAL FINDINGS	DIAGNOSTIC STUDIES
Neuralgia trigeminal	> age 50	Lancinating Stabbing Sudden onset Usually occurs in daytime On surface Usually unilateral Maxillary or mandibular division more common		Touching of trigger points Extremes of temperature	Carbamazepine Phenytoin	Tenderness at trigger points	
Glossopharyngeal		Paroxysmal Recurrent Pain often nocturnal					
Sphenopalatine		Constant Pain "in deep"	Postnasal drip				
Sinusitis		Dull Constant Over affected sinus or behind orbit Recurrent or chronic Gradual onset or chronic	Nasal stuffiness Mucopurulent nasal discharge Upper respiratory infection	Upper respiratory infections Coughing and sneezing Frontal sinusitis pain worsens with recumbency Maxillary sinusitis pain may worsen when erect	Maxillary pain eases when recumbent Frontal pain lessens when erect	Tender to palpation or percussion Decreased transillumination Nasal congestion	Sinus radiographs Nasal endoscopy Sinus CT

Table continued on following page

DIFFERENTIAL DIAGNOSIS OF FACIAL PAIN *Continued*

CONDITION	NATURE OF PATIENT	NATURE OF PAIN	ASSOCIATED SYMPTOMS	PRECIPITATING AND AGGRAVATING FACTORS	AMELIORATING FACTORS	PHYSICAL FINDINGS	DIAGNOSTIC STUDIES
Glaucoma	> age 40 Farsighted	Dull Severe with acute narrow-angle Usually unilateral	Nausea and vomiting			Increased ocular tension Pupil dilated	Tonometry
Acute		Orbital Severe Sudden onset	Halos or rainbows around light Temporary visual obscuration	Darkness Drugs that dilate pupils (e.g., sympathomimetics, some psychotropics, and anticholinergics)		Conjunctival injection with acute glaucoma Steamy cornea	
Subacute		Frontal Dull Gradual onset					
Temporomandibular joint (TMJ) dysfunction	> age 40 Those with rheumatic arthritis	Recurrent or chronic Usually unilateral over TMJ Pain may be in ear, temple, or teeth Worse in morning in night grinders	Tinnitus Clicking Crepitation of TMJ Bruxism	Bruxism Opening mouth widely	Bite plates Correction of malocclusion	Tender to palpation over TMJ Malocclusion Prominent masseter muscles	Radiographs, MRI, and tomograms of TMJ

Condition	Patient characteristics	Symptoms	Precipitating factors	Signs	Treatment	Diagnostic tests
Cluster headache (Horton's cephalalgia) (see Chapter 16)		Eye pain, Frontal headaches		Ipsilateral lacrimentation and rhinorrhea		
Temporal arteritis (see Chapter 16)		Headache, Transient blindness		Temporal artery tender to palpation		Elevated erythrocyte sedimentation rate
Tumors of nasopharynx	Elderly	Constant pain in nose, ethmoid, midface				Skull radiographs and CT scans
Atypical facial pain	Women, Anxious, Similar family history, Often depressed	Pain does not follow any cranial or cervical nerve "Hemicrania"	Large affectual component	Normal	Psychotherapy Antidepressants	
Dental abscess	Any age	Chronic pain in teeth, jaw, or maxillary region	Temperature extremes Mastication	Sensitive to hot or cold, Tender to percussion over teeth		Dental radiographs

Pain in the eye most commonly is due to trigeminal neuralgia, postherpetic neuralgia, sinus disease, or cluster headaches. Less common causes of referred pain to the eye can be observed in patients with hypertension, cranial arteritis, orbital tumors, and ophthalmoplegic migraine (pain with a third nerve palsy), which may be due to an intracranial aneurysm. Direct causes of pain in the orbit include herpetic keratitis, herpes zoster of the ophthalmic branch, narrow-angle glaucoma, acute iritis, and keratoconjunctivitis sicca.

Sialolithiasis may be present if the patient complains of submandibular or parotid pain that is worse on chewing or swallowing, particularly if there is tenderness or swelling in the salivary glands. Exacerbation of the pain and swelling after instillation of lemon juice into the oropharynx or ingestion of lemon juice confirms the diagnosis.

Selected References

Birt, D.: Headaches and head pains associated with disease of the ear, nose, and throat. Med. Clin. North Am. 62:523–531, 1978.

Drinnan, A. J.: Differential diagnosis of orofacial pain. Dent. Clin. North Am. 31:627–643, 1987.

Gerschman, J., Burrows, G. D., and Reade, R. D.: Orofacial pain. Aust. Fam. Physician 6:1219–1225, 1977.

Goodman, B. W.: Temporal arteritis. Am. J. Med. 67:839–852, 1979.

Gray, G.: Sinusitis—or is it? Aust. Fam. Physician 7:121–131, 1978.

Kahn, C. H., and Warfield, C. A.: Orofacial pain. Hosp. Pract. 24:247–248, 253–254, 259, 1989.

Kennedy, D. W., and Loury, M. C.: Nasal and sinus pain: current diagnosis and treatment. Semin. Neurol. 8:303–314, 1988.

Pertes, R. A.: A practical approach to the diagnosis of chronic orofacial pain, Part 1. Somatic Pain Compendium 9:554–555, 558–560, 562, 1988.

Schramm, V. L.: A guide to diagnosing and treating facial pain and headache. Geriatrics 35:78–90, 1980.

Stohoe, N. L.: Ocular pain in the elderly: simple symptom or hidden danger. Geriatrics 35:41–70, 1980.

Sluder, G.: The role of the sphenopalatine ganglion in nasal headaches. N.Y. Med. J. 87:989, 1908.

Thaller, S. R., and Thaller, J. L.: Head and neck symptoms—Is the problem in the ears, face, neck or oral cavity? Postgrad. Med. 87:75–77, 80, 83–86, 1990.

Chapter 14

Fatigue

Fatigue is the seventh most common complaint in primary care. It can be the presenting symptom of almost any disease. A thorough history and physical examination will establish a diagnosis in about 85 per cent of patients. If, in addition to experiencing fatigue, the patient complains of localizing symptoms such as abdominal pain or hemoptysis, the diagnosis is easier. Specific attention then can be focused on abdominal or chest causes, respectively. If the patient's only complaint is fatigue, the diagnosis is more difficult.

Fatigue can be categorized as acute, chronic, or physiologic. *Acute fatigue* is most often a prodrome or sequela of an acute viral or bacterial infectious process. Heart failure and anemia also may present with a sudden onset of fatigue.

Chronic fatigue (of weeks' to months' duration) can be caused by *depression; chronic anxiety* or *stress; chronic infection,* especially *infectious mononucleosis, hepatitis,* or *tuberculosis; cancer; rheumatoid arthritis* and other rheumatologic disorders; *heart failure; serum electrolyte abnormalities* (hyponatremia, hypokalemia, and hypercalcemia); *chronic lung disease;* or *anemia. Drugs* (both prescribed and over-the-counter) are frequent, often unrecognized causes of chronic fatigue. These drugs include antihistamines, tranquilizers, psychotropics, hypnotics, and anti-hypertensives (particularly reserpine, methyldopa, clonidine, and beta blockers).

Patients with *physiologic fatigue* usually recognize the cause of their fatigue and usually do not consult a physician about this problem. Physiologic fatigue can result from overwork (either physical or mental) and insufficient or poor-quality sleep (which may be due to depression, caffeine, drugs, alcohol, or chronic pain).

In about 50 per cent of patients who present with fatigue, the cause is functional (*depression, anxiety,* or *somatoform disorder*) and 50 per cent have an organic cause. It is important for the physician to consider that multiple causes of fatigue may be present. For instance, a patient who complains of fatigue may demonstrate signs and symptoms of depression and have hepatitis, infectious mononucleosis, or bronchogenic carcinoma.

It must be emphasized that depression as a cause of fatigue is NOT a diagnosis of exclusion. Innumerable diagnostic tests to rule out all possible organic causes should not be performed before the diagnosis of depression is made. Rather, if a thorough history and physical examination do not reveal clues to an organic cause yet do uncover symptoms of depression, depression is the probable cause of fatigue.

NATURE OF PATIENT

Fatigue is an uncommon complaint in children and young adults. When it is the presenting symptom, it usually is due to a prodrome or a sequela of an *acute infectious process*. Chronic fatigue in a young person most often is related to *infectious mononucleosis, hepatitis, substance abuse, depression,* or *chronic anxiety.*

Infants and children seldom manifest depression by lowered mood or fatigue; rather, they present with somatic complaints such as headache or acting out. Often, depression is manifested in children and infants by hyperactivity, withdrawal, eating problems, school troubles, sleep disturbances, or vague physical complaints. In adolescents, when fatigue is associated with "acting out" behavior (such as substance abuse or sexual misconduct), depression may be the underlying culprit. Illnesses such as cancer, chronic lung disease, heart disease, and leukemias are quite uncommon in children and adolescents.

As in younger patients, the most common cause of *acute* fatigue in adults is *infection*. The next most frequent causes of fatigue are *depression* and *anxiety*.

In adult patients, particularly the elderly, serious *organic illnesses,* such as circulatory and pulmonary disease, anemia, cancer, and endocrine abnormalities, are more likely to present with fatigue. In the elderly, *masked hyperthyroidism* may present with a chief complaint of fatigue. Patients with this condition do not necessarily show the tachycardia, tremors, and other classic signs of hyperthyroidism. Weakness may be caused by diuretic-induced hypokalemia, psychotropic agents, alcoholism, and neuropathies.

Because fatigue is such a common symptom of depression in adults, it is important for the physician to recognize that the signs and symptoms of depression vary not only with age, but also with sex and socioeconomic status (Table 14–1). Men more commonly manifest depression by guilt, feelings of helplessness, pessimism, and depressed moods. Early signs of depression in women include headache, insomnia, and withdrawal from

TABLE 14–1. Discriminators of Depression by Socioeconomic Class

Low	Middle	High
Affective		
Hopelessness	Loneliness	Decreased social life
Self-accusation	Helplessness	Pessimism
Crying	Guilt	Dissatisfaction
Dissatisfaction	Crying	Anxiety–tension
Guilt	Anxiety–tension	
Depressed mood	Depressed mood	
Somatic		
Palpitation	Decreased sex drive	Fatigue
Headache	Urinary complaints	Insomnia
Anorexia	Trouble falling asleep	
Waking early	Headache	
	Anorexia	
	Waking early	

Data from Rockwell, D. A., and Burr, B. D.: The tired patient. J. Fam. Pract. *5(5)*:853–857, 1977; and Schwab, J., Bralow, M., and Brown, J.: Diagnosing depression in medical patients. Ann. Intern. Med. *67*:695, 1967.

social activities. Depressed patients of lower socioeconomic class are likely to have depressed moods; feelings of guilt, hopelessness, dissatisfaction, and crying spells; and they may complain of palpitations, loss of appetite, early-morning waking, and headaches. Depressed middle-class patients will state that they feel sad or blue, guilty, helpless, lonely, or anxious. They may complain of crying spells, initial insomnia, early waking, loss of appetite, headache, and decreased libido. Patients of the upper socioeconomic class more often complain of fatigue, insomnia, anxiety and tension, dissatisfaction, and decreased interest in work and social life.

NATURE OF SYMPTOMS

The following historical clues suggest fatigue of *organic* origin: Fatigue is of shorter duration, related to exertion, *not* present in the morning but increasingly evident as the day goes on, relieved by rest, and progressive rather than fluctuating over time. Other obvious organic symptoms or signs may be present. The fatigue may be related to a specific muscle group (e.g., weakened arms or drooping eyelids as in myasthenia gravis). Fatigue that increases over several months suggests a progressively deteriorating condition such as anemia or cancer.

Most instances of chronic fatigue in which an organic cause is not initially apparent are probably caused by psychosocial factors. Fatigue of *functional* origin usually is of longer duration than that of organic origin; it often is present—and may be worse—in the morning, but it improves gradually as the day progresses; and it usually is not related to exertion. The cause of functional fatigue may become apparent during the history, especially if the onset of symptoms correlates with emotional stresses, including doubts about job security, major life changes, and significant loss (e.g., death of a spouse, loss of a job, or amputation of a limb). Fatigue that tends to be worse in the morning, even while the patient is in bed, and improves as the day progresses suggests a *depressive* cause. Fatigue that is constant over weeks or months, not aggravated by effort, and associated with numerous somatic complaints, and shows no diurnal variation is probably due to *chronic anxiety*.

Physiologic fatigue that does not represent a pathologic process should be expected in the following situations: prolonged physical activity without adequate rest; insufficient or poor-quality sleep; dieting; sedentary life-style; pregnancy and the postpartum period; and prolonged mental stress.

ASSOCIATED SYMPTOMS

Fatigue associated with dyspnea on exertion or shortness of breath suggests *chronic cardiorespiratory disease*. Fatigue associated with a low-grade fever suggests *infectious processes* such as hepatitis, tuberculosis, or subacute bacterial endocarditis. *Inflammatory diseases* also may present with fatigue and a low-grade fever. Patients with these conditions also may present only with fatigue and no fever.

In adults complaining of fatigue who also have vague gastrointestinal symptoms (e.g., constipation, bloating, and indigestion), skin disorders, and chronic pain syndromes, *depression* may be the cause. Fatigue associated with restlessness, irritability, sweating, palpitations, and paresthesias probably is due to *chronic anxiety, stress,* or, rarely, *hyperthyroidism*.

When fatigue is associated with breathlessness, anorexia, weight loss, and pallor, *anemia* should be suspected. If these symptoms are accompanied by numbness in the legs or arms, *pernicious anemia* should be considered. If fatigue is associated with shortness of breath, swelling of ankles, or paroxysmal nocturnal dyspnea, *congestive heart failure* should be suspected. The presence of diffuse musculoskeletal pain and several tender points suggests *fibromyalgia*.

PRECIPITATING AND EXACERBATING FACTORS

Identifying a precipitating factor is often a major clue in diagnosis. Initiation of medications, increased work load, insomnia, loss of job, and family problems all can be precipitating factors. If the onset of fatigue is associated with psychosocial problems, the cause may be chronic anxiety or stress. It is important for the physician to note that in someone subjected to chronic anxiety or stress, a minimal additional stress may exacerbate anxiety and result in a new complaint of fatigue. It is as important to note, however, that patients with organic disease may erroneously attribute their fatigue to a psychosocial problem.

AMELIORATING FACTORS

Fatigue reduced by rest is probably *physiologic*. If fatigue is improved on weekends and vacations, then *chronic stress* related to employment may be underlying the fatigue. *Drugs* are causal if fatigue disappears after they are stopped. If fatigue abates after a viral illness, the *viral infection* caused the fatigue.

PHYSICAL FINDINGS

The most critical component in examining a patient complaining of fatigue is a thorough history that focuses on the onset of symptoms, relation to exertion, family and social history, a full systemic review, and questions about abuse of drugs or other substances.

Physical findings may provide clues about the cause of fatigue. Coarse hair, loss of the outer third of the eyebrows, hoarse voice, a doughy consistency to the skin, and myoclonic reflexes (particularly the "hung-up" ankle jerk) all suggest *hypothyroidism*. Tachycardia, tremors, fine hair, and warm, moist palms suggest *hyperthyroidism*. Conjunctival or skin pallor suggests *anemia*. Signs of avitaminosis, such as a smooth, glossy tongue and cheilosis suggest a *nutritional deficiency*. Distended neck veins, rales at the lung bases, tachycardia, gallop, and edema suggest that *congestive heart failure* is the cause of fatigue. Auscultation of a midsystolic click or a late systolic murmur suggests *mitral valve prolapse*. This is a fairly common condition in which patients often complain of fatigue that is most often a manifestation of *anxiety*.

When associated with splenomegaly or hepatomegaly, adenopathy (particularly posterior cervical adenopathy) suggests *infectious mononucleosis*. Hepatomegaly (with or without jaundice) and pruritus suggest *hepatitis;* diffuse adenopathy suggests a *lymphoma*, such as *Hodgkin's disease*. An enlarged liver with ascites and spider angiomata suggests *cirrhosis*. Increased bruising sometimes associated with pallor suggests a platelet deficiency, which may be part of some other *hematologic problem*.

Fever suggests an *infectious process*. Rales at the lung apices suggest *pulmonary tuberculosis*. Low blood pressure associated with increased

DIFFERENTIAL DIAGNOSIS OF FATIGUE

TYPE	NATURE OF PATIENT	NATURE OF SYMPTOMS	ASSOCIATED SYMPTOMS	AMELIORATING FACTORS	PHYSICAL EXAMINATION	DIAGNOSTIC STUDIES
Physiologic Prolonged physical activity Overwork Inadequate sleep Dieting Pregnancy and postpartum period	Usually recognizes cause of fatigue and does not complain to physician about it			Rest		Within normal limits
Sedentary life-style				Increased physical activity		
Functional	May appear depressed	Fatigue on arising; may diminish during day Onset with emotional stress (job insecurity, major life changes, significant loss) Often present for a long time	Insomnia Vague gastrointestinal symptoms Chronic pain			
Depression				Improvement in life situations	Flattened affect	
Anxiety			Numerous somatic complaints Irritability Breathlessness	Removal of stress	No physical abnormalities	

Emotional stress	Of longer duration than that of organic origin; Often present or worse in morning; Improves during the day; Unrelated to exertion	Irritability; Breathlessness	Removal of stress	No physical abnormalities	
Organic	Of shorter duration than that of functional origin; Related to exertion; Not present in morning but gets worse as day progresses; Often related to onset of physical ailment	Symptoms of the disease causing the fatigue: dyspnea on exertion (cardiorespiratory disease), fever (infections), muscle weakness (myasthenia), cold intolerance (hypothyroidism)		Signs of organic pathology causing fatigue: pallor (anemia), rales (pulmonary congestion), weight loss (cancer), tachycardia (hyperthyroidism)	If diagnosis is not clinically apparent: CBC with differential, urinalysis, serum glucose, SMA-22, ESR, chest x-ray, PPD, Monospot test, thyroid function tests, serum electrolytes
Acute Viral or bacterial infections	Most common cause of acute fatigue in all age groups; Fatigue usually subsides in 2 weeks	Fever		Signs of particular infection	CBC with differential; Cultures
Depression	Common cause of fatigue in adults	Sleep disturbances		No physical abnormalities	
Anxiety	Tense, nervous	Somatic complaints		May be signs of mitral valve prolapse	
Drugs and medication		Bizarre behavior; Drowsiness		Bradycardia from methyldopa and beta blockers	

Table continued on following page

DIFFERENTIAL DIAGNOSIS OF FATIGUE *Continued*

TYPE	NATURE OF PATIENT	NATURE OF SYMPTOMS	ASSOCIATED SYMPTOMS	AMELIORATING FACTORS	PHYSICAL EXAMINATION	DIAGNOSTIC STUDIES
Acute *Continued* Organic illnesses Anemia		May have acute onset but increases progressively over time	Breathlessness Anorexia and weight loss Pallor Numbness of extremities (with pernicious anemia)	Conjunctival or skin pallor		Hemoglobin, hematocrit
Hypothyroidism			Weight gain		Coarse hair Loss of outer third of eyebrow Hoarse voice "Doughy" skin Myoclonic reflexes (especially "hung-up" ankle jerk)	Thyroid function tests
Serious organic illnesses (e.g., cancer, endocrine disorders)	Rare in children Most common in elderly		Depends on organic illness			

Chronic Depression (not a diagnosis of exclusion)	Does not present with fatigue in children Often overlooked in elderly Adolescents may present with somatic complaints and "acting out" behavior (e.g., abuse or sexual misconduct) Most common cause of chronic fatigue in adults	In adults, worse in the morning, improves as day progresses Signs and symptoms may vary with age, sex, and socioeconomic status	In children: somatic complaints "acting out" hyperactivity school, eating and sleeping problems withdrawal In adults: feelings of guilt, helplessness, pessimism, sadness, loneliness, decreased libido, anxiety, dissatisfaction insomnia early-morning awakening weight loss and decreased appetite social withdrawal crying spells headache vague GI symptoms skin disorders chronic pain syndromes	Patient has "flat" affect	Should not perform innumerable diagnostic studies to rule out all possible organic causes before diagnosing depression

Table continued on following page

DIFFERENTIAL DIAGNOSIS OF FATIGUE *Continued*

TYPE	NATURE OF PATIENT	NATURE OF SYMPTOMS	ASSOCIATED SYMPTOMS	AMELIORATING FACTORS	PHYSICAL EXAMINATION	DIAGNOSTIC STUDIES
Chronic *Continued* Medications	Users of antihistamines, psychotropics, tranquilizers, antihypertensives (reserpine, methyldopa, clonidine, beta blockers)	Onset correlates with beginning of drug ingestion		Cessation of drugs		
Chronic anxiety or stress		Constant over weeks or months Shows no diurnal variation Is not aggravated by effort May be precipitated by psychosocial factors	Somatic complaints Restlessness Irritability Sweating Palpitations Paresthesias		With mitral valve prolapse, there may be midsystolic click or late systolic murmur	
Organic illnesses Congestive heart failure Cancer	Adults		Varies with illness		Varies with illness	
Chronic infection Mononucleosis	Most common in adolescents and young adults				Posterior cervical adenopathy Hepatomegaly Splenomegaly	Monospot test
Hepatitis	Most common in alcoholics and I.V. drug users				Hepatomegaly with or without jaundice	Abnormal liver function tests and hepatitis antigens

skin pigmentation suggests *adrenal insufficiency*. Polyarticular arthritis suggests *rheumatoid arthritis*, whereas migratory arthritis suggests a *connective tissue disorder*.

DIAGNOSTIC STUDIES

Although laboratory tasks seldom yield the cause of chronic fatigue, in cases of fatigue in which the diagnosis is not readily apparent, the following laboratory tests should be performed: complete blood count with differential, urinalysis, serum glucose, SMA-22, erythrocyte sedimentation rate, and chest radiograph. When the patient has a normal sedimentation rate, it is not likely that serious organic disease is present. Depending on the diagnostic considerations, other laboratory tests may be indicated, such as a tuberculin test, a Monospot test, thyroid function tests, and serum electrolyte evaluation. In instances of chronic fatigue, an abnormal laboratory finding does not necessarily indicate the cause of the fatigue.

LESS COMMON DIAGNOSTIC CONSIDERATIONS

The less common causes of fatigue include neoplasia, connective tissue diseases (e.g., disseminated lupus erythematosus, polymyalgia rheumatica, and temporal arteritis), metabolic states (e.g., uremia, hypokalemia, and hyponatremia), endocrine disorders (e.g., hypothyroidism, hyperthyroidism, hypoglycemia, Addison's disease, and diabetes), malnutrition with or without malabsorption, chronic pain, chronic neurologic disorders (e.g., myasthenia gravis and Parkinson's disease), and chronic infections (e.g., brucellosis, subacute bacterial endocarditis, and the postviral fatigue syndrome). The chronic fatigue syndrome, also called myalgic encephalomyelitis, can be totally disabling.

Selected References

Berris, B., and Rachlis, A.: Investigation of fatigue. Can. Fam. Physician *23(465)*:75–76, 1977.

Gordon, M.: Differential diagnosis of weakness—a common geriatric problem. Geriatrics *41*:75–80, 1986.

Kroenke, K.: Chronic fatigue: frequency, causes, evaluation and managment. Compr. Ther. *15*:3–7, 1989.

Lane, T. J., Matthews, D. A., and Manu, P.: The low yield of physical examinations and laboratory investigations of patients with chronic fatigue. Am. J. Med. Sci. *299*:313–318, 1990.

Miller, P. M., Ingham, J. G., and Davidson, S.: Life counts, symptoms and social support. J. Psychosom. Res. *20(6)*:515–522, 1976.

Rockwell, D. A., and Burr, B. D.: The tired patient. J. Fam. Pract. *5(5)*:853–857, 1977.

Zala, J.: Diagnosing myalgic encephalomyelitis. Practitioner *283*:916–919, 1989.

Chapter 15

Fever

This chapter emphasizes fever as the presenting problem rather than fevers of unknown origin (FUO). Only a brief description of FUO will be given here, as excellent, detailed discussions of FUO may be found elsewhere. **Classically, FUO is a temperature greater than 101°F that occurs on several occasions during a 3-week period in an ambulatory patient or during a 1-week period in a hospitalized patient.** Some authors have suggested that the fever need persist only 10 to 14 days in an outpatient. The fever's cause should not be apparent, even after a complete history, physical examination, complete blood count with differential, urinalysis, SMA-22, cardiogram, chest radiograph, Monospot test, and intermediate-strength purified protein derivative test.

In most febrile patients, a diagnosis is readily apparent or becomes evident within a few days. **FUO usually is due to a common disorder that displays atypical manifestations or a benign, self-limiting illness for which no specific cause is found.** Despite this, it is still important for the physician to search for occult sources of infection, especially if a response to antibiotics is possible.

Normal oral temperature is 37°C or (98.6°F), plus or minus about 1°. Body temperature shows a normal diurnal variation: The lowest point is registered in the early-morning hours, and the highest is reached in the late afternoon.

Acute fevers most commonly are due to *upper respiratory infections, tonsillitis, viral syndromes* such as influenza and gastroenteritis, *drug reactions,* and *genitourinary tract infections* (e.g., cystitis, pyelonephritis, and prostatitis). Less commonly, acute fevers accompany meningitis, intra-abdominal abscess, and other forms of sepsis.

Chronic low-grade fevers most commonly are due to *hepatitis, tuberculosis, infectious mononucleosis* (especially in children and young adults), *lymphomas,* and *occult neoplasms* (especially in the elderly). If the source of a fever is not readily apparent on the basis of history,

161

symptoms, or physical examination, the possibility of *drug fever* (particularly that due to penicillins, cephalosporins, antituberculars, quinidine, methyldopa, procainamide, phenytoin, and barbiturates), *sinusitis, dental abscess, prostatitis, tuberculosis, infectious mononucleosis* (especially if there is associated fatigue), and *hepatitis* (both anicteric and icteric) should be considered.

Less common causes of fever whose cause is not readily apparent by presenting symptomatology include diverticulitis, subacute bacterial endocarditis, osteomyelitis, thrombophlebitis, and Crohn's disease.

NATURE OF PATIENT

The most common cause of fever in children is a viral upper respiratory tract infection. Young children usually have signs or symptoms of a respiratory infection but may show only fever. Common causes of fever in children who have no localizing signs or symptoms at the time of examination include *upper respiratory infections, gastroenteritis, tonsillitis, otitis media, urinary tract infections, measles,* and *roseola.* A true FUO in a child has serious implications: In one study, 41 per cent of children with true FUO were found to have a chronic or fatal disease. Fever in children under age 3 months may be the only indication of a serious disease. Unexplained fever in adolescents may be a manifestation of *drug abuse* or *endocarditis.*

A history of urinary tract infection, sinusitis, prostatitis, and recurrent pneumonia on the same side increase the likelihood that the current febrile episode may be similar to those in the past.

In the absence of physical signs or symptoms suggesting the cause of fever, the physician should question specifically about occupational history (particularly exposure or contact with animals or chemicals), drug ingestion, and travel away from the patient's usual residence. In febrile, elderly patients who lack signs or symptoms that suggest a cause, *tuberculosis, occult neoplasm, cranial arteritis,* and *recurrent pulmonary emboli* must be considered. Elderly patients often have a diminished or absent febrile response to infections.

NATURE OF SYMPTOMS

Contrary to common belief, studies have shown that the fever pattern is not likely to be helpful diagnostically, although the magnitude may. Temperatures above 105°F suggest *intracranial pathology, factitious fever, pancreatitis,* or *urinary tract infection,* especially if there are shaking chills as well. A mild fever suggests *upper respiratory infection* or *flulike syndrome.* Low-grade fever (especially when associated with fatigue) may be the initial manifestation of *tuberculosis, infectious mononucleosis,* or *hepatitis.* The fever range may also be helpful. A narrow range of fever, without spikes or chills, may be seen in lymphomas such as *Hodgkin's disease, lymphatic leukemia,* and *hypernephroma.* A fever in an emotionally disturbed patient who is otherwise in good health and is employed in a health care–related position, has no weight loss, and demonstrates no related or proportional increase in pulse rate should make the physician suspect a factitious cause. Some investigators report that this is more likely in female patients. If a factitious cause is suspected, a simultaneous measurement of urine and rectal temperature should be obtained. **The temperature of the urine normally approximates rectal temperature, and a factitious cause should be suspected if the rectal temperature is significantly (usually more than 2.7°C) higher than the urine temperature.** Other clues to a factitious cause include failure of temperature to follow a diurnal pattern, rapid defervescence without sweating, high temperature without prostration, and high temperature without weight loss or night sweats.

Drug fevers usually occur about 7 to 10 days after initial administration but reappear rapidly with subsequent administration.

ASSOCIATED SYMPTOMS

The following clues may help the physician differentiate viral from bacterial infections. **If the fever is high and there appears to be a sparsity of systemic symptoms (e.g., aches, pains, malaise, backache, fatigue), with the more specific findings limited to either the pharynx, abdomen, or chest, a** *bacterial infection* **is more likely. However, if there is a relatively low-grade fever of less than 101.5°F associated with systemic complaints (e.g., aches, pains, backache, fatigue, and headache) and the localizing findings are sparse, a** *viral infection* **is more likely.** For example, the combined findings of a temperature of 103°F, a red, sore throat, hoarseness, and possible dysphagia suggest a bacterial pharyngitis. A viral cause is more likely if the temperature is less than 101°F, the pharynx is injected and edematous but little evidence of follicular tonsillitis is present, and the patient complains of aches, pains, myalgia, and headache.

Shaking chills suggest a bacteremia frequently due to *pyelonephritis.* When fatigue is associated with a low-grade fever, *infectious mononucleosis* or *tuberculosis* is likely. Persistent fever after an upper respiratory infection, occasionally associated with a frontal headache, should suggest the possibility of *sinusitis.*

PRECIPITATING AND AGGRAVATING FACTORS

Contact with people with an upper respiratory infection or influenza or a local endemic increases the likelihood of *upper respiratory infection* or *influenza.* These two conditions are particularly common in the winter and late summer.

In women, a marked increase in sexual activity may precipitate *cystitis* or *urethritis,* referred to as "honeymoon cystitis." In men, a sudden decrease in sexual activity, particularly after an increase in sexual relations (e.g., during a vacation), may precipitate *prostatitis.*

The pain of *sinusitis* may be exacerbated by bending foward, coughing, sneezing, or blowing the nose.

PHYSICAL FINDINGS

In addition to conducting a careful, thorough physical examination, the physician should pay special attention to certain areas when evaluating a patient whose chief complaint is fever. The sinuses should be percussed and transilluminated for evidence of *sinusitis.* The throat should be examined for signs of *bacterial* or *viral infection* as well as the enanthemas of *measles* or *infectious mononucleosis.* Carious teeth should be tapped for signs of *periapical abscess.* All lymph nodes should be palpated. Rectal examination must be performed for evidence of a *perirectal abscess* or *prostatitis.*

If an obvious source of fever is not made apparent by history or physical examination, attention should be focused on sources of fever that initially present without any clue other than fever. This is particularly true in children. Because significant physical findings and symptoms other than fever may be absent in young children, the physician may use the following clues to assess the severity of the illness: decreased playfulness, decreased alertness, reduced motor ability, respiratory distress, and dehydration. It is not uncommon to see fever as an early manifestation of many illnesses, ranging from *teething* to *roseola.* If the source of the fever in a child is not apparent, a urinalysis should be performed; pyuria and albuminuria may be the only manifestations of a urinary tract infection. In teenagers and young adults, *infectious mononucleosis* should be suspected if the fever is associated with any one or more of the following: pharyngitis (either exudative or nonexudative), an enanthema on the soft palate, posterior cervical or generalized adenopathy, hepatosplenomegaly, and exanthema. If these patients are given ampicillin, a rash similar to that seen after administration of penicillin may develop. If this occurs in patients with proven infectious mononucleosis, the likelihood of a true penicillin sensitivity is small.

DIAGNOSTIC STUDIES

Laboratory tests useful in determining the cause of a fever include complete blood count with differential (particular attention should be given to monocytes and atypical lymphocytes), urinalysis, Monospot test, erythrocyte sedimentation rate, SMA-22, antistreptolysin titers, tuberculin test, antinuclear antibodies, febrile agglutinins, and cultures of blood, urine, pharynx, and stools. In certain instances, computed tomography scans, sonograms, technetium, gallium and indium-111 scans, and special radiographic studies may be helpful.

LESS COMMON DIAGNOSTIC CONSIDERATIONS

Uncommon illnesses that cause fever are legion, and include subacute bacterial endocarditis, acute bacterial endocarditis, bacteremia,

TABLE 15–1. Causes of Fever of Unknown Origin in Adults*

Category	Authors				
	Petersdorf and Beeson	Sheon and Van Ommen	Howard et al.	Gleckman et al.	Esposito and Gleckman
Infection	36	21	37	18	36
Tuberculosis	11	5	4	6	8
Abdominal abscess	4	3	9	6	11
Hepatobiliary	7	0	7	0	6
Endocarditis	5	8	9	0	8
Pyelonephritis	3	0	4	0	0
Other	6	5	4	6	3
Neoplasm	19	17	31	9	24
Lymphoma	6	7	22	9	14
Carcinoma					
Renal	1	0	2	0	4
Pancreatic	2	0	0	0	1
Hepatobiliary	0	2	0	0	3
Unknown primary	2	2	2	0	2
Other	8	6	5	0	0
Connective tissue disorder	15	13	19	9	25
Giant cell arteritis	2	0	4	3	17
Systemic vasculitis	0	6	5	3	6
Lupus erythematosus	5	5	3	0	0
Still's disease	0	0	1	3	0
Rheumatic fever	6	2	0	0	1
Other	2	0	6	0	1
Miscellaneous	23	10	8	29	10
Pulmonary emboli	3	0	0	9	5
Factitious fever	3	0	0	0	0
Periodic disease	5	0	0	3	3
Drugs	1	0	2	0	2
Inflammatory bowel disease	0	4	4	3	0
Other	11	6	2	14	0
Undiagnosed	7	39	5	35	5

*All values are expressed as a percentage of total cases.
From Esposito, A. L., and Gleckman, R. A.: A diagnostic approach to the adult with fever of unknown origin. Arch. Intern. Med. *139*:575, 1979. Copyright 1979, American Medical Association.

DIFFERENTIAL DIAGNOSIS OF FEVER

TYPE	NATURE OF PATIENT	NATURE OF SYMPTOMS	ASSOCIATED SYMPTOMS	PRECIPITATING AND AGGRAVATING FACTORS	PHYSICAL FINDINGS	DIAGNOSTIC STUDIES
Acute						
Upper respiratory infections						
viral	Any age	Oral temperature usually <101.5°F	Signs of upper respiratory infection; May be systemic symptoms	Contact with people with upper respiratory infection	Cough; Oropharynx injected but not beefy red	
bacterial	More common in children	Often high fever, >101°F	Marked signs of upper respiratory infection; Sparsity of systemic symptoms; Children are restless	Local endemic	Pharyngotonsillar exudate; Pulmonary findings	Positive culture
Other viral syndromes						
influenza	Any age	Usually mild fever	Muscle aches; Nausea; Vomiting; Cramps; Diarrhea		Minimal	
gastroenteritis	Any age					
Drug reactions	Taking prescription or over-the-counter drug	Often high fever	Occasional rash		Fever abates when patient stops taking drug	
Urinary tract infection	More common in adults	Often high fever with chills	Backache; Urinary frequency and urgency	Obstructive uropathy	Costovertebral angle tenderness	Urinalysis; Urine culture
Prostatitis			Dysuria; Backache	Marked change in sexual frequency	Prostate tenderness	Culture of prostate secretions
Bacterial sepsis		Often high fever with chills				Blood culture; WBC with differential

Chronic Hepatitis	More common in I.V. drug users	Usually low-grade fever	Fatigue, Jaundice, Anorexia	Hepatomegaly, Liver is tender to percussion, Jaundice	Liver function tests, Hepatitis antigens
Tuberculosis	More common in diabetics	Usually low-grade fever		Chest findings	Chest radiograph, Tuberculin test
Infectious mononucleosis	Teenagers, Young adults	Usually low-grade fever	Fatigue	Enanthema, Pharyngitis, Adenopathy (especially postcervical), Splenomegaly	Monospot test
Neoplasm	Adults and elderly	Usually narrow fever range	Weight loss		
Occult infection (e.g., sinusitis, dental abscess, prostatitis, diverticulitis, subacute bacterial endocarditis, osteomyelitis, inflammatory bowel disease)		Usually low-grade fever	Depends on cause	Depends on cause	Many, including radionuclide scanning
Drug reaction	Taking prescription or over-the-counter drug		Occasional rash	Fever abates when drug discontinued	
Factitious fever	May be emotionally disturbed, Associated with health care	Usually >105°F, Can be low-grade	No weight loss, Pulse rate not proportional to fever	Emotional stress	Disparity between rectal or oral temperature and urine temperature	Complete blood count may show hematologic abnormality

disseminated fungal infection, myocarditis, lung abscess, osteomyelitis, encephalitis, neoplasms in any location, retroperitoneal lesions, lymphomas, connective tissue disorders, inflammatory bowel disease, diverticulitis, periodic fever, malaria, rat-bite fever, and pulmonary emboli (Table 15–1). In recent years, cytomegalovirus disease, sinusitis, malignant histiocytosis, juvenile rheumatoid arthritis, Crohn's disease, and cryptic hematoma have been found to cause occult fevers more frequently.

Selected References

Esposito, A. L., and Gleckman, R. A.: A diagnostic approach to the adult with fever of unknown origin. Arch. Intern. Med. *139*:575–579, 1979.

Everett, M. T.: Definition of FUO in general practice. Practitioner *218*:388–393, 1977.

Froelich, J. W., and Swanson, D.: Imaging of inflammatory processes with labeled cells. Semin. Nucl. Med. *14*:128–140, 1984.

Kimmel, S. R., and Gemmill, D. W.: The young child with fever. Am. Fam. Physician *37*:196–206, 1988.

Larson, E. B., Featherstone, H. J., and Petersdorf, R. G.: Fever of undetermined origin: diagnosis and follow-up of 105 cases, 1970–1980. Medicine *61*:269–292, 1982.

Machowiak, P. A., and Le Maistre, C. F.: Drug fever: a critical appraisal of conventional concepts. Ann. Intern. Med. *106*:728–733, 1987.

McCarthy, P. L., et al.: History and observation variables in assessing febrile children. Pediatrics *65*:1090–1095, 1980.

Musher, D. M.: Fever of unknown origin: diagnostic principles. Hosp. Pract. *17*:89–95, 1982.

Nolan, S. M., and Fitzgerald, F. T.: Fever of unknown origin. The general internist's approach. Postgrad. Med. *81*:190–198, 203–205, 1987.

Tabor, P. A.: Drug-induced fever. Drug Intell. Clin. Pharm. *20*:413–420, 1986.

Chapter 16

Headache

About 80 per cent of Americans experience some form of headache each year. Fifty per cent of these patients have severe headaches, and 10 to 20 per cent consult a physician with headache as the chief complaint. The most common type of headache is the *muscle-contraction*, or *tension*, headache. About 10 per cent of the population have *vascular* headaches. Headaches caused by acute *sinusitis* also are fairly common. Less common causes of headaches include glaucoma, temporal arteritis (more common in elderly patients), *cervical arthritis, temporomandibular joint (TMJ) dysfunction*, and *trigeminal neuralgia*. **Eye strain and hypertension are not common causes of headaches. Most patients with hypertension do not have headaches; most patients with headaches do not have hypertension. When headaches and hypertension coexist, the headaches usually are not related to the hypertension.**

To establish a correct diagnosis, the physician must first differentiate acute headaches from recurrent and chronic headaches. Most common headaches are recurrent; a few are chronic. Therefore, the physician should first elicit the "temporal profile" of the particular headache and history of prior headaches. It is important for the examiner to ask any patient who complains of headaches about the number and types of headaches; age and circumstances at the time the headaches began; any family history of headaches; the character of pain (including location of pain, frequency of attacks, duration of headache, and the time of onset of attack); any prodromal symptoms; associated symptoms; precipitating factors; emotional factors; previous medical history (especially past illnesses, concurrent disease, recent trauma or surgery); allergies; and responses to medication. An organic disorder should be suspected if there is an isolated severe headache; consistently localized head pain that prevents sleep; headaches asssociated with straining; headaches accompanied by neurologic signs or symptoms; a change in usual headache pattern; or a chronic, progressively severe headache.

NATURE OF PATIENT

Tension headaches, *vascular* headaches (including migraine), and headaches due to *temporal arteritis* are significantly more common in women, whereas *cluster* headaches are much more common in men (ratio of men to women, 9:1).

Muscle-contraction, or *tension,* headaches are the most common type of headaches in children and adults. These headaches usually are of psychogenic origin and often are induced by situational (home, family, school, or work) problems. Although most children with tension headaches may be suffering from simple anxiety or stress, the headache also may be a manifestation of depression, particularly if it is associated with mood change, withdrawal disturbances, aggressive behavior, loss of energy, self-deprecation, or weight loss. **If a headache has been present continuously for 4 weeks in the absence of neurologic signs, it is probably psychogenic in origin.** Migraine headaches are recurrent.

Studies of young children with *chronic* headaches have revealed that only a small fraction had an organic cause. In children and adolescents, organic headaches most often are due to non—central nervous system infections, fever, trauma, and migraine. In children, acute headaches may be the presenting symptom of a *febrile illness* such as pharyngitis, particularly with otitis media. A child with a sore throat or otitis media, therefore, may present complaining of headache.

Studies have shown that among children up to age 7, there is a 1.4 per cent incidence of *migraine;* among patients who are age 17, the incidence is 5 per cent. Population studies indicate a 12 per cent incidence of migraine in postpubescent males and up to a 20 per cent incidence in postpubescent females. Despite these studies, it is important for one to realize that 20 per cent of all adults who experience migraine headaches have onset of symptoms before age 5, and 50 per cent have onset of migraine symptoms before age 20. **Although combination headaches (i.e., tension and migraine) are common in adults, they are rare in children and their frequency increases with adolescence.**

Sinus headaches are uncommon in children, but they may occur in young patients, particularly in association with persistent rhinorrhea, cough, otitis media, or allergies. The maxillary sinus is most frequently involved in children. Likewise, headaches of ocular origin are uncommon in children; the possibility of *astigmatism, strabismus* or *refractive error* must be considered, however. This is particularly true if the headaches appear to be related to reading or schoolwork or if they occur late in the afternoon or evening.

Increased intracranial pressure should be suspected if a child who complains of headache has other signs of neurologic dysfunction or projectile vomiting without nausea or if the headache is precipitated or exacerbated by coughing or straining. Causes of increased intracranial pressure in children include tumors (the headache usually is progressive and chronic), *pseudotumor cerebri, hydrocephalus* (detected by serial head measurements), *subdural hematoma* (more common in battered children or after trauma), and *brain abscess* (which may be a complication of otitis media). *Malingering* can be the cause of headaches in children as well as in adults.

In *classic migraine,* the aura and prodrome are prominent, and the headaches are throbbing and unilateral. The patient often goes to sleep and, on awakening, frequently finds that the headache has disappeared. *Common migraine* occurs more frequently than classic migraine. In common migraine, the aura may be vague or not present. The prodrome may be vague and manifested only by personality change or malaise, nausea, and vomiting. Common migraine headaches are less often unilateral than classic migraine. It should be noted that cluster headaches are extremely rare in children, although they may occur in teenagers. Cluster headaches have their highest frequency in the fourth to sixth decades of life. A family history of "vascular," "sinus," or "sick" headaches is present in most patients with migraine. A positive family history is not usually present in patients with cluster headaches. Most patients with vascular headaches have a history of headaches caused either by tension or by vascular problems. Prior diagnoses may be incorrect because of an inadequate or an incomplete history.

Because the incidence of significant disease causing the headaches increases with age, the onset of headaches in patients after age 50 requires careful evaluation and differential diagnosis. **Fewer than 2 per cent of patients over age 55 experience new, severe headaches. If patients over age 55 have an acute onset of an unrelenting headache that lasts for hours or days, significant disease such as tumor, meningitis, encephalitis, or temporal arteritis should be suspected.** Headache may precede the onset of neurologic deficit. Sudden new onset of headaches in elderly people occasionally strongly suggests *cerebral ischemia* and *impending stroke* as well as *arteritis.*

In patients over age 50, there are only a few conditions that cause chronic severe headaches. They include *temporal arteritis, cluster headaches, mass lesions, posttraumatic headaches, cervical arthritis,* and *depression.* **Depression is a common cause of chronic headache in patients over age 50, but these patients usually experienced chronic headaches before age 50 as well.** Temporal arteritis, although uncommon, occurs more frequently in elderly women; it should be suspected in elderly patients over age 60 who have unilateral chronic head pain, unexplained low-grade fever, proximal myalgia, markedly elevated erythrocyte sedimentation rate, or an unexplained decrease in visual acuity. Other less common causes of headache in elderly patients include congestive heart failure, glaucoma, trigeminal neuralgia, and

TMJ dysfunction. Iritis, cerebrovascular insufficiency, cerebral hemorrhage, subdural hematoma, and meningitis are even less common but are more serious causes of chronic headache.

NATURE OF PAIN

The type, severity, and location of pain are important in the differentiation of the cause of headaches (Tables 16–1 to 16–3). *Tension, or muscle-contraction,* headaches usually are dull, not throbbing, steady, and of low but persistent intensity. If a patient suffering from chronic tension headaches awakens with a headache, its severity may increase

TABLE 16–1. Causes of Headaches (by Location)

Area of Pain	Possible Cause
Generalized	Muscle tension Hypertension Arteriosclerosis or anemia Central nervous system tumor Head trauma or chronic subdural hematoma Systemic: uremia, thyrotoxicosis
Frontal 　upper	Muscle tension Frontal ethmoid sinusitis Rhinitis
midfacial	Dental disease, maxillary sinusitis, nasal disease Ocular or vascular disease, tumor Neurologic (cranial nerve) or vascular degenerative disease
Lateral 　temporal	Muscle tension Temporomandibular joint disorders, myofascial disease Vascular: arteritis, migraine, cluster headache
facial or ear	Pharyngeal disease (referred pain) Otologic or dental disease; Ramsay Hunt syndrome Myofascial disease
Vertex	Sphenoid or ethmoid disease Hypertension Muscle tension Central nervous system, nasopharyngeal neoplasm
Occipital	Uremia Fibromyositis Subarachnoid hemorrhage Hypertension Muscle tension

From Schramm, V. L.: A guide to diagnosing and treating facial pain. Geriatrics *35*:78–90, 1980.

TABLE 16–2. Diagnosis of Tension Headache Versus Migraine by History

| Characteristics | Tension Headache (Muscle-Contraction) | | | Migraine* Type of Vascular Headache | |
	Description	Percentage of Patients 1970s†	1950	Description	Percentage of Patients 1950
Laterality	Bilateral	86	90	Unilateral	80
Locus	Occipital	25	—	Supraorbital frontal region	55
	Occipital and suboccipital	26	—		
	Frontal and occipital/ frontal	61	<50		
Quality of head pain	Nonthrobbing	73	70	Throbbing or pulsating	80
Onset of head pain	Severity increases gradually	81	—	Severity increases rapidly in classic, steadily in common	
Frequency	≤8 months	54	—	<1 week	60
	Constant or daily	—	50		
Duration	≤7 hours	50	—	<12 hours	50
	1–12 hours	—	33		
	1–3 hours	—	10		
Prodromes	None	88	90	Present	75
Autonomic symptoms	None	75	90	Present	50
Age at onset	15–24 years	52	—		
	Before 20 years	—	30	Before 20 years	55
Family history	No	54	60	Yes	65

*Percentages for common and classic combined.
†Percentages calculated from data of 1420 tension headache patients in three multicenter studies.
From Friedman, A. P.: Characteristics of tension headache. Psychosomatics 20(7):451–457, 1979.

as the day progresses and then decrease toward evening. The pain of *migraine* headaches is severe, initially throbbing, and later boring. The severity of this pain increases rapidly and steadily. The pain of *cluster* headaches is much severer and more stabbing and burning in quality than that of the usual vascular or tension headaches. Acute sinus headache pain usually is described as severe, throbbing, and pressure-like.

Common migraine headaches are usually unilateral, but may be bilateral. Most often they are located in the frontotemporal or supraorbital region. *Classic migraine* headaches are unilateral. *Cluster* headaches are unilateral and periorbital in any given cluster; the pain is described as in the eye and radiating to the front of the face or the temporal regions. *Tension* headaches are most often occipital, suboccipital, and bilateral, and patients describe the pain as similar to that caused by a constrictive band around the head or as tightness of the scalp. These headaches may radiate down the back of the head and neck. The pain of *sinus* headaches is usually over the involved sinus or sinuses: maxillary, ethmoid, or frontal. Some patients with *ethmoid sinusitis*

TABLE 16–3. Factors in Neuralgia and Vascular Pain

Factor	Typical Neuralgia	Atypical Neuralgia	Migraine	Cluster Headache	Temporal Arteritis
Age	50–70 years	30–50 years	15–30 years	30–50 years	50–70 years
Sex	Equal	Predominantly female	About equal	Predominantly male	Predominantly female
Family history	Not significant	60%	Frequent	20%	Not significant
Pain location	Usually limited to one cranial nerve	Deep, diffuse, crosses sensory boundaries	Unilateral head and face	Unilateral face or orbit	Distribution of cranial artery, but may be multiple locations
Pain duration	Short, paroxysmal, seconds to minutes	Fluctuating, hours to days	Minutes to hours	Minutes to hours	Fluctuating, persistent
Pain character	Sharp, localized	Aching, drawing, pulling	Progressive, dull, boring; then throbbing	Repetitive burning or intense throbbing	Intense, deep boring, or throbbing
Precipitating factors	Touch, wind, and others	Variable	None	None	None
Trigger zone	Usual	No	No	No	Artery tenderness only
Autonomic nervous system or other signs or symptoms	Unusual	Occasional lacrimation, flushing	Nausea, photophobia scotomata, hemianopia, paresthesia	Common: lacrimation, rhinorrhea, flushing, congested nose, and conjunctiva; nose, and conjunctiva; occasionally Horner's sign	Fever, malaise, anorexia, progressive decreased visual acuity
Effect of drugs					
vasoconstrictors	None	Occasional relief	Relief	Relief	None
analgesics	Inadequate	Relief with narcotic	Not adequate	Not adequate	Variable
local anesthetics	Relief	Occasional relief	None	None	None
steroids	None	None	None	None	Gradual relief
Effect of surgery					
cranial nerve	Generally effective	Not effective	None	None	None
biopsy	None	None	None	None	Diagnostic

From Schramm, V. L.: A guide to diagnosing and treating facial pain. Geriatrics 35:78–90, 1980.

present complaining of pain behind the eye that intensifies with coughing or sneezing.

Classic migraine headaches usually last for 2 to 8 days. Common migraine lasts for 12 hours to several days. The onset of most migraine headaches is gradual. *Tension* headaches usually persist all day for several days. Some patients state that these headaches are constant. *Cluster* headaches have a much shorter duration than tension headaches or migraines; most cluster headaches last from 20 to 60 minutes. Patients with *trigeminal neuralgia* usually complain of facial pain, but occasionally their presenting symptom is headache. This pain is usually short, sharp, severe, and stabbing. Each episode lasts less than 90 seconds, but repeated pains persist for 2 to 3 minutes. Headaches caused by mass lesions are persistent but intermittent, whereas headaches due to intracranial infections are usually constant.

Headache Patterns

The common varieties of headaches have a typical pattern for each patient. A change in the pattern should suggest the development of a new problem. If a patient who usually has tension headaches in the occipital region or in a bandlike region around the head develops unilateral headaches associated with nausea and vomiting, migraine headaches may have developed as an additional problem. *Migraine* headaches recur at irregular intervals and have no specific pattern; they may recur once or twice weekly or once a year. They often occur around the menstrual period.

The pattern of *tension* headaches varies with the cause of tension. They most often occur daily but may also occur several times a week. **It is not uncommon for a patient with chronic tension headaches to awaken in the morning with a headache, but it is rare for one to be awakened at night by it.** A specific form of muscle-contraction headaches is due to *bruxism* (grinding of the teeth). Patients may present with a constant headache on awakening if they are night grinders. Typically, *hypertensive* headaches also occur in the morning after nighttime recumbency. They are usually throbbing in nature.

The frequency patterns of *cluster* headaches are diagnostic because these types of headaches usually occur in close succession. They often occur at approximately the same time of day for 3 to 8 weeks and may recur one to three times a day. They may have an inexplicable remission for months or years and an equally inexplicable recurrence. Although early-morning onset (1:00 A.M. to 5:00 A.M) is typical of cluster headaches, some attacks occur during the day. If they happen at night, which is rare, they possibly are related to rapid eye movement during sleep. *Sinus* headaches also often begin in the morning, get progressively worse, but tend to get better toward evening.

Migraine headaches have prodromes, which are uncommon in *cluster* headaches; occasionally, some patients experience a burning sensation on the forehead before the onset of pain. The classic migraine prodrome occurs 15 to 30 minutes before the headache. It is abrupt in onset, lasts for 10 to 15 minutes, and is often contralateral to the headache. Visual auras include a variety of scotomata, transient blindness, blurred vision, and hemianopia. Nonvisual auras may include weakness, aphasia, mood disturbances, and photophobia. In contrast to classic migraine, common migraine usually has no specific aura. When prodromes are present, they vary widely and may present as psychic disturbances, fatigue, gastrointestinal symptoms, or mood changes.

ASSOCIATED SYMPTOMS

With *classic migraine,* the most common associated symptoms include anorexia, nausea, vomiting, sonophobia, photophobia, and irritability. Less common are dizziness, fluid retention, abdominal pain, and sleepiness. Symptoms associated with the *common migraine* include all those associated with classic migraine as well as fatigue, chills, diarrhea, and urticaria. Cyclic abdominal pain or vomiting in children and motion sickness in adults are commonly seen in patients with migraine headaches.

Pain in the posterior cervical region that is exacerbated by neck extension often is seen in patients with *tension* headaches. The patients frequently are tense, anxious, significantly depressed, and fatigued. Patients with chronic tension headaches seem to be more emotionally involved in their headache symptoms; they seem to focus on their symptoms more than patients with migraines do. In addition, the intensity of the affective disturbance is more marked in those with tension headaches than in those with migraine.

Patients with acute *sinus* headaches may complain of toothaches; this indicates a maxillary infection. If they complain of pain in the eye, this indicates an ethmoid sinusitis. There frequently are nasal discharge, percussion tenderness over the sinus area, and symptoms of an upper respiratory infection. A *nasal* or *sinus neoplasm* may be present if the physician suspects a sinus headache that does not improve after approximately 2 weeks of appropriate therapy (including antibiotics and nasal decongestants) and if there is blood-tinged rhinorrhea. These symptoms recur despite therapy, and sinus radiographs may show evidence of bone destruction.

The symptoms associated with *cluster* headaches are significantly different, and help the physician establish this diagnosis. Patients may complain of injection of the involved eye, a blocked nose with rhinorrhea, and marked ipsilateral lacrimation. There may be an ipsilateral Horner's syndrome. About 25 per cent of patients with cluster headaches have peptic ulcer disease.

Organic brain disease should be suspected if one or more of the following signs or symptoms are noted:

1. Intermittent or continuous headache that progressively increases in frequency and severity
2. Headache that is exacerbated by coughing or straining at stool
3. Headache that is worse in the morning (note that sinus and hypertensive headaches also may be worse in the morning)
4. Vomiting
5. Headache that disturbs sleep
6. Inequality of pupils
7. Fever
8. Seizures
9. Confusion
10. Recent onset of neurologic deficit
11. Papilledema
12. Onset of severe headaches after age 50

PRECIPITATING AND AGGRAVATING FACTORS

Although migraine headaches may be precipitated by *menstruation,* their frequency increases as estrogen levels fall. Migraine headaches frequently are precipitated by emotional stress. Less frequently, they are precipitated by fatigue, bright lights, fasting, hypoglycemia, odors, exercise, weather changes, and high altitude.

Patients may have a history of headaches that are caused by ingestion of certain *foods* and *beverages* (e.g., aged cheese, chocolate, yogurt, buttermilk, and red wine). Headaches may be precipitated by foods that contain nitrites ("hot dog headache") or monosodium glutamate ("Chinese restaurant syndrome"). *Alcohol* and *caffeine* also are frequent offenders, as is *caffeine withdrawal. Drugs* such as reserpine, vasodilators, and oral contraceptives also may cause headaches. Some patients who have been heavy users of ergot drugs to control migraine may experience migraine headaches when these therapeutic agents are stopped.

Muscle-contraction, or *tension,* headaches can be precipitated by emotional or physical stress, extended periods of mental concentration, and prolonged, somewhat abnormal positions of the neck. Some tension headaches may ocur with cessation of analgesics or tranquilizers used in their treatment. Dental malocclusion may stimulate contraction of the muscles of mastication, thus causing spasm of the muscles and headache. Ill-fitting dentures, particularly if they have been worn for 10 or more years, also may lead to muscle-contraction headaches.

Cluster headaches may be precipitated by short naps, alcohol ingestion, nitroglycerin, tyramine, and emotional stress. *Sinus* headaches may be aggravated by coughing or sneezing, but this is also true of other types of headaches, especially vascular. Eye pain due to *glaucoma* often is precipitated by darkness or sympathomimetic drugs, which cause pupillary dilatation.

AMELIORATING FACTORS

If the patient states that ergot-containing drugs improved the acute headaches, a vascular cause is probable. Likewise, relief with nasal decongestants and antibiotics suggests a sinus cause. A headache that is severe; associated with nausea, vomiting, scotomata, or aura; and relieved by sleep is probably migraine.

PHYSICAL FINDINGS

In patients with *tension* or *migraine* headaches, the physical findings seldom contribute to the differential diagnosis. Patients with *trigeminal neuralgia* may have a trigger point. During an attack of *cluster* headache, there may be ipsilateral lacrimation and rhinorrhea. Patients with acute *sinus* headaches may have a mucopurulent or blood-tinged nasal discharge. In addition, there may be tenderness to percussion or palpation over the involved sinus, which also may demonstrate impaired transillumination. The presence of fever suggests an *infectious process* as the cause of the headache. Severe *hypertension* may suggest that the headaches are of hypertensive origin, although most patients with hypertension do not have headaches. Tenderness to palpation over the temporal artery suggests *temporal arteritis* as a cause.

When nuchal rigidity is found, *meningitis* or a *subarachnoid bleed* should be suspected. Nuchal rigidity must be differentiated from the stiff neck of patients with cervical arthritis (more common in elderly patients). In patients with true nuchal rigidity, the neck is stiff throughout the arc as the examiner flexes it but not in extension or lateral rotation. In contrast, with *cervical arthritis,* the early phase of flexion of the neck is supple; this is followed by a sudden, boardlike rigidity with resistance in other directions of movement as well.

Patients with *psychogenic* or *conversion* headaches may describe the pain in very vivid terms with much affect; the patient does not really appear to be in great pain.

Pain localized to one or both eyes with increased intraocular pressure indicates *glaucoma*. The presence of a jaw click or point tenderness to palpation over the temporomandibular joint suggests that the headache may be due to TMJ dysfunction.

Most patients with headaches do not exhibit any abnormalities on neurologic examination. However, a transient ipsilateral Horner's syndrome may be seen with some migraine headaches.

DIAGNOSTIC STUDIES

There are only a few laboratory tests that help in the differential diagnosis of headaches. Radiographs may confirm *acute sinusitis* if there is a typical fluid level in one or more of the sinuses. Patients may experience sinus headaches and still have normal sinus radiographs. The erythrocyte sedimentation rate is markedly elevated with *temporal arteritis*. A biopsy of the arterial wall showing giant cell infiltration is pathognomonic of arteritis.

If there is sudden onset of headache in patients over age 50, the physician must make a difficult decision regarding whether to perform lumbar puncture. It is indicated in suspected instances of *cerebral hemorrhage* or *bacterial encephalitis,* but it is dangerous in patients with mass lesions or increased intracranial pressure. Noninvasive tests such as a computed tomography scan or magnetic resonance imaging should be done first if intracranial disease is suspected. Arteriograms may show vascular abnormalities and mass lesions.

LESS COMMON DIAGNOSTIC CONSIDERATIONS

Glaucoma, eye strain, and *systemic problems* are less common conditions that also may present with headaches.

Patients with *glaucoma* may complain of pain in one or both eyes; they describe a visual halo around objects; headaches often come on in a darkened environment; and there is increased intraocular pressure and occasionally tenderness to palpation over the globe.

Eye strain is a diagnosis that often is applied incorrectly. Headache from eye strain is unusual. It tends to occur in people who do work that requires close vision. In addition, the headaches tend to occur after a prolonged period of using the eyes.

Systemic causes include *uremia, occult carbon monoxide poisoning, thyrotoxicosis, severe anemia, brain tumors, chronic subdural hematoma, subarachnoid hemorrhage,* and *ocular disease.* Tumors of the eye, ear, nose, or throat also may present with headaches. Occult carbon monoxide poisoning may result from faulty furnaces, space heaters, and kitchen stoves.

The key to diagnosing headaches consists of a careful, detailed

DIFFERENTIAL DIAGNOSIS OF HEADACHE

TYPE	NATURE OF PATIENT	NATURE OF SYMPTOMS	ASSOCIATED SYMPTOMS	PRECIPITATING AND AGGRAVATING FACTORS	AMELIORATING FACTORS	PHYSICAL EXAMINATION	DIAGNOSTIC STUDIES
Tension headaches (muscle-contraction headache)	Most common cause of headache at any age More common in females	Usually of psychogenic origin In children: may be manifestation of stress, anxiety, or depression In adults: usually dull, nonthrobbing, with persistent, low intensity may last a few days severity may increase as day progresses and then decrease toward evening usually occipital, suboccipital, and bilateral described as constrictive band around head or tightness of scalp rarely wakes patient from sleep	Fatigue	Emotional or physical stress Abnormal neck positions (especially neck extension) Prolonged mental concentration Withdrawal of analgesics or tranquilizers Dental malocclusion or ill-fitting dentures Bruxism (nightgrinding of teeth)	Stress reduction		
Vascular headaches	Affect 10% of U.S. population More common in women Family history of headaches			Coughing Sneezing	Ergot-containing drugs Beta blockers		

Type	Incidence/Demographics	Description	Associated Symptoms	Precipitating Factors	Relieving Factors
Common migraine	More frequent in children	Vague or absent aura and prodrome; Gradual onset; Lasts 12 hours to several days; Not always unilateral; Usually in frontotemporal or supraorbital region	Those of classic migraine; General malaise; Fatigue; Chills; Diarrhea; Urticaria; Motion sickness		Sleep
Classic migraine	More common in women; Incidence: 1.4% in children (under age 7 years); 5% in children at age 17 years; 17% in postpubescent males; 20% in postpubescent females; 50% of adults with migraines have symptoms before age 20	Prominent aura; The prodrome: has abrupt onset lasts 10–15 min. precedes headache by 15–30 minutes often contralateral to headache; Headache: severe throbbing unilateral gradual onset intensity increases steadily and rapidly lasts 2–8 days	Visual auras (scotomata, transient blindness, blurred vision, hemianopia); Nonvisual auras (weakness, aphasia, mood disturbances, photophobia); Nausea and vomiting; Anorexia; Sonophobia; Photophobia; Irritability; Dizziness; Fluid retention; Abdominal pain; Sleepiness	Menstruation; Emotional stress; Fatigue; Bright lights; High altitude; Weather changes; Exercise; Certain foods; Fasting; Hypoglycemia	Sleep
Cluster headaches	Highest incidence in fourth to sixth decade; Rare in children; Much more common in men than in women (9:1)	Pain is severer, and more stabbing and burning than that in vascular or tension headache; Unilateral and periorbital in any given cluster	25% of patients have peptic ulcer disease; Injection of involved eye; Rhinorrhea; Marked ipsilateral lacrimation	Short naps; Alcohol; Nitroglycerin; Tyramine; Emotional stress	

Table continued on following page

DIFFERENTIAL DIAGNOSIS OF HEADACHE *Continued*

TYPE	NATURE OF PATIENT	NATURE OF SYMPTOMS	ASSOCIATED SYMPTOMS	PRECIPITAT-ING AND AG-GRAVATING FACTORS	AMELIORAT-ING FACTORS	PHYSICAL EXAMINATION	DIAGNOSTIC STUDIES
Cluster head-aches *Continued*	Family history of cluster head-aches uncom-mon. Recur at same time of day for 3–8 weeks, 1–3 times per day. Typical early-morning onset	May radiate to front of face or to tem-poral regions. Duration ranges from 20–60 minutes	May be ipsilateral Horner's syn-drome				
Headaches due to febrile illnesses	Common cause of headache in children	Headache may be only presenting symptom in chil-dren	Fever	Pharyngitis, espe-cially with oti-tis media		Fever	
Sinusitis (see Chap. 13)	Uncommon in children	Pain: severe, throbbing, and intense pres-sure usually over in-volved sinus begins in morning, grows progres-sively worse dur-ing the day, im-proves toward evening. Maxillary sinus is most often involved in children	Persistent rhinor-rhea. Otitis media. Allergies. Symptoms of up-per respiratory infection. Toothache, with maxillary in-volvement. Eye pain with ethmoid in-volvement	Coughing. Sneezing		Mucopurulent or blood-tinged na-sal discharge. Percussion ten-derness over in-volved sinuses	Transillumination of sinuses. Sinus radiographs
Depression	Common cause of headache in pa-tients > age 50	Constant, chronic headache	Those of depres-sion		Treat depression		

182

Temporomandibular joint (TMJ) dysfunction (see Chap. 13)	Adults	Usually pain in TMJ or ear, but may present with headache (temporoparietal)	Bruxism	Opening mouth too wide	Jaw clicks Point tenderness to palpation over TMJ Prominent masseter muscle	Radiograph of TMJ MRI of TMJ
Temporal arteritis	Most common in elderly women	Unilateral, chronic headache	Unexplained low-grade fever Proximal myalgia Decreased visual acuity		Tenderness to palpation over the temporal artery	Erythrocyte sedimentation rate is markedly elevated
Cervical arthritis	Most common in elderly people	Occipital or nuchal headache			Stiff neck Early phase of flexion is supple but followed by sudden, board-like rigidity with resistance in other directions	Radiograph of cervical spine
Trigeminal neuralgia (see Chap. 13)	Adult	Pain is short, episodic, sharp, severe, and stabbing Each episode lasts < 90 seconds but recurs for 2–3 minutes	Pain in face along distribution of one division of nerve	Trigger point Extremes of temperature	Patient may have a trigger point	
Increased intracranial pressure		Progressive, chronic headache	In children; neurologic dysfunction and projectile vomiting without nausea	Coughing Straining	Papilledema	CT scan Increased cerebrospinal fluid pressure
Glaucoma (see Chap. 13)		Frontal headache	Patient sees halos Pain in eye	Darkened areas Drugs that dilate pupils	Increased intraocular pressure	Tonometry

clinical history and neurologic examination. There is usually time to observe the patient and to evaluate the whole patient in relation to the family and environment, which is helpful in determining the underlying cause of headache. The physician should try to avoid the use of habituating drugs in the treatment of patients with chronic headaches.

Selected References

Appenzeller, O., Feldman, R. G., and Friedman, A. P.: Migraine, headache, and related conditions—Panel 7. Arch. Neurol. *36*:784–804, 1979.

Caviness, V. S., and O'Brien, P.: Current concepts—headache. N. Engl. J. Med. *302*(8):446–450, 1980.

Hecherling, P. S., Leikin, J. B., Maturen, A., and Perkins, J. T.: Predictors of occult carbon monoxide poisoning in patients with headache and dizziness. Ann. Intern. Med. *107*:174–176, 1987.

Kunkel, R. S.: Evaluating the headache patient: history and workup. Headache *19*:122–126, 1979.

Rothner, A. D.: Headaches in children and adolescents. Classification and recommendations. Postgrad. Med. *81*:223–230, 1987.

Schramm, V. L.: A guide to diagnosing and treating facial pain and headache. Geriatrics *35*:78–90, 1980.

Shankland, W. E.: Differential diagnosis of headaches. Cranio *4*:47–53, 1986.

Thompson, J. A.: Diagnosis and treatment of headache in the pediatric patient. Curr. Probl. Pediatr. *10*:1–52, 1980.

Chapter 17

Heartburn and Indigestion

Heartburn and indigestion are common presenting complaints. Because these symptoms are often vague, it is difficult for the physician to determine a precise cause, and therefore, treatment is frequently ineffective. For purposes of this discussion, heartburn is a sensation of burning, warmth, or heat in the retrosternal region between the xiphoid and the manubrium that occasionally radiates toward the jaw or, rarely, the arms. Water brash may be present. Indigestion is a separate entity. Dyspepsia, which is similar to indigestion, has been defined as "episodic or persistent abdominal symptoms often related to feeding which patients or physicians believe to be due to disorders of the proximal portion of the digestive tract." Dyspeptic symptoms include upper abdominal discomfort, postprandial fullness, early satiety, anorexia, belching, nausea, vomiting, bloating, borborygmi, dysphagia, and abdominal burning.

The most common causes of heartburn and indigestion include *reflux esophagitis* (with or without hiatal hernia); ingestion of *drugs* such as aspirin, nonsteroidal anti-inflammatory agents, antibiotics, and theophylline derivatives; *gastritis, non-ulcer dyspepsia;* excessive consumption of *food* or *alcohol; chronic active gastritis; gallbladder disease; pregnancy; aerophagia;* and *functional gastrointestinal disorder.* Although patients with tumors of the gastrointestinal tract may complain of heartburn or indigestion, neoplasms are not a common cause of these symptoms. This chapter focuses on indigestion and heartburn unassociated with abdominal pain. Conditions associated with abdominal pain are discussed in the chapters on abdominal pain.

NATURE OF THE PATIENT

Children rarely complain of indigestion or heartburn, although vague abdominal discomfort may affect children who experience *mal-*

absorption or *food intolerance*. In these conditions, certain foods may cause crampy abdominal pain or diarrhea. Weight loss may be noted if there is significant malabsorption. When children complain of distention or awareness of peristalsis and gurgling, they often have *functional gastrointestinal disease*. If these complaints are intermittent and not disabling, if the patient is otherwise healthy, and if the results of the physical examination are normal, an emotional cause should be suspected. Questioning the child may reveal depression or other emotional problems. These problems frequently occur with external environmental stress, such as divorce, birth of a sibling, illness in a family, starting school, and problems with boyfriend or girlfriend.

In adults, heartburn is almost always due to *reflux esophagitis*. This is more common in pregnant women, particularly during the later months. Patients with esophagitis may complain of severe heartburn that is relieved by alkali and aggravated by recumbency. Although *hiatal hernia* is three times more common in multiparous patients than in primigravid women, it should be remembered that the *symptoms of heartburn are due to esophageal reflux and not to the hiatal hernia.* Pregnant patients have delayed gastric emptying, increased intra-abdominal pressure, and increased estrogen levels, all of which facilitate esophageal reflux. Thirty to 50 per cent of adults demonstrate hiatal hernias on radiographs; only 5 per cent of this population report symptoms of heartburn.

Indigestion due to gastritis occurs frequently in patients who ingest large quantities of *alcohol* or *drugs* such as salicylates, corticosteroids, nonsteroidal anti-inflammatory agents, theophylline, quinidine, and some antibiotics.

Elderly patients are more likely to complain of vague feelings of indigestion, possibly related to bloating. Many of the symptoms of indigestion and abdominal bloating are due to excessive amounts of *intestinal gas*. Virtually all intestinal gas is the result of bacterial fermentation, although the amount of discomfort is not necessarily proportional to the amount of gas in the intestines. The complaints of indigestion and bloating are more common in elderly patients because of relative gastric and intestinal stasis, hypomotility of the gut, altered intestinal bacteria, increased incidence of constipation, and lack of exercise, all of which tend to facilitate the production of intestinal gas.

Tense and *anxious patients* are more likely to be aware of normal intestinal movement and are also more likely to complain about these feelings. Many patients with *gallbladder disease* and *ulcers* complain of vague abdominal discomfort and occasional distention.

NATURE OF SYMPTOMS

Heartburn is a burning sensation that occurs in the xiphisternal region with occasional proximal radiation. It may vary in intensity from a mild feeling of warmth to extreme pain. Occasionally, the pain may be indistinguishable from that of severe angina pectoris; it is therefore important for the physician to note that heartburn has *no relation to physical activity*. The pain is usually caused by esophageal spasm, is intermittent over several minutes, and recurs over long periods of time. Pain may radiate into the neck and occasionally into the arms, back, or jaw. According to one study, the pain radiated to the back in 40 per cent of patients with proven *esophageal reflux* but radiated to the arms or neck in only 5 per cent.

Initially, the pain of heartburn may be felt only after heavy meals or while the patient is lying down or bending over. In more advanced cases, the pain is more easily provoked, lasts longer, and is accompanied by dysphagia.

Patients with *gastritis* may have abdominal pain, vague indigestion, or heartburn as a presenting complaint. Epigastric discomfort that is worse after eating, loss of appetite, a sense of fullness, nausea, and occasional vomiting are also common complaints in patients with gastritis. These same symptoms may be seen in patients with chronic active gastritis caused by *Helicobacter pylori*. Heartburn is also a common complaint in patients with *bile gastritis,* which often occurs after gastric resection or pyloroplasty. In these cases bile refluxes into the stomach and subsequently into the distal esophagus, causing heartburn. Some patients who have *peptic ulcer* do not complain of the classic symptoms but only of vague indigestion that is sometimes relieved by vomiting.

Gastrointestinal symptoms in patients with *functional gastrointestinal disorders* are often vague and nonspecific. Patients do not get consistent relief with any medication or therapeutic regimen. Other neurotic symptoms are often present, and there is no evidence of systemic disease or weight loss despite a long history of vague symptoms. Because various patients who present with an organic pathology (e.g., peptic ulcer, gallbladder disease, or colonic tumors) may also have vague symptoms, a specific workup will be required in some cases. When these vague symptoms occur in young adults, it is unlikely that a malignant process is present. Likewise, if the symptoms have been present for many years without any significant progression or evidence of systemic disease, a major disease process is also unlikely.

Other distinguishing characteristics often help the physician differentiate functional from organic pain. With functional illness, patients may present with severe and continuous pain but will not experience significant weight loss. The patients often give exaggerated descriptions of their pain and have a significant emotional investment; they may come into the office with a list of their symptoms written on a piece of paper—"Le malade avec le petit morceau de papier." With organic disease, the pain, although severe, is often periodic and not uncommonly associated with weight loss.

ASSOCIATED SYMPTOMS

Patients with *peptic esophagitis* frequently have chest pain. They may complain of heartburn or chest pain when there is esophageal spasm. In some instances, the patients will complain only of substernal pain, which may radiate into the neck, jaw, or upper arms.

Belching secondary to *aerophagia* is often seen in patients with reflux esophagitis and in patients with functional gastrointestinal disease. If indigestion is associated with nausea, right upper quadrant pain, or pain in the right shoulder (particularly the inferior angle of the right scapula), duodenal *loop distention* or *cholelithiasis* should be considered. Hematemesis suggests *peptic ulcer disease* or *variceal bleeding,* regardless of how vague the other symptoms are.

PRECIPITATING AND AGGRAVATING FACTORS

In many patients whose symptoms are due to *reflux esophagitis,* coronary artery disease or hysteria has been previously diagnosed. **Clues to the correct diagnosis of esophagitis are that the pain is not usually brought on by exercise, frequently occurs in the recumbent position, and is often relieved by antacids.** Anything that distends the lower third of the esophagus, irritates its mucosa, or reduces lower esophageal pressure can precipitate *reflux esophagitis.* This includes recumbency, acidic foods, gastric stasis, large meals, and fatty foods (which delay gastric emptying). Several studies show that in addition to gastric juices, bile and other duodenal juices may play a role in the pain of reflux esophagitis. Conditions that increase intra-abdominal pressure (e.g., pregnancy and marked ascites) can facilitate regurgitation of gastric or duodenal contents into the distal esophagus. Caffeine frequently causes heartburn in susceptible people. Certain spices, carminatives (e.g., oil of spearmint and peppermint), garlic, onions, chocolate, fatty foods, alcohol, and carbonated beverages may reduce lower esophageal pressure and thus facilitate reflux. Cigarette smoking also reduces lower esophageal pressure and stimulates gastric acidity. It is important for the physician to remember that certain drugs (particularly theophylline derivatives, isoproterenol, and anticholinergics) lower esophageal pressure and may precipitate reflux and heartburn. Other precipitating factors include straining, recumbency, lifting, and ingestion of orange juice, tomato juice, and spicy foods and drinks.

In some patients who swallow air, chew gum, or eat rapidly, heartburn develops as a result of belching and subsequent regurgitation of gastric juices into the distal esophagus. Although there are some instances in which patients with hiatal hernia have heartburn or chest pain, the presence of a hiatal hernia does not establish the presence of esophagitis.

AMELIORATING FACTORS

In general, avoidance of the aforementioned precipitating factors reduces and may eliminate the discomfort. In addition, raising the head of the bed (by tilting the entire bed, not by merely using another pillow), retiring with an empty stomach, sucking on antacid tablets, eating small, frequent meals, following a low-fat diet, and avoiding tight garments may help.

The pain of peptic esophagitis is frequently relieved by antacids. These substances reduce gastric acidity and re-establish more normal lower esophageal sphincter pressure, thus reducing reflux. It is particularly important for the physician to remember that the pain of peptic esophagitis may be relieved by nitrates, ordinarily thought to relieve only the pain of angina pectoris. **Relief of substernal pain by nitroglycerin does not necessarily establish the diagnosis of angina pectoris, as this drug can also relieve the pain of lower esophageal spasm.** In fact, patients with peptic esophagitis who obtain inadequate relief from the usual therapeutic measures (antacids, bethanechol, cimetidine, and metoclopramide) may receive additional relief from nitroglycerin. **If the pain is relieved by ingesting viscous lidocaine (Xylocaine Viscous), it is probably due to peptic esophagitis.** Some authors suggest using this procedure as a diagnostic tool because studies have shown that when chest pain was relieved by ingestion of Xylocaine Viscous, it usually was due to peptic esophagitis. There were a few false-positives, however, among patients who had chest pain of coronary origin. Therefore, this test is useful but will not rule out coronary artery disease with absolute certainty.

Once the diagnosis of serious disease is excluded, patients with vague symptoms of indigestion and functional gastrointestinal complaints should be treated with reassurance and, occasionally, tranquilizers. In some instances, antispasmodics and digestants may be helpful.

PHYSICAL FINDINGS

Most patients who complain of indigestion or heartburn demonstrate no abnormal physical findings, despite a careful examination. Auscultation of peristalsis in the chest should suggest a large diaphragmatic hernia. Mild, diffuse, abdominal tenderness associated with abdominal distention sometimes is observed with *pancreatitis* or *excessive swallowed air* in the intestinal tract. A succussion splash can often be elicited in

DIFFERENTIAL DIAGNOSIS OF HEARTBURN AND INDIGESTION

CAUSE	NATURE OF PATIENT	NATURE OF SYMPTOMS	ASSOCIATED SYMPTOMS	PRECIPITATING AND AGGRAVATING FACTORS	AMELIORATING FACTORS	PHYSICAL FINDINGS	DIAGNOSTIC STUDIES
Reflux esophagitis	Adults More common in pregnant women in later months	Severe heartburn Water brash often occurs with recumbency Recurrent pain radiates to back (40%), arms, or neck (5%) Not induced by exercise	Chest pain Dysphagia Belching (due to aerophagia) Cough Asthma, especially nocturnal	Recumbency Straining or lifting Drinking alcoholic, caffeinated, or carbonated beverages Eating heavy meals or fatty, spicy, or acidic foods Smoking Pregnancy	Raising head of bed Antacids Nitrates Small, frequent, low-fat meals Avoidance of tight garments		Pain often relieved by ingestion of viscous lidocaine Esophagoscopy Upper GI radiograph Esophageal pH monitoring
Gastritis	Alcoholics	Abdominal pain Vague indigestion Heartburn	Decreased appetite Sense of fullness Nausea and vomiting	Alcohol Meals Drugs (aspirin, nonsteroidal anti-inflammatory agents, corticosteroids, antibiotics, antiasthma agents)	Bile gastritis may be relieved by vomiting	Tenderness to abdominal palpation or epigastric percussion	Endoscopy Upper GI radiograph Gastric biopsy and culture for *Helicobacter pylori*
Active chronic gastritis (B)	Especially older adults	Indigestion			Bismuth compounds (Pepto-Bismol) Antimicrobials		Gastric mucosal biopsy and culture for *Helicobacter Pylori*
Non-ulcer dyspepsia		Diffuse abdominal pain or discomfort	Nocturnal pain uncommon		Pain not usually relieved by antacids		Endoscopy

Disorder	Age group	Symptoms	Social/environmental stresses	Relieving/associated	Diagnostic findings
Functional gastrointestinal disorder	Children and adults	Distention Awareness of peristalsis and gurgling Intermittent symptoms Vague, nonspecific symptoms No weight loss Continuous pain Significant emotional investment Other neurotic symptoms Belching (secondary to aerophagia)			No signs of systemic disease Studies normal
Excessive intestinal gas	Common in elderly	Vague feelings of indigestion Abdominal bloating Belching Passing flatus	GI stasis Hypomotility of gut Changed intestinal bacteria Constipation Lack of exercise	Belching Passing flatus	
Gas entrapment (hepatic or splenic flexure syndrome)		Abdominal discomfort Pain often referred to chest Chest pain	Bending over Wearing a tight garment	Passing flatus	Flexion of thigh on abdomen replicates symptoms Abdominal radiograph shows trapped gas in hepatic or splenic flexure
Gallbladder disease		Vague abdominal discomfort Occasional distention Indigestion Nausea Pain in right shoulder	Fatty foods		Cholecystograms Sonograms

patients with *gastric dilatation,* whether due to reflex or secondary to pyloric obstruction. Some patients with *gastritis* will have tenderness on abdominal palpation, whereas others may have no physical findings other than midepigastric tenderness to percussion. The same is true for patients with *peptic ulcer disease.* Patients with *cholelithiasis* may have no symptoms, although there occasionally may be right upper quadrant tenderness to palpation or percussion. In some patients with *hydrops of the gallbladder,* a dilated gallbladder is palpable or ballotable.

DIAGNOSTIC STUDIES

Endoscopy is the most reliable diagnostic technique for establishing the cause of upper gastrointestinal symptoms. Esophageal reflux can be observed on upper gastrointestinal radiographs. Esophagitis can be detected by esophagoscopy, and its symptoms can be produced by instillation of dilute hydrochloric acid in the distal esophagus (Bernstein test). Esophageal pH monitoring is the most sensitive test.

Gastritis is best diagnosed by gastroscopy.

Gallbladder disease can be diagnosed by sonography, cholecystography, and isotopic studies.

LESS COMMON DIAGNOSTIC CONSIDERATIONS

When the patient finds that abdominal discomfort is intensified by bending over or wearing a tight garment, gas entrapment (e.g., hepatic or splenic flexure syndrome) should be suspected. Sometimes this discomfort is relieved by passage of flatus. Gas entrapment can be confirmed if flexion of the right or left thigh on the abdomen replicates the pain or if an abdominal radiograph shows a large bubble of trapped gas in the hepatic or splenic flexure. The pain of gas entrapment in the hepatic or splenic flexure is often referred to the chest, and the patient may present with a complaint of chest pain.

Heartburn may be caused by viral esophagitis and moniliasis of the esophagus. Disseminated sclerosis that invades the esophagus may also cause severe heartburn. Indigestion may be the presenting symptom in uremia, pulmonary tuberculosis, migraine, gastric dilatation, glaucoma, hypercalcemia, diabetes, and coronary artery disease.

Selected References

Barbara, L., Camilleri, M., Corinaldesi, G. P., et al.: Definition and investigation of dyspepsia. Consensus of an international ad hoc working party. Dig. Dis. Sci. *34*:1272–1276, 1989.

Chamberlain, C. E., and Peura, D. A.: *Campylobacter (Helicobacter) pylori.* Is peptic disease a bacterial infection? Arch. Intern. Med. *150*:951–955, 1990.
Hunt, T.: Indigestion in Harvey's time. Am. J. Med. *85*:891–893, 1978.
Long, W. B., and Cohen, S.: The digestive tract as a cause of chest pain. Am. Heart J. *100*:567–572, 1980.
Reed, P. I.: Oesophageal reflux. Practitioner *224*:357–363, 1980.
Talley, N. J., and Phillips, S. F.: Non-ulcer dyspepsia: potential causes and pathophysiology. Ann. Intern. Med. *108*:865–879, 1988.
Thompson, W. G., and Heaton, K. W.: Functional bowel disorders in apparently healthy people. Gastroenterology *79*:283–288, 1980.
Volpicelli, N. A., Yardley, J. H., and Hendrix, T. R.: The association of heartburn with gastritis. Dig. Dis. *22*:333–339, 1977.

Chapter 18

Insomnia

Of all the sleep problems, disorders of initiating and maintaining sleep (insomnias) are the most common. Studies have shown that hypnotics are used on a regular basis by about 20 per cent of the adult population. Insomnia includes the following problems: delay in falling asleep, poor quality of sleep (deficiency of deep and rapid eye movement [REM] sleep), frequent awakening, and early-morning wakefulness. Insomnia can be caused by *physical disorders* (e.g., congestive heart failure, pregnancy, hyperthyroidism, nocturnal asthma, or nocturnal seizures); *painful* or *uncomfortable syndromes* (e.g., toothache, arthritis, or restless legs syndrome); *psychiatric illnesses* (e.g., depression, anxiety, schizophrenia, or mania); the use or withdrawal of *drugs* (e.g., caffeine, alcohol, antidepressants, sympathomimetics, beta blockers, or hypnotics) and *situational stressors*. Insomnia may be transient or chronic.

NATURE OF PATIENT

Nocturnal enuresis (bedwetting), *sleepwalking, talking while asleep,* and *night terrors* are thought to be arousal disorders because they usually occur with emergence from deep non–REM sleep. Children who experience nocturnal enuresis and sleepwalking often have difficulty sleeping. Bedwetting is the most common sleep–arousal disorder in children between ages 3 and 15. It is more prevalent in males than in females. When there is no obvious organic or psychological cause, bedwetting usually occurs in the first part of the night as the child emerges from delta sleep and before the first REM sleep. The change of sleep state often is accompanied by body movements and increased muscle tone; urination occurs during this period. Although most of these problems have a psychological cause, many investigators believe that such disorders stem from a basis that is psychophysiologic rather than from one that is strictly psychological.

Nightmares and night terrors often disturb sleep. Nightmares, in both children and adults, occur during REM sleep. Night terrors, characterized by sudden screams and arousal, occur during deep sleep. **Insomnia in children is most often due to psychological stress, although occasionally it can be due to organic disease (e.g., a disorder of the hip).**

Some patients who *snore* have *sleep-induced apnea,* which causes nocturnal wakefulness and daytime drowsiness. These patients commonly are obese males. Typically, their sleep companions complain that they snore loudly. These loud snorers may have as many as 100 episodes of sleep apnea each night; many episodes lead to brief arousal.

Sleep patterns often change with aging; many elderly people require less sleep than they did in their younger years. Elderly patients often complain of both delay in falling asleep and poor sleep quality.

Many patients who ingest products that contain *caffeine* (e.g., coffee, tea, and cola) complain of insomnia. Even those patients who previously tolerated caffeine well may develop sleeping problems. Because the half-life of caffeine may range from 2 to more than 6 hours in different people, the ingestion of caffeine, especially after 6 P.M., may contribute significantly to insomnia. Patients may or may not be aware that caffeine is the cause of their insomnia. People who drink *alcohol,* even in moderate amounts (i.e., two drinks at night), as well as cured alcoholics, often experience poor sleep quality with frequent awakening.

Poor sleep at night may be related to napping or dozing during the day, which is more common in elderly people. Elderly patients with *dementia* are often restless and wakeful at night. *Depression,* a common cause of sleep disturbances, is frequently undiagnosed in the elderly.

Depressed (unipolar affective disorder) patients of all ages frequently experience insomnia characterized by delayed sleep onset (prolonged latency), frequent awakening, and, classically, early-morning wakefulness. Patients with *manic depression (bipolar affective disorder),* may experience marked insomnia, especially just before and during the manic phase. Patients who suffer from *anxiety* may have trouble falling asleep but seldom experience early-morning wakefulness.

NATURE OF SYMPTOMS

Patients usually describe insomnia rather loosely as "trouble sleeping." A patient may have one or more types of insomnia. Therefore, the physician must question specifically for each type of insomnia to diagnose the cause correctly and to provide effective, specific therapy. Short-term (less than 2 weeks) insomnia is most often due to a life stress, such as emotion, noise, pain, stimulation, grief, anxiety, jet lag, or a change in working hours. Chronic insomnia may be due to psychiatric disorders (depression or dysthymic disorder), conditioned insomnia, psychophysiologic drugs, caffeine, or alcohol. It is very helpful to ask patients what they are thinking about before they fall asleep and what they are thinking about on awakening. This often provides significant clues to the cause of their insomnia. It is also important to interview the sleep partner of an insomniac about snoring, apnea, leg twitches, seizures, and unusual sleep postures.

Prolonged sleep latency (the time from turning the lights out until stage 1 sleep) is most common in anxious patients, caffeine and alcohol users, and elderly patients, especially those who sleep during the day. Most patients overestimate the latency period. Some complain of a poor quality of sleep when they do not feel rested despite an adequate amount of sleep; this is usually due to a deficiency of deep REM sleep and is particularly common in patients with painful syndromes, pregnant women, people who consume alcohol, and cured alcoholics. Some patients, particularly alcoholics, complain of frequent awakening; this is usually from stage 2 sleep. **Early-morning awakening from which a patient cannot return to sleep is most common and particularly characteristic of depressed patients.** Some studies show depressed patients to have prolonged sleep latency, decreased total sleep, increased intermittent awakening, and less deep sleep than other patients.

ASSOCIATED SYMPTOMS

Painful and *uncomfortable conditions* such as pleurisy, peptic esophagitis, toothaches, pregnancy, and even severe itching can interfere with normal sleep. Paroxysmal nocturnal dyspnea, nocturnal asthma, hyperthyroidism, alcoholism, use of caffeine or other drugs, recent cessation of hypnotics or antidepressants, and severe snoring may also contribute to sleeping problems. **The most common causes of insomnia are ingestion of caffeine, alcohol consumption, anxiety, and depression.**

Although anxiety and depression often cause insomnia, patients with these conditions usually have additional symptoms. *Anxious patients* often have somatic complaints such as headaches, chest pain, palpitations, dizziness, gastrointestinal distress, nervousness, and feelings of foreboding. *Depressed patients* frequently complain of decreased appetite, weight loss, lack of energy, lack of interest in activities, decreased libido, constipation, and vague aches and pains. Patients with fibrositis and insomnia (which some investigators attribute to depression) may obtain excellent relief of their aches, pains, and insomnia with antidepressant medication.

DIFFERENTIAL DIAGNOSIS OF INSOMNIA

CAUSE	NATURE OF PATIENT	NATURE OF SYMPTOMS	ASSOCIATED SYMPTOMS	PRECIPITATING AND AGGRAVATING FACTORS
Bedwetting (nocturnal enuresis). Nightmares and night terrors	Children (especially ages 3–15) More common in males More common in children	Arousal after deep sleep Arousal during REM sleep	Sleepwalking	Environmental or psychological stresses and fears
Painful or uncomfortable conditions Physical disorders	Any age	Delayed latency Poor sleep quality	Symptoms related to physical disorder or painful or uncomfortable condition	Toothache Pleurisy Arthritis Pregnancy Esophagitis Nocturnal asthma or seizures Congenital hip lesions Hyperthyroidism Nocturia
Change in sleep habits	Elderly people	Delayed sleep latency Poor sleep quality	Daytime naps or dozing	
Unipolar depression	Depressed	Delayed sleep latency Early morning wakefulness	Anorexia Fatigue Lack of interest in activities Decreased libido Constipation Vague aches and pains	Conditions, medications, and situations that produce depression
Bipolar depression	Manic Manic-depressive	May not sleep at all during manic phases	Agitation Hyperactivity Flight of ideas	Worse just before and during manic phase

	Age	Sleep pattern	Symptoms	Situations
Anxiety	Any age	Delayed sleep latency	Somatic complaints Headaches Chest pain Palpitations Dizziness GI symptoms Nervousness Feelings of foreboding	Situations that produce anxiety
Sleep apnea	Adults Often obese males	Frequent awakening Poor sleep quality	Snoring Excess daytime sleepiness	Sleep apnea Obstruction Central apnea
Caffeine	Any age	Delayed sleep latency Poor quality sleep	May have previously tolerated caffeine well	Use of caffeine (especially after 6 P.M.)
Alcohol	Teenagers Adults Elderly	Delayed latency Frequent awakening	Nervousness Signs of alcoholism	Alcohol Alcoholic withdrawal "Cured" alcoholics
Withdrawal of antidepressants or hypnotics	Any age	Similar to prior symptoms	May redevelop symptoms of anxiety, depression	
Medications and drugs	Any age	Poor sleep quality Prolonged sleep latency	Depends on drug responsible	Psychotropics Beta blockers Bronchodilators Sympathomimetics Diuretics Hypnotics Appetite suppressants Amphetamines Cocaine

PRECIPITATING AND AGGRAVATING FACTORS

Patients who complain of insomnia should be questioned about whether certain situations (e.g., death in the family, financial concerns, family crises, school examinations, changes in life patterns, alterations in work schedules, or changes in drug habits) coincided with the onset of insomnia. So-called rebound insomnia often occurs with cessation of benzodiazepine drugs, especially at higher dosage levels. Paradoxically, these drugs may have originally been used as hypnotics. The patient should also be questioned about prior episodes of insomnia and what may have precipitated them. Transient insomnia may occur in anticipation of a joyous event or during periods of excitement.

According to one study of patients referred to a sleep center, the most common cause of insomnia is ingestion of caffeine in any form. Many of these patients previously tolerated caffeine well. The second most common cause is alcohol. Although small amounts of alcohol may facilitate sleep onset for some patients, it may also cause early awakening or nightmares, contrary to common belief. These patients often note poor quality of sleep and frequent awakening.

In evaluating sleep disturbances, physicians should have patients keep a sleep diary for 1 week. Patients should note the time they retire; their latency period; number of awakenings; time of last awakening; any sleep events such as dreams, nightmares, and the need to urinate; and any comments made by the sleep partner. It is particularly important for patients to note their thoughts during latency and on awakening, as these may help establish the cause of their insomnia.

Other precipitating and aggravating factors in insomnia include fear of illness, and even pruritus. Although these factors may be tolerated during the day when the patient is active, they may be distracting enough to cause insomnia when the patient is at rest.

AMELIORATING FACTORS

Hypnotics, including over-the-counter preparations, are occasionally helpful for short periods of insomnia. However, their continued use (for more than 1 week) may exacerbate insomnia, particularly if REM sleep has been suppressed. Hypnotics are *rarely* indicated to treat the symptom insomnia. **One must treat insomnia by dealing with its cause.** Daytime naps or pain can be identified as the probable cause of insomnia if cessation of the former or relief of the latter results in improved sleep. If avoidance of caffeine (in all forms) after noon permits the return of normal sleep patterns, caffeine was probably responsible for the insomnia. When changes in work shifts are associated with insomnia, patients should be advised to try to return to their original sleep schedule to determine whether this eliminates their insomnia. Avoidance of noisy or extremely warm environments and strenuous exercise at night also may facilitate a return to normal sleep patterns.

PHYSICAL FINDINGS

The physical examination is usually not helpful in determining the cause of insomnia. Occasionally, medical conditions that contribute to insomnia may yield abnormal physical findings; this occurs in hyperthyroidism, congestive heart failure, peptic esophagitis, pulmonary disease, ulcer disease, seizure disorders, and prostatism. Any condition that causes frequent nocturia may interfere with normal sleep patterns.

DIAGNOSTIC STUDIES

When the cause of insomnia cannot be determined and the patient cannot be relieved of this symptom, he should be referred to a sleep center for sleep studies. Centers are located in many regions and are discussed by several other authors (Reynolds et al., 1979).

LESS COMMON DIAGNOSTIC CONSIDERATIONS

Conditions that occur less frequently include nocturnal myoclonus, painful erections, central sleep apnea, and restless legs syndrome. The last two conditions are more common in elderly people. Sleep apnea often is exacerbated by hypnotics and alcohol.

Selected References

Doghramje, K.: Sleep disorders: a selective update. Hosp. Community Psychiatry *40*:29–40, 1989.

Gillen, J. C., and Byerly, W. F.: The diagnosis and management of insomnia. N. Engl. J. Med. *322*:239–248, 1990.

Hauri, P. J., and Esther, M. S.: Insomnia. Mayo Clin. Proc. *65*:869–882, 1990.

Kales, A., Soldatos, C. R., and Kales, J. D.: Sleep disorders: insomnia, sleepwalking, night terrors, nightmares and enuresis. Ann. Intern. Med. *106*:582–592, 1987.

Kales, A., et al.: Insomnia and other sleep disorders. Med. Clin. North Am. *66*:5, 1982.

Kogeorgos, J., and Scott, D. F.: Sleep and sleep disorders. Practitioner *224*:717–721, 1980.

Mathis, J. L.: Insomnia. J. Fam. Pract. *6*:873–876, 1978.

Pring, P. N., Vitiello, M. V., Raskind, M. H., and Thorpy, M. J.: Geriatrics: sleep disorders and aging. N. Engl. J. Med. *323*:520–526, 1990.

Reynolds, C. F., et al.: Sleep and its disorders. Symposium on psychological issues in primary care. Prim. Care *6*:417–438, 1979.

Chapter 19

Menstrual Irregularities

ABNORMAL BLEEDING

Menstrual irregularity is especially common in the perimenarchal and perimenopausal years. Bleeding from the vagina is considered abnormal whenever it occurs at an unexpected time of life (before menarche or after menopause) or when it varies from the norm in amount or pattern. *Spontaneous abortions, pregnancy complications,* and *bleeding from polyps* or other pathologic processes account for approximately 25 per cent of the cases of abnormal vaginal bleeding.

Dysfunctional uterine bleeding is a somewhat confusing nonspecific diagnostic term. It has been defined as abnormal uterine bleeding not due to organic gynecologic disease. Therefore, this diagnosis may be reached only by a process of exclusion. With advances in the understanding of the neuroendocrinologic basis of the menstrual cycle, diagnosis and therapy have become more specific. The reader can find detailed reviews of these developments in several excellent articles (see references). To understand and diagnose the various causes of menstrual irregularities, one must have a thorough knowledge of normal physiology (Fig. 19–1). **Although the history is important, it seldom is diagnostic and serves only as a guide to the origin of the bleeding. In most instances, hormonal or cytologic studies are necessary to establish the correct diagnosis.**

Anovulatory Bleeding

Hormonal mechanisms of endometrial bleeding include *estrogen-withdrawal bleeding, estrogen-breakthrough bleeding, progesterone-withdrawal bleeding,* and *progesterone-breakthrough bleeding.* **Anovulatory,**

203

Figure 19–1. Physiology of the normal ovulatory menstrual cycle. (From Lopez, R. I.: Menstrual irregularities in teenage girls. Drug Therapy, April 1981, p. 47.)

hormone-related bleeding is most common. This form of dysfunctional uterine bleeding is due to estrogen-withdrawal or estrogen-breakthrough bleeding.

Estrogen-Withdrawal Bleeding. In instances of estrogen-withdrawal bleeding, the endometrium proliferates and remains stable as long as the estrogen level remains above the threshold. When the estrogen falls below the threshold, there is bleeding. When this occurs in the absence of progesterone, the endometrium is not in the secretory phase, and bleeding is often prolonged and profuse. This type of bleeding often occurs during adolescence and the climacteric.

Estrogen-Breakthrough Bleeding. This type of bleeding has been divided into two categories. The first is associated with low but constant levels of estrogen (near the threshold). This causes portions of the endometrium to degenerate and results in spotting. **This type of threshold-breakthrough bleeding occurs with the use of low-dose oral contraceptives.** The second type of estrogen-breakthrough bleeding occurs when estrogen levels are initially well above the threshold. This causes the endometrium to proliferate and become hyperplastic; areas of endometrium outgrow their blood-borne hormone supply, with degeneration and irregular, prolonged bleeding resulting.

Progesterone-Withdrawal Bleeding. As in polycystic ovarian syndrome, this type of bleeding occurs only with an estrogen-primed endometrium. When estrogen therapy is continued as progesterone is withdrawn, progesterone-withdrawal bleeding occurs. This type of bleeding is observed when intramuscular progesterone or oral medroxyprogesterone acetate (Provera) is administered as a test for the presence of endogenous estrogen.

Progesterone-Breakthrough Bleeding. This is a form of estrogen-breakthrough bleeding that occurs when a high dose of a progestational drug is given.

Ovulatory Dysfunctional Bleeding

Ovulatory dysfunctional bleeding may be suspected by history and confirmed with simple investigations (Table 19–1). Ovulatory bleeding is usually associated with a regular cycle length, occasional ovulation pain (mittelschmerz), premenstrual symptoms (e.g., breast soreness, bloating, weight gain, and mood changes), and a biphasic basal body temperature. *Anovulatory bleeding* causes an irregular cycle in which bleeding is not preceded by or associated with subjective symptoms. In such cases, there is a monophasic basal body temperature pattern.

Bleeding Patterns

Recognition of particular bleeding patterns is another way of considering cases of abnormal vaginal bleeding (Table 19–2). *Menorrhagia,* or *hypermenorrhea* (excessive menstrual bleeding), is often due to local gynecologic disease (e.g., polyps, cancer, salpingitis, and uterine fibroids). It also commonly occurs in association with intrauterine devices. *Metrorrhagia* (intermenstrual spotting between otherwise normal periods) is also often caused by local disease. It frequently is associated with exogenous estrogen therapy. *Menometrorrhagia* is bleeding that is unpredictable with regard to amount and frequency; it can be caused by local lesions, complications of early gestation, or endocrine dysfunction (e.g., dysfunctional bleeding). *Polymenorrhagia* is excessive cyclic hem-

TABLE 19–1. Differentiation of Ovulatory and Anovulatory Bleeding

Criteria	Ovulatory Bleeding	Anovulatory Bleeding
History	Regular cycle length, ovulation pain (mittelschmerz), premenstrual molimina (breast soreness, bloating, weight gain, mood change), dysmenorrhea (cramps up to 12 hours before flow and/or for first 2 days of flow)	Irregular cycles in which bleeding is not preceded by or associated with subjective symptoms
Basal body temperature record	Biphasic pattern	Monophasic pattern
Cervical mucus	Preovulatory: Thin, clear, watery mucus with stretchability (spinnbarkeit) and ferning Postovulatory: Thick, cloudy, cellular mucus that lacks stretchability and ferning	Always dominated by estrogen
Maturation index	Preovulatory: Dominated by superficial cells Postovulatory: Shift to high percentage of intermediate cells	Always a marked right shift due to high estrogen level
Premenstrual endometrial biopsy	Secretory endometrium	Proliferative and possibly hyperplastic changes
Serum progesterone level	Preovulatory: <1 ng/mL Postovulatory: >5 ng/mL	Never exceeds 5 ng/mL; usually preovulatory values

From Strickler, R. C.: Dysfunctional uterine bleeding—diagnosis and treatment. Postgrad. Med. 66:135–146, 1979.

TABLE 19–2. Nomenclature to Describe Menstrual Disturbances

Term	Bleeding Pattern
Menorrhagia	Excessive flow (amount and/or duration) with normal cycle (21–35 days)
Polymenorrhea	Normal flow with cycle less than 21 days
Polymenorrhagia	Excessive flow with cycle less than 21 days
Metrorrhagia	Excessive flow that is acyclic
Metrostaxis	Continuous bleeding
Ovulation bleeding (pseudopolymenorrhea)	Spotting or light flow at time of midcycle estrogen nadir
Premenstrual staining	Spotting or light flow up to 7 days before menstruation in ovulatory cycle

From Strickler, R. C.: Dysfunctional uterine bleeding—diagnosis and treatment. Postgrad. Med. 66:135–146, 1979.

orrhage occurring at intervals of 21 days or less. This type of bleeding is most commonly the result of anovulatory cycles.

Nature of Patient

Before menarche, there is a characteristic sequence of events that begins at about age 8 (Fig. 19–2): Breast buds develop, pubic hairs appear, breasts enlarge, axillary hairs appear, and finally a height spurt occurs. Menstrual function usually begins after the height spurt. About 6 months before menarche, there is a physiologic leukorrhea. One must remember that in the first year after menarche, 55 per cent of menses are anovulatory, with a sharp decline to about 7 per cent by 8 years after menarche. Usually 15 months are required for completion of the first 10 menstrual cycles. This means that when menses begin, it is unusual for them to occur at regular monthly intervals.

The average age at which girls begin to menstruate is 12 years. The characteristics of normal menstruation are shown in Table 19–3. Bleeding that occurs before ages 9 to 10 years of age is abnormal, and local pathology as well as adrenal and ovarian tumors must be suspected. Because some teenage girls are reluctant to volunteer information about their menstrual periods, it is essential that physicians routinely ask a series of questions: (1) When did your menses begin? (2) How often do your menstrual periods occur? (3) On what date did your last period occur? (4) Is there any pain associated with menstruation? (5) Are you sexually active? (6) Are you practicing any form of birth control? These questions must be asked in a nonthreatening way so that the patient feels at ease and understands that the physician is willing to listen. Likewise, when asking questions about sexual activities, it is essential that the physician remain nonjudgmental. The teenager should be reassured that any discussion of this nature will remain a private matter between patient and physician.

The adolescent commonly has cycles of variable length. Anovulation may be associated with both short and long cycles together with short follicular and luteal cycles. Another important point is that menarche may be delayed in underweight adolescents. In some teenage girls who are on strict diets to remain fashionably thin and in athletes with normal body weight but low body fat, menarche may be delayed. Likewise, there is often a familial pattern of menarche: It is common for girls to start menstruating at about the same age as their mothers and sisters did.

There are several significant age-associated conditions that can cause abnormal vaginal bleeding. In children, insertion of *foreign bodies* into the vagina may cause bleeding. During the reproductive years, *dysfunctional uterine bleeding* and bleeding from *pregnancy complications, tumors,* and *fibroids* may occur (Table 19–4). Anovulatory *estrogen-withdrawal bleeding* is the most common cause of irregular menses

Stage	Description

Breast development

B1	Preadolescent: elevation of nipple only
B2	Breast-bud stage: elevation of breast and nipple as a small mound
B3	Further enlargement of breast and areola with no separation of contours
B4	Projection of areola so as to form a secondary mound
B5	Mature stage: nipple projects from general contour of breast

Pubic hair development

PH1	None
PH2	Sparse growth of long straight hair along labia; no hair on mons pubis
PH3	Thicker, coarse, curled hair on mons pubis
PH4	Adult-type hair on mons pubis but not reaching the medial aspect of thighs
PH5	Hair reaches the medial surface of thighs

Figure 19–2. Relationship of pubertal events in adolescent girls. (From Lopez, R. I.: Menstrual irregularities in teenage girls. Drug Therapy, April 1981, p. 49.)

TABLE 19–3. Characteristics of Menstruation*

Characteristics	Range	Average
Menarche (age of onset)	9–17 yr	12.5 yr
Cycle length (interval)	21–35 d	28 d
Duration of flow	1–8 d	3–5 d
Amount of flow	10–80 mL	35 mL
Onset of menopause	45–55 yr	47–50 yr

*Range and averages for American women.
From Hamilton, C.: Vaginal bleeding: evaluation and management. Resident and Staff Physician, November 1981, pp. 62–64.

TABLE 19–4. Causes of Vaginal Bleeding in the Reproductive Years

Menstruation and Variations
  Ovulational spotting (midcycle)
Pregnancy Complications
  Early (< 20 wk)
    Implantational bleeding
    Abortion
    Ectopic pregnancy
    Trophoblastic disease
  Late (> 20 wk)
    Placenta previa, vasa previa, other
  Postpartum
    Uterine atony
    Retained products
Normal Delivery
Disorders of the CNS-Hypothalamic-Ovarian-Pituitary Axis
  Dysfunctional uterine bleeding
    Anovulatory (80%–90%)
    Ovulatory
  Functioning ovarian cysts or tumors
  Emotional stress
  Anticholinergic drugs
Exogenous Hormones
  Estrogen
  Estrogen-progestin oral contraceptives
Trauma
Anticoagulant Drugs
Organic Gynecologic Disease
  Pelvic infections
  Neoplastic diseases
    Benign
    Malignant
  Adenomyosis
Systemic Disease
  Generalized bleeding disorders
  Thyroid disease

From Hamilton, C.: Vaginal bleeding: evaluation and management. Resident and Staff Physician, November 1981, pp. 62–64.

during the reproductive and perimenopausal years and accounts for 40 per cent of menstrual disturbances that occur in the perimenopausal years. Other less common causes of abnormal vaginal bleeding in perimenopausal women include organic lesions (neoplasm or inflammatory diseases of the cervix, vagina, and endometrium), constitutional diseases (hypothyroidism, hyperthyroidism, Cushing's disease, cirrhosis, thrombocytopenia, and complications of pregnancy), and certain drugs (Table 19–5). In postmenopausal women, bleeding may result from *endometrial* and *cervical cancers*.

Nature of Symptoms

Prolonged irregular and profuse bleeding may occur with either estrogen-breakthrough or estrogen-withdrawal bleeding. The bleeding may be spotty (threshold-breakthrough bleeding). Anovulatory bleeding is usually unexpected and painless. Anovulatory cycles may result in *polymenorrhagia*. With ovulatory menstrual abnormalities, there may

TABLE 19–5. Common Drugs That May Alter Menstrual Bleeding

Generic Name	Trade Name
*Amphetamines	*Desoxyn, Obetrol
Anticoagulants	Coumadin, Heparin
*Benzodiazepines	
Diazepam, Oxazepam	*Valium, Serax
Benzomide derivatives	Pronestyl, Matulane
*Butyrophenones	*Haldol, Inapsine
Cannabis	Marijuana
Chlordiazepoxide	Librium
*Cimetidine	*Tagamet
Ethyl alcohol	Whiskey, wine, beer
*Isoniazid	*INH
*Methyldopa	*Aldomet
Monoamine oxidase inhibitors	Eutonyl, Nardil
*Opiates	*Morphine, Heroin, Methadone
*Phenothiazines	*Compazine, Thorazine, Phenergan
Prostaglandin inhibitors	Motrin, Indocin
Rauwolfia	Raudixin
*Reserpine	*Serpasil
*Spironolactone	*Aldactone
Steroids	
Gonadal	
*Estrogens	*Premarin, oral contraceptives
*Progesterones	*Provera, oral contraceptives
*Testosterone	*Android
Thyroid hormones	Synthroid, Cytomel
*Thioxanthenes	*Navane
*Tricyclic antidepressants	*Elavil

*May also produce galactorrhea.

From Murata, J. N.: Abnormal genital bleeding and secondary amenorrhea. Common gynecological problems. J. Obstet. Gynecol. Neonatal Nurs. *19*:26–36, 1990.

be a short luteal phase, in which case menstrual cycles may be variable in length with excessive flow. Patients with these problems may also complain of premenstrual bleeding or staining. When *menorrhagia* is present, *tumors, fibroids, cancer, polyps, salpingitis,* or *intrauterine contraceptive devices* may be the cause. *Endometriosis, salpingitis,* and *cancer* may also cause minimal bleeding and should be suspected if there is also a purulent discharge. The symptoms of endometriosis are reviewed in detail in Chapter 20.

During the reproductive years, abnormal vaginal bleeding often represents *pregnancy complications.* There may be a history of sexual activity without adequate contraceptive measures. In addition, symptoms of pregnancy such as missed periods, morning sickness, and breast tenderness, may be present. In these cases, the uterine bleeding initially results from endometrial sloughing, and therefore spotting rather than amenorrhea may occur before gross hemorrhage.

Gross hemorrhage may be concealed or visible. *Ectopic pregnancy* is strongly suggested by an adnexal or cul-de-sac mass in a pregnant woman who has a normal or only slightly enlarged uterus. Concealed pelvic hemorrhage from a ruptured ectopic pregnancy can occur either with or without vaginal bleeding. This diagnosis should be suspected when there is amenorrhea, pelvic or abdominal fullness, abdominal pain (particularly if the pain is unilateral or referred to the shoulder), tenesmus, and urinary frequency or urgency. Fever, signs of peritoneal irritation, purulent vaginal discharge, and pain can be seen in patients with ectopic pregnancy or salpingitis. **It is axiomatic that copious vaginal bleeding is most often the result of pregnancy complications and less often due to local gynecologic disease or dysfunctional bleeding.** Bright red hemorrhage with clots suggests a brisk nonmenstrual flow. A darker tint of blood implies slower hemorrhage acted on by cervical or vaginal secretions. Irregular bleeding during pregnancy may be due to separation of the placenta or the embryo from its attachment, but malignant cervical erosions, polyps, and local vaginal lesions must be excluded.

Menorrhagia during puberty is usually due to anovulation. This gradually abates within several months of the onset of the menarche. Menorrhagia during the reproductive years can also be due to anovulation, as can *polymenorrhagia.* Menorrhagia that occurs during the reproductive years may be caused by *fibromyomas.* **The chief characteristic of a uterine fibroid is an asymmetrically enlarged uterus.** There may be more than one fibroid in the uterus, and the shape can be extremely irregular. As a rule, the consistency of the fibroid is hard and unyielding. Usually the cervix and uterine fibroid move together.

In some instances, it is difficult for the physician to distinguish a fibromyoma from an *ovarian cyst.* **A helpful point in the differentiation of fibroids from ovarian cysts is that ovarian cysts almost**

never cause menorrhagia. Ovarian tumors usually create no menstrual disturbances. *Adenomyoma* of the uterus usually causes symmetrical uterine enlargement, but absolute differentiation must be accomplished by pathologic examination.

Chronic salpingo-oophoritis (hydrosalpinx, tubo-ovarian abscess, or *chronic salpingitis)* as well as *ovarian endometriosis* can cause menorrhagia, and congestive (premenstrual) dysmenorrhea is usually present as a prominent symptom. Menorrhagia can also be caused by intrauterine devices, thrombocytopenia, and other coagulation defects.

Irregular menstrual bleeding may be divided into three groups: (1) irregular bleeding during menstrual life, (2) bleeding before puberty and after menopause, and (3) bleeding during pregnancy.

Irregular Bleeding During Menstrual Life
(Table 19–5)

Metrorrhagia. The lesions of the reproductive organs that cause metrorrhagia include *cervical carcinoma, benign* and *malignant uterine tumors, endometritis*, and, rarely, *tuberculous endometritis*. Usually *fibromyomas* cause menorrhagia but occasionally can cause metrorrhagia. Fibroids tend to produce irregular bleeding when they are submucosal or in the process of extrusion. A carcinoma can develop in a patient known to have uterine fibroids, and a fibroid occasionally can undergo sarcomatous degeneration. Rapid enlargement of the uterus associated with irregular bleeding is very suggestive of a *sarcoma.* However, several fibroids can be present in the same uterus and are a common cause of rapid uterine enlargement. *Choriocarcinoma* is a rare cause of uterine enlargement that follows a *hydatidiform mole* in about 50 per cent of the recorded cases. It should be suspected during early pregnancy in women in whom there is a threat of abortion and in whom the uterus is extremely enlarged. Choriocarcinoma is also likely in women who have persistent uterine enlargement.

Cervical erosions usually do not bleed. If there is irregular bleeding from the erosion or if the cervix bleeds during an examination, cancer should be excluded.

Menorrhagia. *Polyps* and *fibroids* are common causes of menorrhagia. *Dysfunctional uterine bleeding* can occur at any age. Fifty per cent of cases occur in women between ages 40 and 50, about 10 per cent develop at puberty, and the remaining 40 per cent occur between puberty and age 40. Bleeding related to dysfunctional uterine bleeding—frequently due to an anovulatory cycle—usually is in the form of menorrhagia, although the interval between periods may be shortened.

Women who are using *estrogen preparations* to control menstrual symptoms or to prevent conception may develop menorrhagia while the drugs are being taken or following their withdrawal. The menorrhagia is often related to the dosage of estrogen.

Bleeding associated with *ovulation* is uncommon; when it occurs, it is midway between the periods (approximately at the time of ovulation). Mid–menstrual cycle bleeding accompanied by lower abdominal pain is referred to as *mittelschmerz*.

Bleeding Before Puberty and After Menopause

When vaginal bleeding occurs in neonates, it is usually due to a temporarily *high concentration of estrogen* in the *fetal circulation*. Postmenopausal bleeding may be due to *malignant growths, polyps, senile endometritis,* or *cervicitis*. *Carcinoma of the body of the uterus* seldom causes much uterine enlargement, and any increase in size usually occurs slowly. It should be noted that the postmenopausal uterus decreases considerably in size. Thus, a uterine size that would be regarded as normal in a younger woman indicates abnormal enlargement in a postmenopausal woman.

Bleeding During Pregnancy

It is important for the physician to differentiate the uterine hemorrhage of extrauterine gestation from that due to threatened abortion. Bleeding can be caused by *placenta previa* and by *abruptio placentae*.

Associated Symptoms

Ovulatory irregular bleeding is often associated with midcycle ovulation pain (mittelschmerz), premenstrual symptoms, and dysmenorrhea. Fever, purulent vaginal discharge, and pain may be clues to pregnancy complications, including spontaneous and induced abortion. These same signs and symptoms may be observed in cases of ectopic pregnancy and salpingitis. Irregular menses associated with galactorrhea suggests a prolactinoma. Anovulatory irregular bleeding associated with hirsutism and occasionaly hypertension suggests *polycystic ovarian syndrome*.

Precipitating Factors

Anovulatory irregular menstrual bleeding often occurs during the first 12 to 18 months after menarche. It is seen most commonly in obese patients; in women who have adrenal disease, pituitary tumors, polycystic ovary syndrome, Cushing's disease, diabetes, malnutrition, chronic illness, or hypothyroidism; and in patients who use phenothiazines or opiates.

Physical Findings

Physical examination should be complete and include thorough pelvic and abdominal evaluations. It should be directed at detection of systemic diseases such as *endocrinopathies*, including adult-onset adrenal hyperplasia, Cushing's disease, thyroid dysfunction, polycystic ovaries, and obesity. Vaginal examination must be thorough.

Diagnostic Studies

Diagnostic tests that are useful in the differential diagnosis of patients with abnormal vaginal bleeding include a complete blood count, reticulocyte count, platelet count, coagulation studies, thyroid-stimulating hormone test, follicle-stimulating hormone test, luteinizing hormone test, plasma glucose, and urinalysis. Other diagnostic tests that help the physician evaluate the cause of abnormal vaginal bleeding include uterine curettage, endometrial, vaginal, and cervical biopsies, and a Papanicolaou test for detection of cancer; Gram's stain and culture for determination of infections; and serum and urine pregnancy tests for confirmation or exclusion of pregnancy.

Pelvic ultrasonography helps the physician diagnose ectopic pregnancies, ovarian cysts, and tumors. Because most patients of reproductive age who have severe uterine bleeding are pregnant, human chorionic gonadotropin (HCG) levels should be determined. HCG is produced during uterine or ectopic pregnancy, development of hydatidiform moles, and formation of choriocarcinoma. The most sensitive test for detecting early pregnancy is radioimmunoassay for the beta subunit of HCG. This test often will allow the physician to detect pregnancy as early as 1 week after fertilization, whereas less sensitive urine tests may not confirm a normal pregnancy until the seventh week. This test is particularly important, since the physician cannot exclude the possibility of an ectopic pregnancy on the basis of a negative urine test. However, a negative serum radioimmunoassay for the beta subunit of HCG will almost always exclude an ectopic pregnancy. Although ectopic pregnancy accounts for only 0.5 per cent of all pregnancies, it is the cause of 10 to 15 per cent of maternal deaths. More than 90 per cent of ectopic pregnancies are due to tubal implants that rupture during the first trimester. Major risk factors for ectopic pregnancy include history of a previous ectopic pregnancy, salpingitis, previous tubal procedure, and pregnancy that occurs when an intrauterine contraceptive device is in place. The physician is unlikely to miss a catastrophic rupture; however, some ectopic pregnancies leak slowly over several days, so they may go unrecognized until the patient's second or third visit. Ultrasonography helps rule out an ectopic pregnancy by confirming the presence of a uterine gestational sac with an intrauterine pregnancy. When there is a positive culdocentesis or a suspicious sonogram, laparoscopy must be performed, followed by surgical exploration if an ectopic pregnancy is seen. A negative radioimmunoassay for the beta subunit of HCG essentially excludes any pregnancy complication.

Less Common Diagnostic Considerations

Patients with endometriosis may have abnormal vaginal bleeding, but usually these women have dull backaches and dyspareunia associated with their congestive dysmenorrhea. Cervical erosions can be detected on physical examination. Bleeding disorders, including idiopathic thrombocytopenic purpura, may present with menometrorrhagia. Thrombocytopenia is often seen in patients with disseminated lupus.

Because clear cell adenocarcinoma of the vagina or cervix can be fatal, the possibility of this tumor must always be considered. It is most common in daughters of the 2 to 3 million women who took diethylstilbestrol (DES) as a fertility drug. These "DES daughters" also may have congenital abnormalities of the cervix, uterus, and upper vagina. In addition, they demonstrate an increased risk of pregnancy complications (e.g., threatened, or spontaneous or induced incomplete abortion and ectopic gestation). Abnormal vaginal bleeding may also be a sign of a coagulation defect, especially platelet deficiency, von Willebrand's disease, or leukemia.

AMENORRHEA

The average age of menarche in the United States is 12.7 years, and the age range for menarche is 11 to 15 years. Primary amenorrhea refers to the condition in women who fail to menstruate at all. Most young patients simply have delayed menarche. Because weight loss and severe malnutrition can result in delayed menarche, it is particularly important for the physician to determine the patient's diet. In addition, substances such as amphetamines, cannabis, estrogens, and phenothiazines may interfere with the onset of menstruation (Table 19–6). Primary amenorrhea is rare; it usually is associated with an endocrine imbalance or congenital abnormalities. In patients with this condition, it is particularly important for the physician to rule out chromosomal aberrations and genital malformations. In all these cases, a chromatin analysis of a buccal smear should be performed (Table 19–7). Age is a significant factor in the diagnosis. For example, a 15-year-old girl who has not yet menstruated usually has a delayed menarche, whereas a 17-year-old girl who has not begun to menstruate is considered to have primary amenorrhea (Fig. 19–3).

Patients with *secondary amenorrhea* have menstruated but then

TABLE 19–6. Common Drugs That May Cause Amenorrhea

Generic Name	Trade and Common Names
Amphetamines	Desoxyn, Obetrol
Benzodiazepines	
Diazepam, oxazepam	Valium, Serax
Benzomide derivatives	Pronestyl, Matulane
Butyrophenones	Haldol, Inapsine
Cannabis	Marijuana
Cimetidine	Tagamet
Isoniazid	INH
Methyldopa	Aldomet
Monoamine oxidase inhibitors	Eutonyl, Nardil
Opiates	Morphine, heroin
Phenothiazines	Compazine, Thorazine, Phenergan
Rauwolfia	Harmonyl, Raudixin
Reserpine	Serpasil
Spironolactone	Aldactone
Steroids	
Gonadal	Ingredients of birth control
Estrogens	or contraceptive pills
Progesterones	
Thyroid hormones	Synthroid, Cytomel
Thioxanthenes	Navane
Tricyclic antidepressants	Elavil

From Murata, J. N.: Primary amenorrhea. Pediatr. Nurs. *15*:125–129, 1989.

TABLE 19–7. Diagnostic Scheme for Evaluation of Primary Amenorrhea

```
                       Anamnesis ———— Physical examination
                                    ┬
Positive————————————————Chromatin analysis (buccal smear)————— Negative
   │                                                              │
Hypogonadotropic amenorrhea        Gonadal dysgenesis——→     Turner's syndrome X0
Primary ovarian failure            Testicular feminization XY Mosaicisms X0/XY,
                                                                 X0/XX
Central nervous system tumor or trauma   Pure gonadal dysgenesis
Congenital adrenogenital hyperplasia     (Swyer syndrome XY)
Congenital absence of uterus and/or vagina            │
Endocrine active ovarian tumors          Quinacrine staining for Y chromosomes
Psychogenic amenorrhea                        │                   │
                                         Positive            Negative
                                              │                   │
                                         Testicular feminization  Gonadal dysgenesis
                                         Pure gonadal dysgenesis  (Turner's syndrome)
Endocrine diagnostic                     Mosaicisms (XX/XY)       Mosaicisms (X0/XX)
```

From Lehmann, F.: Diagnostic approach to ovarian dysfunction. Hormone Res. *9*:319–338, 1978.

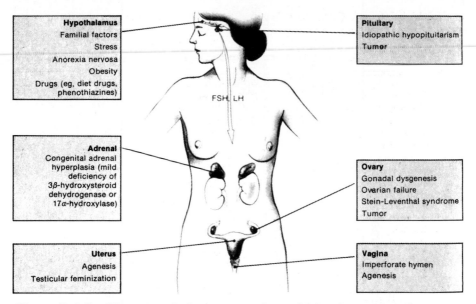

Figure 19–3. Possible causes of primary amenorrhea and delayed menarche. (From Lopez, R. I.: Menstrual irregularities in young girls. Drug Therapy, April 1981, p. 42.)

stop. **During the reproductive years, the most common cause of secondary amenorrhea is pregnancy.** An endocrine imbalance may be an associated factor, but tumors seldom cause secondary amenorrhea. A vaginal smear and evaluation of the cervical mucus will help in determining whether there is ovarian estrogen production. Various endocrinologic tests help determine whether there is normal ovarian progesterone production and whether there are normal or elevated levels of ovarian androgen. If a patient with secondary amenorrhea has galactorrhea, a prolactinoma is probable. The various causes of secondary amenorrhea are shown in Table 19–8.

Diagnostic studies that are useful in the evaluation of amenorrhea include buccal chromatin analysis, blood and urine hormone estimation, chromosomal analysis, basal body temperature, vaginal smear, tomographs of the pituitary fossa, computed tomography scans, and a progesterone withdrawal test for determination of whether estrogen is being manufactured.

Less Common Diagnostic Considerations

Less common causes of amenorrhea include nutritional disorders and strict dieting; systemic disorders such as tuberculosis, diabetes, prolactinoma, hypothyroidism, hyperthyroidism, and psychogenic disturbances, including severe stress and anorexia nervosa. Polycystic ovarian

Text continued on page 223

TABLE 19–8. Possible Causes of Secondary Amenorrhea

	Ovarian Hormone Production		
Normal (Cyclic)	Decreased (Acyclic)		Increased (Acyclic)
Asherman's syndrome	High gonadotropin levels	Low or normal gonadotropin levels	Polycystic ovary syndrome
Endometrial destruction			Virilizing ovarian tumors
infective (tuberculosis,	Premature ovarian failure	Functional aberrations of the	(arrhenoblastoma, hilus cell
schistosomiasis)		hypothalamic-pituitary axis	tumor)
iatrogenic (curettage,	Castration (surgical	Psychogenic factors	Feminizing ovarian tumors
irradiation)	or radiation)	Nutritional factors	(granulosa cell tumor, theca
		Nongonadal endocrine disorders	cell tumor)
		(thyroid, adrenals, pancreas)	
		Systemic infections and chronic	
		diseases	
		Pharmacologic factors (psychotropic	
		drugs, post-pill oversuppression,	
		drug addiction)	
		Central nervous system disease	
		(tumor or trauma)	

From Lehmann, F.: Diagnostic approach to ovarian dysfunction. Hormone Res. 9:319–338, 1978.

DIFFERENTIAL DIAGNOSIS OF MENSTRUAL IRREGULARITIES

CAUSE	NATURE OF PATIENT	NATURE OF SYMPTOMS	ASSOCIATED SYMPTOMS	PRECIPITATING AND AGGRAVATING FACTORS	PHYSICAL FINDINGS	DIAGNOSTIC STUDIES
Dysfunctional Uterine Bleeding (Hormonal Causes)	Can occur at any age 10% of cases occur at puberty 50% of cases occur between ages 40 and 50	Usually due to anovulatory cycles Menorrhagia Interval between periods may be decreased				Diagnosis may be reached only by a process of exclusion
Anovulatory cycles	Normal occurrence in 55% of girls within first year of menarche	Irregular cycle length Polymenorrhagia Bleeding not preceded by or associated with subjective symptoms		Obesity Adrenal or pituitary disease Polycystic ovaries Diabetes Malnutrition Chronic illness Hypothyroidism Use of phenothiazines or opiates		Monophasic basal body temperature Serum progesterone level never exceeds 5 ng/mL
Estrogen-withdrawal bleeding	Most common cause of irregular menses in reproductive years, especially adolescence and climacteric	Prolonged, irregular, profuse bleeding	Painless			
Estrogen-breakthrough bleeding Threshold bleeding		Spotty bleeding		Low-dose oral contraceptives		
With estrogen levels above threshold		Prolonged, irregular, profuse bleeding				

Table continued on following page

DIFFERENTIAL DIAGNOSIS OF MENSTRUAL IRREGULARITIES *Continued*

CAUSE	NATURE OF PATIENT	NATURE OF SYMPTOMS	ASSOCIATED SYMPTOMS	PRECIPITATING AND AGGRAVATING FACTORS	PHYSICAL FINDINGS	DIAGNOSTIC STUDIES
Dysfunctional Uterine Bleeding *Continued* Progesterone-breakthrough bleeding Progesterone-withdrawal bleeding				High doses of progestational drugs Intramuscular progesterone or oral medroxyprogesterone acetate (Provera) administered as test for presence of endogenous estrogen		
Ovulatory cycles		Cycle length is usually regular Premenstrual staining or bleeding Dysmenorrhea	Mittelschmerz Premenstrual syndrome (PMS)			Biphasic basal body temperature Serum progesterone level >3 ng/mL
Complications of Pregnancy	Reproductive age	Spotting precedes gross hemorrhage (may be visible or concealed)	Missed periods Morning sickness Breast tenderness			
Ectopic pregnancy	Increased risk for women with previous ectopic pregnancy, salpingitis, previous tubal procedure or pregnancy that occurs with intrauterine devices	Amenorrhea Pelvic or abdominal fullness Abdominal pain (usually unilateral) May refer to shoulder May or may not be vaginal bleeding Purulent vaginal discharge	Tenesmus Increased urinary frequency or urgency		Adnexal or cul-de-sac mass Normal or slightly enlarged uterus Peritoneal irritation	Positive HCG Pelvic sonogram

Condition	Age / Occurrence	Bleeding	Associated Symptoms	Physical Findings	Diagnostic Tests
During uterine pregnancy		Irregular bleeding due to separation of placenta or embryo from its attachment			
Spontaneous abortion		Hemorrhage (sometimes with clots)	Fever, Purulent vaginal discharge or pain		
Endometriosis (see Chap. 20)		Slight bleeding	Dysmenorrhea, Purulent vaginal discharge, Dull backache	Implants may be palpable	
Endometrial and Cervical Cancer	Postmenopausal women	Extent of bleeding may vary	Purulent vaginal discharge		Dilation and curettage, Biopsy, Pap test
Fibroids	Women of reproductive age	Menorrhagia, occasionally metrorrhagia, Irregular bleeding		Uterus is asymmetrically enlarged; Fibroids are hard and unyielding; Cervix and fibroids usually move together	Pelvic sonogram
Intrauterine device		Menorrhagia	Cervical discharge	Intrauterine device	
Salpingitis	Usually occurs in reproductive years	Menorrhagia or slight bleeding	Purulent discharge, Fever, Abdominal pain, Dysmenorrhea	Signs of peritoneal irritation	

Table continued on following page

DIFFERENTIAL DIAGNOSIS OF MENSTRUAL IRREGULARITIES *Continued*

CAUSE	NATURE OF PATIENT	NATURE OF SYMPTOMS	ASSOCIATED SYMPTOMS	PRECIPITATING AND AGGRAVATING FACTORS	PHYSICAL FINDINGS	DIAGNOSTIC STUDIES
Insertion of Foreign Body into Vagina	Most common cause of abnormal vaginal bleeding in children				Foreign body	
Amenorrhea Primary	In girls up to age 17, delayed menarche is the most common cause; Girls age 18 or older who have not yet menstruated (rare)			Severe malnutrition; Weight loss; Vigorous exercise; Amphetamines; Phenothiazines; Cannabis; Endocrine and congenital abnormalities; Chromosomal aberrations	Abnormal pubertal development; Abnormal external or internal genitalia; Short stature	Chromatin analysis
Secondary	Patients have menstruated and then stop menstruating			Pregnancy; Endocrine imbalance; Tumors; Breast-feeding; Oral contraceptives; "Post-Pill" amenorrhea		Vaginal smear and evaluation of cervical mucus to determine whether there is ovarian estrogen production and to determine other hormone levels
Prolactinoma			Galactorrhea			Serum prolactin levels; CT scan of sella

syndrome should be suspected in obese young women who have normal sexual development, hypertension, and hirsutism. They may have secondary amenorrhea or oligomenorrhea. In early polycystic ovarian syndrome, there may be severe dysfunctional bleeding and serum gonadotropin levels may be elevated. The patient also may have severe acne.

Congenital adrenal hyperplasia (virilizing tumor) is also manifested by hirsutism and severe acne. Secondary amenorrhea has been reported in female marathon runners, a finding that probably is related to the marked decrease in total body fat in these women. It also has been reported in competitive swimmers and ballet dancers for the same reason. Asherman's syndrome is amenorrhea due to destruction of the basal layer of the endometrium and adhesions following "overenthusiastic" uterine curettage.

Selected References

Altchek, A.: Dysfunctional uterine bleeding in adolescence. Clin. Obstet. Gynecol. *20*:633–650, 1977.

Burnett, R. G.: Diagnostic strategies for amenorrhea. Postgrad. Med. *87*:241–247, 250, 1990.

Dewhurst, J.: Secondary amenorrhea. Pediatr. Ann. *10(12)*:38–42, 1981.

Goldfarb, J. M., and Little, A. B.: Abnormal vaginal bleeding. N. Engl. J. Med. *302*:666–669, 1980.

Hamilton, C.: Vaginal bleeding: evaluation and management. Resident and Staff Physician, November 1981, pp. 62–64.

Kustin, J., and Rebar, R. W.: Menstrual disorders in the adolescent age groups. Prim. Care *14*:139–166, 1987.

Lehmann, F.: Diagnostic approach to ovarian dysfunction. Hormone Res. *9*:319–338, 1978.

Marul, E. L., and Dawood, M. Y.: Amenorrhea. Clin. Obstet. Gynecol. *26(3)*:749–761, 1983.

Nesse, R. E.: Abnormal vaginal bleeding in perimenopausal women. Am. Fam. Physician *40*:185–192, 1989.

Reindollar, R. H., Novack, M., Tho, S.P.T., and McDonnough, P. G.: Adult onset amenorrhea: A study of 262 patients. Am. J. Obstet. Gynecol. *155*:531–543, 1986.

Soules, M. R.: Adolescent amenorrhea. Pediatr. Clin. North Am. *34*:1083–1103, 1987.

Spellacy, W. N.: Abnormal bleeding. Clin. Obstet. Gynecol. *26(3)*:702–709, 1983.

Strickler, R. C.: Dysfunctional uterine bleeding—diagnosis and treatment. Postgrad. Med. *66*:135–146, 1979.

Taber, B.: Manual of Gynecologic and Obstetric Emergencies. 2nd ed. Philadelphia, W. B. Saunders Co., 1984.

Chapter 20

Menstrual Pain

Dysmenorrhea is the term used to describe painful menstruation. Approximately 50 per cent of postpubescent women experience dysmenorrhea; 10 per cent of these women are incapacitated by pain for 1 to 3 days per month. As the greatest single cause of lost working hours and school days among young women, dysmenorrhea has been found to be associated with substantial economic losses to the entire community as well as to the patient. In some instances, anticipatory fear of the next menstrual period can cause anxiety during the intermenstrual period.

In evaluating a patient with pelvic pain at time of menstruation, the physician must first decide whether the patient has *premenstrual syndrome (PMS)* or dysmenorrhea. **PMS usually begins 2 to 12 days before the menstrual period and subsides at the onset or early in the course of menstruation.** The major symptoms of PMS are a diffuse, dull pelvic ache, mood changes (irritability, nervousness, headaches, and depression), swelling of the breasts and extremities, occasional weight gain, and a sensation of abdominal bloating. The diagnostic process is sometimes more difficult when, as is commonly the case, the symptoms of PMS overlap or are followed by those of dysmenorrhea.

It is helpful to classify dysmenorrhea as primary or secondary. *Primary dysmenorrhea* is the most common menstrual disorder and occurs in 30 to 50 per cent of young women. Dysmenorrhea is classified as primary (intrinsic, essential, or idiopathic) if it occurs in a woman who has no pelvic abnormality. About 95 per cent of female adolescents have primary dysmenorrhea, and this problem is a major cause of school absenteeism. *Secondary dysmenorrhea* (extrinsic or acquired) results from organic pelvic diseases such as fibroids, endometriosis, bacterial infections, and infections caused by intrauterine contraceptive devices (IUDs). Because effective therapy is now available for primary and secondary dysmenorrhea, it is not sufficient merely to diagnose "dysmenorrhea." The physician must distinguish among PMS, primary dysmenorrhea, and secondary dysmenorrhea.

Some women will not initiate a discussion of dysmenorrhea with their physician. They may have been taught that it is normal or that relief cannot be obtained. It is therefore essential that the practitioner ask the patient whether dysmenorrhea is a problem.

NATURE OF PATIENT

Severe *primary dysmenorrhea* is common in young women during the first hours of their menstruation. **When dysmenorrhea begins within the first 2 to 3 years of menarche, primary dysmenorrhea is the most likely diagnosis.** Primary dysmenorrhea usually occurs with ovulatory cycles; these normally begin 3 to 12 months after menarche, when ovulation occurs regularly. Primary dysmenorrhea usually begins a few months after menarche and becomes progressively more severe. If a patient has gradually increasing monthly pain without menstruation, a *congenital abnormality* obstructing menstrual flow must be considered. These rare abnormalities may lead to hematocolpos, hematometra, and eventually intraperitoneal bleeding.

Secondary dysmenorrhea usually begins many years after menarche. Dysmenorrhea that develops after age 20 is usually of the secondary type. Dysmenorrhea often can be caused by an *IUD*. If dysmenorrhea develops after cervical conization, cautery, or radiation, *acquired cervical stenosis* or *cervical occlusion* may be the cause. Dysmenorrhea after uterine curettage may be due to *intrauterine synechiae* (Asherman's syndrome). Secondary dysmenorrhea due to *endometriosis* is usually late in onset (beginning when the patient is in her 30s) and worsens with age. Endometriosis is uncommon in teenagers. *Adenomyosis* may be a cause of secondary dysmenorrhea, particularly in parous women over age 40, especially if menorrhagia is present.

NATURE OF SYMPTOMS

Pain that begins with menstrual flow or a few hours before flow commences and lasts for 6 hours to 2 days is most characteristic of *primary dysmenorrhea*. In teenagers, endometriosis may mimic the pain of primary dysmenorrhea in that the pain may be limited to the first day of menstruation. The pain of primary dysmenorrhea is usually crampy but may be a dull ache. It is normally located in the midline of the lower abdomen just above the symphysis. It occasionally radiates down the anterior aspect of the thighs or to the lower back.

The pain of *secondary dysmenorrhea* often begins several hours or even a few days before menses and is often relieved by the menstrual flow. This pain is usually a dull, continuous, diffuse, lower abdominal pain but may be crampy. Like the pain of primary dysmenorrhea, it can radiate down the thighs and into the back.

When *pelvic inflammatory disease* causes dysmenorrhea, the pain is greatest premenstrually and is relieved with the onset of vaginal bleeding. A common cause of secondary dysmenorrhea that deserves special attention is *endometriosis*. Symptoms in these patients become progressively more severe with each cycle; the pain usually begins (and increases in severity) 2 to 3 days premenstrually and persists for more than 2 days after the onset of flow. It is most severe on the first and second days of bleeding, and the usual drop in basal body temperature, which normally occurs 24 to 36 hours after menses, is delayed until the second or third menstrual day.

Despite the differences between primary and secondary dysmenorrhea, their symptoms can overlap, and vary greatly in intensity, and do not necessarily occur with every menstrual period. It is important for the physician to recognize that patients with primary dysmenorrhea may develop pelvic pathology and have additional, superimposed symptoms of secondary dysmenorrhea. These patients can have constant, crampy pain beginning 1 to 2 days before menstrual flow and continuing for 2 to 3 days after menstrual flow.

ASSOCIATED SYMPTOMS

Systemic symptoms such as nausea, vomiting, diarrhea, headache, fatigue, nervousness, and dizziness are more characteristic of primary dysmenorrhea than of secondary dysmenorrhea. If menorrhagia and colicky pain are associated with menstruation, *uterine fibroids* should be suspected, although fibroids seldom are responsible for menstrual pain. If a nonpregnant patient with an enlarged, soft uterus complains of menorrhagia and dysmenorrhea, *adenomyosis* should be suspected. Bleeding from glandular tissue located deep within the myometrium has been implicated as the cause of the pain.

The pain of *endometriosis* may continue into the intermenstrual period. Rectal pain on defecation during the menstrual period also suggests endometriosis as a cause of dysmenorrhea. When dysmenorrhea is associated with dyspareunia, rectal pain, tenesmus, backache, and urgent micturition, endometriosis should be suspected.

PRECIPITATING AND AGGRAVATING FACTORS

Primary dysmenorrhea is aggravated by *PMS*. *IUDs* may cause secondary dysmenorrhea and, in some instances, aggravate preexisting primary dysmenorrhea. *Menstrual flow* that continues longer than 8

DIFFERENTIAL DIAGNOSIS OF MENSTRUAL PAIN

CAUSE	NATURE OF PATIENT	NATURE OF SYMPTOMS	ASSOCIATED SYMPTOMS	AMELIO-RATING FACTORS	PRECIPITAT-ING AND AGGRAVATING FACTORS	PHYSICAL FINDINGS	DIAGNOSTIC STUDIES
Premenstrual syndrome		Begins 2–12 days before menses and subsides at onset or during first days of period Diffuse, dull, pelvic ache May coexist with dysmenorrhea	Irritability Nervousness Headaches Swelling of breasts and extremities Bloating and weight gain Breast tenderness	Menses	Emotional stress Dysmenorrhea	Breasts tender to palpation	
Primary dysmenorrhea	30–50% of young women 95% of adolescents	Most common menstrual disorder, especially in adolescents Begins within 3–12 mo of menarche with ovulatory cycles Becomes severer with age Pain: just precedes or begins with menstrual flow lasts for 6 hs to 2 days is crampy or a dull ache is usually in mid-line of lower abdomen may radiate down thighs and to lower back	Nausea and vomiting Diarrhea Headache Fatigue Nervousness Dizziness	Pain may lessen as menstrual cycles become regular Pregnancy Oral contraceptives NSAIDs	Premenstrual syndrome IUD Emotional stress	None	

Secondary dysmenorrhea	Over age 20 Often a history of recurrent pelvic inflammatory disease	Secondary to organic disease Begins years after menarche; may occur with anovulatory cycles Pain: begins several hours before menses is a dull, continuous, diffuse, lower abdominal pain may be crampy can radiate down thighs and into back		Menses	Cervical stenosis secondary to cervical conization or radiation IUD	Depends on cause of secondary dysmenorrhea	Papanicolaou test Gonorrhea culture Laparoscopy Ultrasound for myomas and ovarian cysts
Endometriosis	Usually over age 30 Uncommon in teenagers	Symptoms worsen with each cycle Pain: begins 2–3 days before menses and persists for 2 days after may continue into intermenstrual period	Rectal pain with defecation Dyspareunia Tenesmus Backache Urgent micturition	Pregnancy Birth control pills		Pelvic examination best done in late luteal phase Nodularity felt in uterosacral ligaments or other sites of endometrial implants	Fern test Basal body temperature Laparoscopy Ultrasonography
Fibroids	Uncommon cause of dysmenorrhea		Menorrhagia			Uterine mass	Ultrasonography
Pelvic inflammatory disease	Pain is greatest premenstrually		Menorrhagia		Onset at menses	Cervical discharge Chandelier sign	Gonorrhea culture Leukocytosis Chlamydial culture

days and *emotional stress* also appear to intensify dysmenorrhea. By itself, retroversion does not cause dysmenorrhea; however, some conditions that cause retroversion also cause dysmenorrhea.

AMELIORATING FACTORS

Dysmenorrhea is not consistently alleviated by any known physical measure. Some patients may state that lying on the floor in the knee–chest position gives some relief. Dysmenorrhea that occurs soon after the onset of menarche frequently disappears as the menstrual cycles become more regular. Pregnancy often relieves primary dysmenorrhea and secondary dysmenorrhea due to endometriosis. The pain may be alleviated for several months or, on occasion, permanently. Birth control pills often alleviate the pain of primary dysmenorrhea and endometriosis. Spontaneous alleviation of dysmenorrhea may occur with advancing age, but this is not usually the case.

PHYSICAL FINDINGS

In patients who have primary dysmenorrhea, no physical abnormalities are usually found. In patients who have secondary dysmenorrhea, physical findings depend on the specific cause.

The practitioner must perform a careful physical examination to check for pelvic infection, endometriosis, pelvic mass, uterine enlargement, and other pelvic disease. When evidence of endometriosis is being sought, the pelvic examination should ideally be performed in the late luteal phase, immediately before menstruation, when the endometrial implants (often in the uterosacral ligaments) are largest and therefore most palpable. Using a laxative to promote bowel evacuation facilitates pelvic examination for endometrial implants. **Special attention should be paid to genital development, vaginal discharge, stigmata of pelvic infection, appearance of the cervix, and the size, shape, consistency, and position of the uterus.**

DIAGNOSTIC STUDIES

A Papanicolaou test and chlamydial and gonococcal cultures should be obtained for all patients with secondary dysmenorrhea. A fern test and basal body temperature may help diagnose endometriosis. Uterine curettage, laparoscopy, and sonography are often useful diagnostic tools.

LESS COMMON DIAGNOSTIC CONSIDERATIONS

Less common causes of dysmenorrhea include congenital malformations, uterine hypoplasia, and true cervical stenosis or obstruction that occurs as the result of cauterization, conization, or radiation therapy. Endometrial carcinoma and tuberculosis are rare causes of secondary dysmenorrhea. A foreign body (e.g., an IUD or any object inserted into the vagina) can cause dysmenorrhea.

Selected References

Avant, R. E.: Dysmenorrhea. Prim. Care *15*:549–559, 1988.
Coupey, S. M., and Ahlstrom, P.: Common menstrual disorders. Pediatr. Clin. North Am. *36*:551–571, 1989.
Dawood, M. Y.: Dysmenorrhea. Clin. Obstet. Gynecol. *33*:168–178, 1990.
Friederich, M. A.: Dysmenorrhea. Women and Health *8(2–3)*:91–106, 1983.
Heinrichs, W. L., and Adamson, G. D.: A practical approach to the patient with dysmenorrhea. J. Reprod. Med. *25*:236–242, 1980.
Renaer, M., and Guzinski, G. M.: Pain in gynecologic practice. Pain *5*:305–331, 1978.
Ylikarkala, O., and Dawood, M. Y.: New concepts in dysmenorrhea. Am. J. Obstet. Gynecol. *130*:833–847, 1978.

Chapter 21

Nausea and/or Vomiting Without Abdominal Pain

Nausea is a vague, unpleasant sensation; it may herald the onset of vomiting or occur without vomiting. *Vomiting* is the forceful expulsion of gastric contents through the mouth and must be differentiated from *regurgitation.* The latter is an effortless backflow of small amounts of ingested food or liquid during or between meals or feedings. Dribbling of milk from a child's mouth is an example of regurgitation. When a patient complains of vomiting, it is helpful for the physician to distinguish acute from chronic vomiting.

The most common cause of acute nausea and vomiting in adults and children is *gastroenteritis.* Other common causes of acute nausea and vomiting include *gastritis, excessive alcohol ingestion,* certain *drugs, motion sickness,* and, in children, *otitis media.* Common causes of chronic nausea and vomiting include *gastritis, drugs* (especially codeine, digitalis glycosides, quinidine, salicylates, theophylline, chemotherapeutic agents, and antibiotics), *uremia,* and *hepatic failure.* Recurrent nausea that occurs without vomiting is often a reaction to *environmental* or *emotional stresses.* This form of nausea is temporally related to the stressful period and usually disappears when the stress is removed.

NATURE OF PATIENT

In neonates, vomiting with the first feeding is suggestive of *esophageal atresia* or some other congenital gastrointestinal anomaly (malrotation, Hirschsprung's disease). The most common causes of vomiting in the first year are *feeding problems, gastrointestinal* or *urinary tract infection,* and *septicemia.* When projectile vomiting occurs in infants less than age 3 months (usually ages 2 to 3 weeks), *pyloric stenosis* must be considered. Although uncommon, recurrent vomiting of bile-stained material in neonates may indicate *intestinal obstruction* due to atresia, stenosis, or volvulus of the small bowel.

The most common causes of vomiting in children are *viral* and *bacterial infections, high fevers* of any cause, and *otitis media.* Otitis media has its highest incidence in young children and may present with unexplained vomiting and fever.

In adults, the common causes of acute nausea or vomiting are *gastritis* (alcohol- or drug-induced), *viral gastroenteritis, psychogenic conditions,* and occasionally *labyrinthine disorders.* Nausea and vomiting can also be the presenting symptoms in patients with *hepatitis, myocardial infarction,* and *diabetic ketoacidosis.* Chronic vomiting in adults is usually due to *gastritis, mechanical obstruction, gut motility disorders,* (including *diabetic gastroparesis*), *achalasia, drugs, labyrinthine disorders,* and *uremia.* Both *food contamination* and *chemical poisoning* must be considered as causes of vomiting, particularly if several people are affected at the same time; in cases of food poisoning, usually more than one person is experiencing symptoms. Nausea and vomiting of *pregnancy* must be considered in women of reproductive age; some pregnant women experience morning sickness in the first trimester of pregnancy, often before they are aware of their condition.

Self-induced vomiting should be suspected in neurotic patients. If these patients are questioned carefully, they may admit to a feeling of nausea, which they attempt to relieve by gagging themselves to produce vomiting. If an elderly patient presents with persistent vomiting, gastric or intestinal obstruction secondary to *neoplasm* should be suspected.

NATURE OF SYMPTOMS

When vomiting is painless or has preceded abdominal pain by a considerable amount of time, a surgical lesion is unlikely. Repeated episodes of unexplained vomiting and nausea may indicate *pancreatitis,* which is not always associated with abdominal pain. Persistent vomiting without any bile staining is an indication of *pyloric obstruction.* In children this may be due to *pyloric stenosis;* in adults pyloric obstruction may be secondary to ulcer scarring or tumor. Vomiting or regurgitation of undigested food indicates *esophageal obstruction.* Vomiting secondary to *increased intracranial pressure* is often projectile and not preceded by nausea. Nausea and vomiting are frequent manifestations of *digitalis toxicity.* These symptoms are not necessarily due to high serum levels of the digitalis glycoside; a gastrointestinal adverse effect of the drug may occur at normal serum levels. Although many patients with *gastritis* have abdominal pain, it is not uncommon for these patients to present with unexplained nausea or vomiting without pain. *Substance abuse* (alcohol, caffeine, and recreational drugs) also may be associated with unexplained nausea or vomiting.

The timing of vomiting may be of diagnostic importance. Patients with *uremia, pregnant* women, and *chronic alcoholics* often experience early-morning nausea and vomiting. Vomiting immediately before food is ingested may be a manifestation of *neurosis,* whereas vomiting shortly after eating may be a consequence of *gastric outlet obstruction* caused by a pyloric channel ulcer, adenocarcinoma, or other infiltrative lesions.

Postprandial vomiting may also be of *functional origin,* although organic gastric disease should be suspected. Vomiting soon after eating occurs frequently in patients with *gastritis* and in those with *digitalis toxicity*. Vomiting that begins 20 to 40 minutes after meals suggests *gastric atony* associated with diabetes, prior gastric surgery, or peritonitis. If vomiting begins 1 to 2 hours after a meal, disease of the biliary tract or pancreas may be the cause. In these latter instances, pain usually is not relieved by vomiting. Recurrent vomiting that occurs 1 to 4 hours after eating may be due to gastric or duodenal lesions causing *gastric outlet obstruction*. Vomiting that follows and relieves an episode of epigastric pain is usually due to an *intragastric lesion* or *pyloric spasm.*

The odor of vomitus may also provide a clue to the cause. If the vomitus lacks the pungent odor of gastric acid, a *dilated esophagus* (possibly due to a stricture or achalasia) may be the cause. Patients frequently vomit in the morning and not uncommonly will vomit or regurgitate undigested food. If vomitus has a fecal odor, *intestinal obstruction* or *gastrocolic fistula* should be suspected.

ASSOCIATED SYMPTOMS

If headache (especially a unilateral one) is associated with nausea or vomiting, *migraine* should be suspected. Occasionally, nausea and vomiting may be the only manifestation of migraine (i.e., acephalic migraine). If vertigo and tinnitus are associated with nausea and vomiting, *Meniere's disease* or other middle ear disturbances should be considered. If symptoms of depression are present and there is little or no weight loss despite a history of long-standing emesis, psychogenic vomiting is probable. As in *anorexia nervosa,* women experience psychogenic vomiting more often than men. If chest pain or other symptoms of myocardial infarction are associated with vomiting, the vomiting is probably due to myocardial infarction. Nausea and vomiting often precede the development of chest pain. Rarely, chest pain and vomiting are caused by a strangulated diaphragmatic hernia. In these instances, electrocardiographic abnormalities may be erroneously suggestive of a posterior infarction.

Acute nausea and vomiting associated with diarrhea and occasionally abdominal pain are most commonly due to *gastroenteritis*. When vertigo accompanies vomiting, *labyrinthine disorders* should be suspected. When vomiting, without vertigo, is induced by a recumbent posture, a *posterior fossa lesion* should be suspected. Vomiting may be the initial manifestation of *diabetic ketoacidosis*. It is a particularly common presentation in juvenile (insulin-dependent) diabetics.

PRECIPITATING AND AGGRAVATING FACTORS

Nausea and vomiting are frequently precipitated by medications such as digitalis, theophylline, quinidine, potassium preparations, chemotherapeutic agents, antibiotics, and antihypertensives. Iron preparations, salicylates, and nonsteroidal anti-inflammatory agents also cause nausea and occasionally vomiting. Nicotine poisoning and excessive use of Nicorette gum may cause vomiting. Radiation therapy may also cause nausea and vomiting. *Anticipatory nausea and vomiting* may occur before radiation therapy or chemotherapy, especially in anxious patients. If vomiting is preceded by a cough, it may be the primary manifestation of *asthma* when wheezing is trivial or not present.

AMELIORATING FACTORS

Vomiting usually relieves the symptoms of fullness and pain caused by pyloric obstruction. Vomiting relieves nausea if it is being caused by nauseating substances in the stomach. It does not usually alleviate nausea caused by gastroenteritis, gastritis, uremia, or drugs that cause nausea through a central effect.

PHYSICAL FINDINGS

The presence of fever in a vomiting patient suggests that *infection* is causative. In children, physical findings of *otitis media* suggest that this is the probable cause of the vomiting. A walnut-size mass may be palpable in the epigastrium of infants with hypertrophic pyloric stenosis. A cloudy sensorium or papilledema suggests an *intracranial lesion*, whereas nystagmus suggests a labyrinthine cause. Jaundice or hepatomegaly suggests *hepatitis* or *cirrhosis* as the cause. A distended abdomen accompanying nausea and vomiting may indicate paralytic ileus or mechanical obstruction of the intestine. Abdominal tenderness, distention, and occasionally visible peristalsis suggest *gastrointestinal obstruction*. The location of abdominal pain may provide clues about which organ is responsible for the symptoms.

Chronic vomiting results in weight loss. If a patient's weight is maintained despite a history of chronic nausea and vomiting, the origin of symptoms is probably psychogenic. Decreased skin turgor suggests that the vomiting has caused significant fluid loss. Physical findings consistent with congestive heart failure (e.g., tachycardia, gallop, and peripheral edema) suggest that nausea may be from hepatic capsule distention and mesenteric congestion.

DIAGNOSTIC STUDIES

Studies to confirm a visceral origin of nausea and vomiting include survey films of the abdomen, upper gastrointestinal series, cholecystography, and endoscopy. Detailed neurologic studies, including spinal tap and computed tomography scan, should be performed only if an intracranial process is suspected. A metabolic cause may be suspected if laboratory tests indicate abnormal serum levels of substances such as urea nitrogen, creatinine, glucose, bilirubin, and calcium. An elevated serum amylase level suggests pancreatitis. Digitalis excess may be diagnosed on the basis of elevated serum digitalis levels. Toxicology screening may detect toxins and drugs that cause vomiting.

More sophisticated tests include radioisotope studies of liquid and solid gastric emptying, esophageal and gastrointestinal manometry, and electrogastrography (Table 21–1). Psychiatric assessment, including the Minnesota Multiphasic Personality Inventory test, may also be helpful.

LESS COMMON DIAGNOSTIC CONSIDERATIONS

Several authors have categorized the causes of vomiting as follows: allergies, cerebromedullary factors, toxins, visceral problems, deficiency states, and motion sickness. Gastrointestinal allergies should be considered if sudden nausea or vomiting consistently follows ingestion of specific food. The less common cerebromedullary causes include increased intracranial pressure, trauma, cerebral tumors, abscesses, hydrocephalus, intracranial hemorrhage, and acephalic migraine. Hepatic coma and Addison's disease are less common causes of nausea and vomiting. Disorders of the gastrointestinal tract such as ulcers, obstructive tumors (particularly those of the stomach and proximal small bowel), adhesive bands, volvulus, and gastritis may also cause nausea and vomiting. Blood in the gastrointestinal tract also causes nausea and vomiting. Patients with pyelonephritis and pelvic inflammatory disease may pre-

DIFFERENTIAL DIAGNOSIS OF NAUSEA AND/OR VOMITING WITHOUT ABDOMINAL PAIN

CAUSE	NATURE OF PATIENT	NATURE OF SYMPTOMS	ASSOCIATED SYMPTOMS	PRECIPITATING AND AGGRAVATING FACTORS	PHYSICAL FINDINGS	DIAGNOSTIC STUDIES
Gastroenteritis	Most common cause at any age	Acute nausea and vomiting	Diarrhea Fever Abdominal pain		Hyperactive peristalsis	
Gastritis		Acute or chronic nausea and vomiting occur postprandially	Abdominal pain	Viral infection Alcohol- or drug-induced		Endoscopy
Viral or bacterial infection	Common cause of vomiting in children	Acute nausea and vomiting	Fever		High temperature	
Drugs		Acute or chronic nausea and vomiting Postprandial vomiting		Cytotoxic Codeine Digitalis glycosides Quinidine Salicylates Theophylline Antihypertensives Antibiotics Iron preparations Nonsteroidal anti-inflammatory agents Nicotine and Nicorette gum		Serum drug levels
Otitis media	Children	Acute nausea and vomiting	Fever Earache			
Excessive alcohol ingestion	Alcoholics Social drinkers	Early-morning vomiting				

238

Condition	Clinical setting	Symptoms	Physical findings	Diagnostic test
Uremia		Chronic nausea and vomiting; Usually in early morning		Elevated blood urea nitrogen and creatinine levels
Morning sickness	Pregnant females	Early-morning nausea and vomiting; Usually in first trimester		Serum HCG
Environmental or emotional stresses		Episodic nausea usually without vomiting		
Diabetic gastroparesis	Diabetic		Succussion splash	Radiograph of abdomen
Pyloric obstruction	In infants aged <3 mo may be due to pyloric stenosis; In adults may be secondary to ulcer scarring or tumor	Projectile vomiting; Abdominal pain	Palpable mass; Succussion splash	
Esophageal obstruction and achalasia		Vomiting or regurgitation of undigested food; Odorless vomitus; Usually occurs in early morning or after large meals		Esophageal radiograph; Endoscopy
Increased intracranial pressure		Projectile vomiting not preceded by nausea	Papilledema	Neurologic examination; Spinal tap; Computed tomography scan
Pancreatitis	Alcoholics	Repeated episodes of unexplained nausea and vomiting; Abdominal pain	Excessive alcohol intake	Elevated serum amylase level; Computed tomography scan of pancreas

TABLE 21–1. Tests That May Be Necessary in Diagnosis of Unexplained Vomiting

History, including psychiatric assessment and family history
Physical examination, with particular attention paid to
  Orthostatic hypotension
  Succussion splash, rash, Raynaud's phenomenon
  Neurologic assessment, especially cranial nerves, vestibular and pupillary function,
    peripheral neuropathy, extrapyramidal signs
Laboratory tests
  Routine hematologic and biochemical screening
  Amylase
  Drug screening, such as digoxin levels
  Hormonal levels: thyroxine, thyroid-stimulating hormones; plasma cortisol
    (0900 h, 2400 h), orthostatic catecholamines
  Serum (and urine) protein electrophoresis
  Immunologic tests: rheumatoid factor, DNA-binding titer, autoantibody screening
  Gastric intubation for residual volume after overnight fast
Radiologic tests
  Plain abdominal radiograph
  Gastrointestinal tract contrast series
  Intravenous urogram
  Computed tomography scan of abdomen and head
Upper gastrointestinal tract endoscopy
Gastric emptying tests
  ^{99m}Tc chicken liver (absorbable solid)
  ^{131}I-fiber (nondigestible solid)
  ^{111}In-pentetic acid (aqueous phase)
Conventional esophageal and anorectal manometry
Gastrointestinal manometry and electrogastrography
  Manometry: low compliance perfusion system (peroral or intraoperative)
  Electrogastrography: internal, external, intraoperative
Formal psychiatric assessment, such as Minnesota Multiphasic Personality Inventory
  and inpatient evaluation
Laparotomy and full-thickness biopsy of small bowel, including electrophysiologic study
  of muscle

From Malagelada, J. R., and Camilleri, M.: Unexplained vomiting: a diagnostic challenge. Ann. Intern. Med. *101*:211–218, 1984.

sent with a chief complaint of vomiting, particularly if they also have reflex ileus. Patients with anorexia nervosa, particularly in the early stages, may practice vomiting. Because anorectic patients seldom complain of this symptom, however, it may be difficult for the physician to diagnose the condition before pronounced weight loss has occurred. Vomiting may also be caused by conditions that alter neural control of gut motility.

Selected References

Bockus, H.: Gastroenterology. 4th ed. Philadelphia, W.B. Saunders Co., 1985.
Bramble, M. G., and Record, C. O.: Drug-induced gastrointestinal disease. Drugs *15*:451–463, 1978.

Bruppacher, R., Gyr, N., and Fisch, T.: Abdominal pain, indigestion, anorexia, nausea and vomiting. Baillieres Clin. Gastroenterol. 2:275–292, 1988.

Christian, P. E., Moore, J. G., Sorenson, J. A., et al.: Effects of meal size and correction techniques on gastric emptying time. Studies with two tracers and opposed detectors. J. Nucl. Med. 21:883–885, 1980.

Fuchs, S., and Jaffe, D.: Vomiting. Pediatr. Emerg. Care 6:164–167, 1990.

Hanson, J. S., and McCallum, R. W.: The diagnosis and management of nausea and vomiting: a review. Am. J. Gastroenterol. 80:210–218, 1985.

Katelares, P. H., and Jones, D. B.: Chronic nausea and vomiting. Dig. Dis. 7:324–333, 1989.

Malagelada, J. R., and Camilleri, M.: Unexplained vomiting: a diagnostic challenge. Ann. Intern. Med. 101:211–218, 1984.

Rosenthal, R. H., et al.: Diagnoses and management of persistent psychogenic vomiting. Psychosomatics 218:722–730, 1980.

Toccalino, H.: Vomiting and regurgitation. Clin. Gastroenterol. 6:267–282, 1977.

Valman, H. B.: The first year of life—vomiting. Br. Med. J. 280:620–623, 1980.

Chapter 22

Pain in the Foot

Foot pain is usually due to local disease or abnormality but occasionally results from referred pain. Therefore, examination of the foot should begin with the spine and proceed distally. Foot pain is most commonly due to *muscular* or *ligamentous strain* associated with *trauma,* unaccustomed or strenuous *physical activity,* and *sport.* New shoes or change in heel size also may cause foot pain. Other common causes include *gout, plantar warts, callosities,* and *metatarsal fracture (march fracture).* Isolated pain in the heel can result from a *calcaneal spur, arterial insufficiency, Achilles tendinitis* or *bursitis,* and *jogger's trauma.* In adolescents, pain in the heel may be caused by *calcaneal apophysitis.*

NATURE OF PATIENT

Foot pain in children is rare. When it occurs it is usually due to acute bone and ligament injuries or chronic bone–tendon disorders. Rarely, it is due to tumors, infections, or arthritis. Because foot pain is usually due to *muscular* or *ligamentous strain,* it is more likely to occur in people who are physically active, particularly those who are unaccustomed to physical exercise and muscular strain in their feet, such as unconditioned athletes and weekend sportsmen. *Gout* is more common in men over age 40 but does occur in women, especially those who are postmenopausal. The patient may present with a history of previous attacks of painful joints or urolithiasis. Often a family history of gout may be elicited.

Pain in the heel caused by a *calcaneal spur* and its associated soft-tissue irritation is most common in patients over age 40. When adolescents complain of pain in the heel, it most likely is caused by *calcaneal apophysitis. Achilles tendinitis,* which also causes heel pain, is usually due to trauma (e.g., injury from jogging), although the trauma may not be recalled by the patient. It is interesting to note that Achilles tendinitis

243

is more common in patients with Reiter's syndrome and ankylosing spondylitis who are HLA-B27–positive, even without a history of trauma.

NATURE OF SYMPTOMS

As with other types of pain, a careful history of the location and quality of the pain, how it began, and what intensifies it is most helpful in determining its cause.

If the foot pain is described as a dull ache, it is most likely due to *foot strain.* This is more likely to occur in older adults, overweight people, people wearing new shoes, and those who are on their feet for a large part of the day. It is critical that the physician establish the precise location of the ache because this will determine which ligaments, tendons, or fascia are involved (torn or under strain). For example, pain below the ankle on the inner aspect of the heel suggests a tear or strain of the ligamentous fibers attached to the internal malleolus.

Plantar warts and *callosities* can cause severe pain, particularly with weight bearing. These commonly are located on the plantar surface of the foot in the metatarsal region. Pain from a *calcaneal spur* or *plantar fasciitis* is usually continuous, although it may worsen with weight bearing. The spur is usually located in the center of the under-surface of the heel, about 2.25 cm from the back of the foot; the pain, however, may be more toward the back of the heel. The condition called *jogger's foot* may produce complaints of a burning pain in the heel, aching in the arch, or diminished sensation in the sole behind the large toe.

The pain of *Achilles tendinitis* is usually over the Achilles tendon and may be associated with tenderness to palpation and swelling.

With *gout,* the pain is usually acute, frequently recurrent, and often agonizing, although atypical cases of gout may present with less severe symptoms. The attacks usually have a sudden onset and characteristically start during the early hours of the day, while the patient is still in bed. Before a patient knows that he suffers from gout, he may attribute the bouts of pain to minor trauma such as "stubbing the toe" or "spraining the involved joint." Once the diagnosis of gout has been established, the patient usually recognizes subsequent attacks. Although the metatarsophalangeal joint of the big toe is classically affected, one or more other joints, including the ankle, may also be affected.

PRECIPITATING AND AGGRAVATING FACTORS

Most foot pain is precipitated by *trauma,* unaccustomed or *strenuous physical activity,* and *sport.* Change in occupation or work that involves constant jarring of the foot, walking on concrete floors, or standing may lead to foot strain. Constant vibration or jarring frequently leads to heel pain that may result from calcaneal periostitis. Likewise, new shoes or change in heel size can lead to foot strain. Gouty pain in the foot may have no particular precipitating factors, although several reports have indicated that a gouty diathesis may be caused by minor trauma to the involved joint.

PHYSICAL FINDINGS

In addition to careful examination of the foot for local discoloration, swelling, and areas tender to palpation, patients who complain of foot pain should have a careful examination of the lower back and legs, as foot pain may result from referred pain.

The following are some clues to the cause of foot pain. When pain is due to *foot strain,* the forefoot may flatten on weight bearing, and calluses under the metatarsal heads may be present. When the pain is due to gout, there is usually a warm, violaceous, tender, swollen joint (commonly the metatarsophalangeal joint of the big toe or the ankle). Tophi may be present in the foot, other joints, or the ear lobe. When the pain is due to a *calcaneal spur* or *plantar fasciitis,* there may be spot tenderness with deep palpation, particularly on the undersurface of the heel. If this is associated with radiographic evidence of calcaneal spur, the diagnosis is obvious. In cases in which there is no radiographic confirmation of a calcaneal spur, this pain may be due to plantar fasciitis.

Although the diagnosis of *ankle sprain* is usually obvious by history, patients may not remember the traumatic incident. Sprained ankles are most commonly due to an inversion injury and have tenderness and swelling over the anterior talofibular ligament. Likewise, *fractures* are usually associated with a history of significant trauma. A radiograph is usually necessary to diagnose small fractures of the ankle. In patients with a history suggesting a sprained ankle, the physician should suspect an associated fracture if the swelling appears disproportionate to the severity of the sprain.

Bunions can also cause foot pain, particularly at the metatarsophalangeal joint. This pain is usually worse with extension of the big toe. *Heel fasciitis,* also called *calcaneal periostitis,* may produce chronic pain in the bottom of the foot. Patients with this condition usually have pain and tenderness localized to the insertion of the long plantar tendon into the base of the calcaneus. When *peripheral ischemia* gives rise to isolated heel pain without other evidence of peripheral vascular disease, there is often cornification of the heel skin and coolness in this area.

DIAGNOSTIC STUDIES

Doppler studies help the physician detect arterial insufficiency. Radiographs may demonstrate calcaneal spurs and fractures, including small stress fractures. Quantitative scintigraphs help the physician identify abnormal weight distribution and its associated fasciitis. Occasionally, computed tomography scans, magnetic resonance imaging, or arthroscopic examination is helpful. Bone scans may detect avascular necrosis, stress fracture, or osteomyelitis.

LESS COMMON DIAGNOSTIC CONSIDERATIONS

Metatarsalgia is not a cause but a symptom of pain in the forefoot (Table 22–1). Primary metatarsalgia is pain in the forefoot due to a

TABLE 22–1. Twenty-three Diagnoses in Ninety-eight Patients with Pain in the Forepart of the Foot

Diagnosis	Number
Primary metatarsalgia	
Static disorders	12
Iatrogenic (postoperative)	12
Secondary to hallux valgus	9
Hallux rigidus	3
Morton's foot	3
Congenital	3
Long first ray	2
Freiberg's disease	1
Total	45
Secondary metatarsalgia	
Rheumatoid arthritis	11
Sesamoiditis	10
Posttraumatic	4
Neurogenic	3
Stress fractures	2
Gout	1
Short ipsilateral lower limb	2
Total	33
Pain under the forepart of the foot	
Morton's neuroma	5
Plantar fasciitis	3
Causalgia	2
Tarsal tunnel syndrome	2
Tumors	2
Intermittent claudication	1
Buerger's disease	1
Plantar verrucae (warts)	4
Total	20

From Scranton, P. E.: Metatarsalgia: diagnosis and treatment. J. Bone Joint Surg. *62*:723–732, 1980.

NEUROMA

COMMUNICATING BRANCH
LATERAL PLANTAR NERVE
MEDIAL PLANTAR NERVE

TIBIAL NERVE

Figure 22–1. Anatomy of Morton's neuroma. (From Morris, M. A.: Morton's metatarsalgia. Clin. Orthop. Rel. Res. *127*:203–207, 1977.)

chronic disorder of weight distribution across the metatarsophalangeal joints. Pain in the metatarsal region can be due to other local processes (e.g., plantar warts, tarsal tunnel syndrome, and plantar fasciitis) or systemic disease (e.g., rheumatoid arthritis, sesamoiditis, and gout). Neuralgia and polyneuritis from alcohol ingestion, lead poisoning, or diabetes may produce pain in one or both feet. In addition, these patients frequently complain of burning sensations or paresthesias of the soles. Decreased tactile and vibratory sensations may be observed on physical examination.

If foot pain is precisely located on the plantar surface between a pair of metatarsal heads, *Morton's neuroma* should be suspected (Fig. 22–1). This relatively rare condition is more common in women than in men. The usual history is foot pain for 2 or more years that is relieved by shoe removal and unchanged by conservative measures. This pain is often described as "burning," "shooting," "needles," "daggers," or "like walking on a stone." It may radiate to the toes. Patients may complain of numbness and tingling. Physical findings include pain with compression of the toes, a palpable click after the release of pressure in the affected area, occasional swelling, and some sensory changes. The pain is precipitated by walking and is aggravated by compression of the toes and weight bearing.

Patients with Raynaud's disease, in addition to having tingling and numbness, may present with pain in the toes that often is associated with pain in the fingers. These pains may be precipitated by exposure to cold, emotional stress, beta blockers, and cigarette smoking. Some

DIFFERENTIAL DIAGNOSIS OF FOOT PAIN

CAUSE	NATURE OF PATIENT	NATURE OF SYMPTOMS	PRECIPITATING AND AGGRAVATING FACTORS	PHYSICAL FINDINGS	DIAGNOSTIC STUDIES
Muscular and ligamentous strain	Physically active, especially those unaccustomed to exercise	Pain in region of strained muscles or ligaments	Trauma Unaccustomed or strenuous physical activity	Localized tenderness on palpation	
Foot strain	Older adults Overweight patients	Dull ache in foot, especially forefoot	New shoes Change in heel size Prolonged standing	Forefoot may splay with weight bearing	
Plantar warts and callosities		Pain in plantar surface in metatarsal region	Weight bearing	Plantar callosities	
Jogger's foot	Joggers	Burning in heel Aching in arch		Decreased sensation behind big toe	
Fractures	Patients with history of trauma Joggers		Trauma		May need radiographs or magnetic resonance imaging to diagnose small fractures of ankle and march fractures of metatarsals

Condition	Typical patient	Symptoms	Precipitating factors	Physical findings	Diagnostic tests
Calcaneal spur or plantar fasciitis		Pain on undersurface of heel Continuous One inch from back of heel	Worse with weight bearing	Worse with dorsiflexion of toes	Radiograph may show calcaneal spur
Achilles tendinitis or bursitis	Joggers	Heel pain over Achilles tendon	Trauma Running	Swelling and tenderness over Achilles tendon	
Apophysitis of calcaneus	Adolescents	Pain in back of heel	Running and jumping	Pain on palpation of Achilles insertion	
Arterial insufficiency	Older adults Diabetics	Rest pain in heel or toes		Coolness Decreased pulses Cornification of heel skin	Arteriography
Gout	Males, especially over age 40 Postmenopausal females	Acute severe pain in big toe metatarsophalangeal joint, occasionally other toes or ankle	Trauma	Warm, violaceous, tender, swollen joints	Uric acid Radiographs

patients with rheumatoid arthritis have marked prominence of the metatarsal heads with pain in this region. Foot ulcerations, which are not necessarily associated with significant pain, can occur in patients with diabetes mellitus, tabes dorsalis, leprosy, paraplegia, Raynaud's disease, and thromboangiitis obliterans. These conditions should be suspected whenever there is an ulcer without much pain. They may all cause some degree of neuropathy that interferes with pain perception.

Erythromelalgia is painful dilatation of the superficial vessels of the foot. The pain is burning in quality and may be severe. It may be seen in patients with lead poisoning, polycythemia, or syringomyelia and in some psychologically disturbed patients.

Selected References

Maurice, H. D., Newman, J. H., and Watt, I.: Bone scanning of the foot for unexplained pain. J. Bone Joint Surg. *69*:448–452, 1987.

Rask, M. R.: Medial plantar neuropraxia (jogger's foot): report of three cases. Clin. Orthop. *134*:193–195, 1978.

Scranton, P. E.: Metatarsalgia: diagnosis and treatment. J. Bone Joint Surg. *62*:723–732, 1980.

Stern, S. H.: Ankle and foot pain. Prim. Care *15*:809–826, 1988.

Swell, J. R., et al.: Quantitative scintigraphs in diagnosis and management of plantar fasciitis (calcaneal periostitis). Con. Comm. J. Nucl. Med. *21*:633–636, 1980.

Wilkins, K. E.: The painful foot in the child. Intr. Course Lect. *37*:77–85, 1988.

Chapter 23

Pain in the Lower Extremity in Adults

To diagnose pain in the lower extremity accurately, the physician must determine whether the pain is *articular* (hip, knee, or ankle), or whether it is *nonarticular* (muscular, vascular, or neurologic). In addition, it is particularly helpful for the examiner to note whether the pain is present at rest or whether it is primarily associated with exercise. The most likely causes of pain in a child's leg are different from those in an adult. Therefore, lower-extremity pain in adults and lower-extremity pain and limp in children are reviewed in separate chapters.

In adults, the most common causes of leg pain include *muscular* and *ligamentous strains, degenerative joint disease* (particularly of the hip and knee), *intermittent claudication* due to arterial insufficiency, *sciatica, night cramps, varicose veins, thrombophlebitis, gout,* and *trauma.* **The major clues to diagnoses are (1) the location of the pain, (2) the age of the patient, and (3) whether the pain is related to exertion.**

NATURE OF PATIENT

The most common cause of leg pain is *muscular* or *ligamentous strain,* seen frequently in weekend athletes. Questioning usually reveals a history of unusual or strenuous exercise. The usual causes of leg pain in joggers and runners are *shin splints, stress fractures,* and *compartment syndromes.* The most common is shin splints, a musculotendinous inflammation of the anterior tibia that occasionally involves the periosteum. The pain is usually on the anterior aspect of the tibia, particularly the distal third along the medial crest, but it can occur on the lateral aspect of the tibia as well. Shin splints are most common in less well conditioned athletes and are most frequently reported early in the running season. Skiers often develop anterior knee pain due to *patellofemoral problems.*

Patellar problems are more common in young women—often beginning in adolescence. During pregnancy, the common causes of painful legs include *venous insufficiency, postphlebitic syndrome, thrombophlebitis, muscle cramps,* and *trauma.*

Degenerative joint disease (DJD) is uncommon in patients under age 40 unless it has been facilitated by unequal leg length (causing DJD of the hip) or prior trauma, such as athletic injuries of the knee. After age 40, pain in the hip or knee is commonly due to DJD.

In patients age 50 or older, calf pain precipitated by walking or exercise that abates with rest is most likely due to *peripheral arterial insufficiency.* **Intermittent claudication pain in the hip is seen in patients with aortoiliac disease.** When exercise-induced calf pain occurs in younger adults—frequently with a history of phlebitis—*venous claudication* is probable. *Gout* is most common in older men but can occur in women, particularly those who have had an early menopause (natural or surgically induced). Patients with gout may or may not have a family history of the condition. Often a history of a prior attack can be elicited. Classic gouty pain occurs in the big toe, but it may occur in other toes or in ankles or knees; it is rare in the hip.

NATURE OF SYMPTOMS

Anterior knee pain is most often due to patellar tendinitis, prepatellar bursitis, or *chondromalacia patellae.* Sharp pain in the knee suggests *synovial impingement* or structural difficulties such as loose bodies. Aching joint pain is usually seen in inflammatory conditions with diffuse involvement of the synovium, such as in *rheumatoid arthritis.*

DEGENERATIVE JOINT DISEASE. When the knee or hip joints are painful and stiff in the morning, improve during the day, and worsen toward the end of the day, DJD is probable. These pains may be exacerbated by certain activities (e.g., descending stairs). Patients with osteoarthritis of the hip may present with pain in the groin or the knee. Therefore, the diagnosis of DJD of the hip must be considered in patients who present with knee or groin pain when no pathology is noted in these areas. With DJD of the hip, hip motion is usually restricted and radiographs are abnormal. Involvement of the *obturator nerve* also can cause pain in the groin and medial aspect of the thigh and knee. A hernia may be suspected because of groin pain; if no hernia is found, obturator nerve involvement should be considered.

Osteoarthritis of the hip also may present with pain in the buttock; therefore, causes of buttock pain must be considered in the differential diagnosis. Buttock pain caused by *lumbar disc disease* is worse with extension of the spine and relieved by rest in the fetal position. Buttock pain caused by osteoarthritis of the hip is not usually exacerbated by spinal extension or relieved by rest in the fetal position. Likewise, there is usually no evidence of nerve root compression with osteoarthritis of the hip.

SCIATICA. Typical sciatica causes pain in the buttock that radiates down the posterolateral aspect of the leg. It may radiate into the dorsum of the foot and tends to follow standard dermatome patterns. Sciatic pain may be sharp or burning. Frequently, it is made worse by coughing, straining at stool (if sciatica is caused by a herniated disc), or walking down steps; it may be precipitated by sudden strenuous movements. The patient may present with pain initiated by an attempt to lift a heavy object or by vigorous turning or twisting with the back flexed (e.g., pulling the rope on a lawn mower or outboard engine).

EFFECTS OF EXERCISE AND REST ON PAIN. Leg pain that develops during walking occurs in patients with arterial insufficiency, venous insufficiency, spinal stenosis, and thrombophlebitis.

Arterial Insufficiency. The pain of arterial insufficiency (intermittent claudication) usually is described as soreness, a cramp, or a burning sensation in the calf. The discomfort also may be described as a tightness, heaviness, tiredness, or achiness rather than pain. The discomfort usually is precipitated by walking and relieved by rest. It rarely occurs while the patient is at home. It usually develops after the patient has walked a predictable (by the patient) distance and is relieved by rest in a standing position after a predictable (by the patient) period of time. After resting, the patient can resume walking and walk a similar distance before the pain starts again; relief is achieved again after resting. A common mistake is the diagnosis of osteoarthritis of the hip when gluteal claudication is the actual problem. This error is more likely if buttock pain is not associated with pain in the calf. Some patients with vascular disease of the iliac artery complain only of the symptoms of gluteal claudication, which are usually felt when the patient walks outside.

Rest pain (often nocturnal) in the toes or heel is almost pathognomonic of arterial insufficiency. With arterial insufficiency there may be pallor on elevation, rubor on dependency, and loss of hair on the toes. Some men with aortoiliac disease may present with pain in the upper leg or the buttock and an inability to develop or sustain an erection. Intermittent claudication pain is usually unilateral but can be bilateral. When the pain is present bilaterally, it seldom occurs in both legs simultaneously. Not uncommonly, the onset of pain in one leg prevents the patient from walking to the point at which symptoms develop in the other leg. Physical examination for evidence of arterial insufficiency must be performed on both legs, not only on the one about which the patient complains.

Venous Insufficiency. Venous claudication is difficult to distinguish from claudication due to arterial insufficiency. In both conditions, walking causes calf pain that may be severe enough for the patient to stop walking. In cases of venous claudication, there usually are no physical signs of arterial insufficiency.

Spinal Stenosis. Spinal stenosis is another cause of leg pain that is exacerbated by exercise. The pain is similar to that associated with arterial insufficiency; it also occurs more frequently in older men. The first clue that the pain in the leg is not due to arterial insufficiency is the presence of normal pedal pulses. **Although both the pain of spinal stenosis and the pain of arterial insufficiency begin with exercise, the former is less typically relieved by rest (Table 23–1).** The pain of intermittent claudication is relieved within a few minutes, whereas the pain of spinal stenosis requires 10 to 30 minutes to subside. Some patients with calf pain from spinal stenosis state that they must sit or lie down with the thighs flexed to relieve the discomfort. The pain of spinal stenosis is caused by a localized narrowing of the spinal canal

TABLE 23–1. Comparison of Symptoms and Signs in Vascular and Spinal Claudication

	Vascular Claudication	Cauda Equina Claudication
Backache	Uncommon, occurs in aortoiliac occlusion	Common but need not be present
Leg symptoms	Quantitatively related to effort	May be brought on by effort; directly related to posture of extension of spine
Quality	Cramplike, tight feeling; intense fatigue; discomfort; pain may be absent	Numbness, cramplike, burning, paresthetic; sensation of cold or swelling; pain may be absent
Relief	Rest of affected muscle group	Rest not enough; postural alteration of spine to allow flexion is necessary in most
Onset	Simultaneous onset in all parts affected	Characteristic march up or down legs
Urinary incontinence	Does not occur	Very rare
Impotence	Common in aortoiliac disease (failure to sustain erection)	Very rare (failure to achieve erection?)
Wasting of legs	Global in aortoiliac disease	Cauda equina distribution in severe cases
Trophic changes	May be present; absent in aortoiliac disease	Absent but may be present in combined disease
Sensory loss	Absent	Not uncommon; common after exercise
Ankle jerks	Often absent in patients over 60 years	Common, particularly after exercise
Straight-leg raising	Full	Often full

From DeVilliers, J. C.: Combined neurogenic and vascular claudication. S. A. Med. J. *57:*650–654, 1980.

due to a structural abnormality that results in cauda equina compression. With spinal stenosis, the patients occasionally complain of backache or buttock pain as well as numbness and tingling in the feet with walking. Walking uphill is easier than walking downhill for these patients. They have no problem riding a bicycle, probably because the stooped position that they assume during this activity reduces the amount of cauda equina compression. It must be remembered that vascular claudication and spinal stenosis can coexist.

Thrombophlebitis. Unilateral pain and swelling in the calf commonly is due to thrombophlebitis. The pain is usually present at rest and seldom is worsened by exercise. In a patient with thrombophlebitis who experiences calf pain when walking, there is an acute exacerbation of the calf pain immediately after he places his foot on the ground. Although the history and physical examination of thrombophlebitis are well known to most physicians (i.e., pain, swelling, tenderness to palpation, and occasionally a history of prior trauma or previous bouts of phlebitis), this relatively common cause of leg pain often is misdiagnosed. Several studies have suggested that venography should be used to confirm the clinical diagnosis because thrombophlebitis has often been incorrectly diagnosed in the absence of venographic evidence.

Other Conditions. Other causes of painful swelling of the calf include traumatic *rupture of the plantaris tendon* or the *medial head of the gastrocnemius, muscle trauma, muscle stiffness* after unaccustomed exercise, and popliteal *(Baker's) cyst.* The last condition has been called the "pseudothrombophlebitis syndrome" because it causes painful swelling of the calf, thus mimicking thrombophlebitis. Therefore, all patients with painful calf swelling should be examined for a popliteal cyst. In one large series, most patients with painful popliteal cysts also had inflammatory joint disease of the knee, usually rheumatoid arthritis (Table 23–2).

Diffuse aching in one or both calves with no relation to exercise suggests *varicose veins.* Patients with this condition frequently complain that their legs hurt when they go to bed at night, and they often

TABLE 23–2. Disease Entities Associated with Pseudothrombophlebitis Syndrome

Rheumatoid arthritis	Traumatic arthritis
Psoriatic arthritis	Meniscal injury
Osteoarthritis	Osteochondritis dissecans
Juvenile rheumatoid arthritis	Villonodular synovitis
Reiter's syndrome	Systemic lupus erythematosus
Gonococcal arthritis	Ankylosing spondylitis
Gouty arthritis	Mixed connective tissue disease

From Katerndahl, D. A.: Calf pain mimicking thrombophlebitis. Postgrad. Med. *68(6)*:107–115, 1980.

complain of night cramps. The pain of venous insufficiency is vague, nonspecific, and unrelated to any specific muscle groups. Superficial varicosities may suggest the diagnosis, but deep venous insufficiency may be present without noticeable superficial serpiginous varicosities.

A first attack of *gouty arthritis* of the knee (or, rarely, of the hip) may be difficult to diagnose unless there is a warm, swollen joint in the big toe (podagra) and a prior history of gout. When the first attack is a warm, swollen, painful knee, the diagnosis is less apparent and may be confused with *pyogenic arthritis*. Patients with gout do not usually have as many systemic signs and symptoms (rash, malaise, and fever) as do patients with pyogenic arthritis. With gouty arthritis, there is often a hot, red, tender, swollen joint. The involved joint is sensitive to external pressure; some patients cannot even tolerate the weight of a sheet or blanket on the joint.

ASSOCIATED SYMPTOMS

Patients with *degenerative joint disease* often have pain and stiffness in other joints. A limp may be present in cases of DJD of the hip. Patients with *sciatica* may have numbness, paresthesia, weakness, and sensory deficits as well as abnormal knee or ankle jerks (hyperactive early; diminished to absent later). Patients with *intermittent claudication* may complain of numbness in the foot, which may erroneously suggest a *peripheral neuropathy*. If they also report *impotence,* an *aortoiliac lesion* is probable.

Night cramps, edema of the legs, and stasis abnormalities suggest *chronic venous insufficiency*.

PRECIPITATING AND AGGRAVATING FACTORS

Pain during activity usually is seen with structural abnormalities, whereas pain at rest or after activity suggests inflammatory processes. Bone pain occurs at rest and increases with weight bearing. The pain of *DJD* worsens with exercise and prolonged weight bearing. *Sciatic* pain is aggravated by coughing, straining at stools, sneezing, walking, stooping, lifting, and spinal extension. As mentioned before, both the pain of *intermittent claudication* and the pain of *spinal stenosis* are brought on by walking and exercise. Pain in the knee after sitting for a while suggests patellofemoral disorders.

AMELIORATING FACTORS

Patients with *DJD* will report that their morning stiffness, aches, and pain often abate during the day as they move the joint. *Sciatic* pain often is alleviated by recumbency in the fetal position. The pain of *intermittent claudication* abates within a few minutes after cessation of walking; the pain of *spinal stenosis* is relieved more slowly and by spinal flexion. The pain of *varicose veins* usually is alleviated somewhat by elevation of the involved limb; the resting (nocturnal) pain of *arterial insufficiency* often is relieved by lowering of the involved limb. **Relief of symptoms with an adequate dose of colchicine is pathognomonic of gout.**

PHYSICAL FINDINGS AND DIAGNOSTIC STUDIES

A careful history and physical examination are essential in all patients who complain of pain in the extremities. During the history, special attention should be paid to any history of previous joint disease, precipitating events, previous diagnoses, and medications, particularly oral contraceptives, which are associated with a higher incidence of thrombophlebitis. Physical examination should include observation of gait, attempts to reproduce the pain by palpation or maneuver, examination and determination of range of motion of all joints, measurement of both calves and both thighs, and inspection and palpation for arterial insufficiency. Examination of the knee and popliteal space should be performed in both the supine and the erect position: Joint effusions are more readily detected in the supine position, whereas cysts are more prominent when the patient is erect.

MUSCULAR AND LIGAMENTOUS STRAINS AND TEARS. When patients complain of pain in the knee, the joint should be palpated (Fig 23–1). Tenderness at the joint line suggests damage to the medial or collateral ligaments, the capsular ligament, or the meniscus. Radiographs, magnetic resonance imaging, and arthroscopic examination may be needed for an accurate diagnosis. The stability of the knee ligaments should be determined by careful physical examination. Tenderness above or below the joint line suggests a muscle pull or strain. With acute muscle tears, there usually are local tenderness, bruising, and possibly a gap in the muscle. With *acute gouty arthritis,* the joint is usually warm, red, tender, and swollen. Although pain can be as severe as that seen in pyogenic arthritis, patients with gouty arthritis do not have comparable systemic symptoms. The serum uric acid level usually is elevated, and uric acid crystals may be seen in the joint aspirate.

DEGENERATIVE JOINT DISEASE. The major physical findings that suggest DJD include joint crepitus, limitation of joint movement, and elicitation of presenting symptoms at extremes of joint movement. In advanced cases, there may be fixed flexion contractures, joint effusions, and radiographic evidence of arthritis. Patients with DJD are often in the same age group as those with vascular insufficiency, in whom the

Figure 23–1. Major landmarks in examination of the knee. (From Smith, J. B.: Knee problems in children. Pediatr. Clin. North Am. *24*:4, 1977.)

symptoms are referable to soft tissue. **It is essential that the physician remember that both conditions can coexist. A good axiom to keep in mind is that if a careful examination reveals no swelling of the joint, there probably is no serious problem inside the joint.**

SCIATICA. Some common physical findings in sciatica include restriction of spinal movement (hyperextension often reproduces sciatic pain), limitation of straight-leg raising, and spasm over the sacrospinal muscles (which may be tender to palpation). There may be changes in reflex activity as well as sensory or motor loss over the involved segments. Myelograms and computed tomography scans are rarely necessary for diagnosis. They are used to determine the extent of the spinal cord compression.

INTERMITTENT CLAUDICATION. Physical findings in intermittent claudication include pallor on elevation, rubor on dependency (most noticeable in the toes and sole), loss of hair on the toes, and diminished arterial pulsations. The presence of normal pedal pulses at rest and after walking virtually rules out arterial insufficiency.

Patients with *venous claudication* usually have varicose veins. Occasionally, they can identify a tender point in the calf, but examination is nonrevealing. In such cases, the patient should be exercised to the point of discomfort, at which time a group of varices may be noted. Venography may be required for diagnosis.

THROMBOPHLEBITIS. The classic findings in patients with thrombophlebitis are swelling and a measurable increase in calf circumference when compared with that of the opposite side. The clinician often can palpate a tender cordlike vein between the heads of the gastrocnemius muscle. There may be dilation of other veins, edema, erythema, and Homans' sign. These findings are variable and not always reliable for the diagnosis of thrombophlebitis. Inflation of a sphygmomanometer around each calf until pain is produced is a sensitive test for the pain of thrombophlebitis. The single most important test is venography. **Because thrombophlebitis may coexist with a popliteal (Baker's) cyst, a venogram should be obtained for all patients with popliteal cysts.**

OTHER CONDITIONS. The diagnosis of *joint sprain* is made by demonstrating instability of the joint. Tears of joint ligaments often can be demonstrated by the use of stress-view radiographs of the joint involved. With suspected *fractures,* a radiograph including the joints at both ends of the fractured bone always should be performed. Instability of joints suggests ligamentous tears. Angulation in valgus or varus with knee slightly flexed suggests either medial or lateral ligament instability. Abnormal forward or backward shift of the tibia on the femur is indicative of anterior cruciate or posterior cruciate ligament instability, respectively. Occasionally, abnormal rotations may be present; these suggest a complicated combination injury of the knee.

If the diagnosis is still unclear after a complete physical examination is conducted with special attention given to the musculoskeletal, vascular, and nervous systems, noninvasive and invasive studies of the vascular system, electromyography, CT scanning, and myelography may be helpful.

LESS COMMON DIAGNOSTIC CONSIDERATIONS

Sudden onset of pain that sometimes is associated with paralysis, paresthesia, pallor, or absence of arterial pulsation suggests acute arterial embolism. The likelihood of this diagnosis is increased by the presence of atrial fibrillation. Vague arthralgias and muscle aches often are seen with viral and flulike infections, but no joint abnormality can be detected on physical examination in these cases. Primary bone tumors are rare in adults; pain from metastatic bone disease, however, frequently is seen in patients with breast, lung, and prostatic tumors.

Because cellulitis of the calf can mimic thrombophlebitis, the two conditions must be differentiated. In patients with cellulitis, the pain is described as being on the surface, no palpable cord is present, and Homans' sign is absent. Careful examination will reveal that the pain of cellulitis is induced by light palpation rather than deep palpation over the course of the vein. Likewise, the area of erythema is more clearly demarcated, and there occasionally is an associated open wound. An inflated sphygmomanometer requires high pressure to reproduce the pain, and often there is no difference between the two calves. These findings contrast with those reported in patients with thrombophlebitis.

Chondromalacia patellae, although more common in adolescents than in adults, may be seen in patients in their 40s and 50s. These patients characteristically have pain, stiffness, grating, or locking of the knee. The pain is worse when the knee is weight bearing in flexion. Crepitation and pain with manipulation of the patella over the femoral condyle are characteristic. Pain is exacerbated when the patient tenses the quadriceps with the knee in free extension while the examiner depresses the upper pole of the patella.

Meralgia paresthetica, which is slightly more common in men than in women, is caused by entrapment of the lateral femoral cutaneous nerve by the tensor fasciae latae. The patient complains of pain, burning, or tingling over the lateral aspect of the thigh that occasionally is worse at night or after exercise. It is alleviated by rest, particularly in the sitting position.

Peripheral neuropathies are more common in diabetic patients but may be seen in nondiabetics. Patients complain of burning, tingling, and numbness, particularly in the feet. They may have a sensation of coldness, but no decrease in vascular pulsations is noted in those with a pure peripheral neuropathy. Diabetics with a peripheral neuropathy often have an associated vascular insufficiency. Physical findings include sensory loss (often symmetrical), muscle wasting, weakness, decreased tendon reflexes, and signs of arterial insufficiency.

Obturator hernias, an uncommon cause of pain, occur more frequently in elderly debilitated women than in other patients. The female-male ratio is 6:1. Patients usually present with pain along the anteromedial aspect of the thigh. This pain is increased by adduction of the thigh. Pain also may be felt in the hip or knee. The pain may be associated with intermittent bouts of nausea, vomiting, abdominal pain, and distention—all signs of small bowel obstruction. **Obturator hernia should be given particular consideration in elderly women who complain of pain in the hip or knee when there is no objective**

evidence of DJD or other common causes of pain in the hip or knee.

Pseudothrombophlebitis due to a popliteal (Baker's) cyst has been discussed previously. Fifty per cent of patients with this syndrome have rheumatoid arthritis. It is notable that among patients in whom a popliteal cyst has been confirmed, only 50 per cent had palpable masses, and 12 per cent had masses below the popliteal space. **A Baker's cyst should be suspected in all patients with thrombophlebitis and rheumatoid arthritis and in all patients in whom thrombophlebitis is suspected but for whom no evidence of phlebitis is found on venography.** An arthrogram is essential to the diagnosis of a popliteal cyst. Ultrasonography may help the physician diagnose an intact cyst, but it is not often useful in the diagnosis of a ruptured popliteal cyst.

Rheumatoid arthritis is a relatively uncommon cause of pain in the lower extremity. The joint pain usually lasts for a few weeks, and there is characteristic morning stiffness, joint tenderness, and pain with motion. Frequently, there is joint effusion, soft-tissue swelling, and synovial thickening. As already mentioned, pseudothrombophlebitis should be suspected when calf pain occurs in any patient with rheumatoid arthritis, especially if active inflammation of the knee is present.

Spinal stenosis (neurogenic claudication, cauda equina claudication) is often difficult to differentiate from intermittent claudication due to arterial insufficiency. The patient's history is particularly important because both conditions affect the same age group. Patients with calf pain due to spinal stenosis state that the pain starts insidiously, is exacerbated by walking, and is particularly related to extension of the spine. They may have associated backache or buttock pain, which is relatively uncommon in patients with intermittent claudication. A paresthetic quality to the pain suggests a neurogenic origin. Patients with spinal stenosis do not experience prompt relief of pain with cessation of exercise (as do those with arterial insufficiency); they feel greater relief when they lie or sit down with their thighs flexed. It is noteworthy that patients with spinal stenosis do not have pain when riding a bicycle because the spine is in a flexed position. In any case that involves a patient who has signs of intermittent claudication and who rides a bicycle without difficulty, spinal stenosis should be suspected.

Rupture of the gastrocnemius or the plantaris tendon, particularly during athletic activities such as jogging, running, and tennis, is characterized by a sudden onset of pain in the leg ("felt like I got a shot in the leg"). Frequently, the physician can palpate the retracted end of the plantaris muscle.

Trochanteric bursitis, a relatively uncommon cause of leg pain, usually presents with pain over the greater trochanter, in the buttock, and in the lateral thigh along the distribution of the second lumbar dermatome. On physical examination, the patient may limp, and there

DIFFERENTIAL DIAGNOSIS OF LOWER EXTREMITY PAIN IN ADULTS

CAUSE	NATURE OF PATIENT	NATURE OF SYMPTOMS	ASSOCIATED SYMPTOMS	PRECIPITATING AND AGGRAVATING FACTORS	AMELIORATING FACTORS	PHYSICAL FINDINGS	DIAGNOSTIC STUDIES
Muscular or ligamentous strain	Weekend athletes Those with trauma			Unaccustomed or strenuous muscular activity		With ligamentous injury of joint may be tenderness at the joint line and swelling of joint Local tenderness	Magnetic resonance imaging for injury of knee, especially meniscal and ligamentous
Degenerative joint disease	> age 40 (except those with prior trauma)	Knee or hip pain Morning stiffness Gradual onset	Pain and stiffness in other joints Occasional limp	Standing and weight bearing Descending stairs	Movement	Buttock pain not worse with hyperextension No evidence of nerve root compression Crepitation of joint Joint limitation of movement and/or effusion	Radiographs Arthroscopy of knee Magnetic resonance imaging
Lumbar disk disease (sciatica)	More common in men over age 40	Pain in buttock and posterolateral aspect of leg Acute onset Lancinating or like toothache Less severe previous episodes	Paresthesias Dysesthesias Weakness	Lifting Turning Twisting Spinal extension Coughing Straining	Fetal position	Spasm of hamstrings Positive straight- or flexed-leg signs Neurologic signs in lower leg Reversal of lordotic curve Pain of sciatic distribution with spinal hyperextension Asymmetrical limitation of motion	CT scan Electromyography Magnetic resonance imaging

Varicose veins		Diffuse aching of one or both calves Worse at night	Edema and stasis abnormalities		Elevation of limb	Varicose veins may or may not be apparent	Venography Doppler studies
Thrombophlebitis	History of phlebitis Use of oral contraceptives	Unilateral Pain at rest	Swelling	Placing foot on ground		No evidence of arterial insufficiency Swelling of calf with tenderness and warmth Palpable cord	Venography Doppler studies
Arterial insufficiency	> age 50, earlier in diabetics	Pain in calf with walking Intermittent claudication of hip with aortoiliac disease Rest pain in calf, toes, or heel suggests severe arterial insufficiency Usually unilateral	Impotence with aortoiliac disease	Walking	Rest Dependency of involved limb	Decreased pulses Pallor on elevation, rubor on dependency Cool Loss of hair on toes	Arteriography Doppler studies Magnetic resonance imaging
Spinal stenosis	Older men	Calf pain induced by walking and/or leg exercise	Paresthesias Backache Buttock pain	Exercise Not precipitated by exercise with spine flexed (bicycling)	Not quickly relieved by rest Spinal flexion	Good pedal pulses Transient neurologic deficit	Electromyography Computed tomography Magnetic resonance imaging
Gout	More common in men	Acute onset Toe and knee pain Rare in hip		Occasionally precipitated by trauma		Joint warm, swollen, exquisitely tender	Serum uric acid test Uric acid crystals in joint aspirate

usually is marked point tenderness over the greater trochanter. The differential diagnosis consists of arthritis of the hip or lumbar spine problems. The major factors in differential diagnosis include pain with palpation over the trochanteric bursa and the absence of sensory loss that would be seen with lumbar disc disease. The pain is not exacerbated by coughing and sneezing but by squatting, climbing stairs, and sitting with the painful leg crossed over the other one. It is alleviated by infiltration of the trochanteric bursa with local anesthetics or steroids or both.

THE LEG AND SPORTS MEDICINE

The most common causes of chronic leg pain in runners include *shin splints, stress fractures,* and *compartment syndromes.* Shin splints represent muscle tenderness, inflammation, and probably subclinical periosteal reaction. With stress fractures there is usually point tenderness over the involved bone, and the diagnosis may be confirmed radiographically. Stress fractures are more common in experienced long-distance runners, particularly in those who attempt to run more than 20 to 30 miles per week. These fractures may occur in the tibia, fibula, or the metatarsus. "Compartment syndromes" occur when the fascial compartment is too small to accommodate the approximately 20 per cent increase in muscle size that occurs with strenuous exercise. This results in a limited venous outflow and tends to produce an ischemic pain of the involved tissue. Patients with compartment syndromes usually present with a gradual onset (over 1 or more years) of pain that is progressive, dull, aching, and particularly worse after long runs. Paresthesias also may be present. The anterior compartment of the leg usually is affected. The next most likely compartment to be affected is the posterior compartment, followed by the posterior superficial compartment. Physical findings include tenderness in the muscle mass itself but not as much in the bone and tendons. Elevated compartment pressures are diagnostic.

Selected References

Detmer, D. E.: Chronic leg pain. Am. J. Sports Med. *8(2)*:141–144, 1980.

Goodreau, J. J., et al.: Rational approach to the differentiation of vascular and neurogenic claudication. Surgery *84(6)*:749–757, 1978.

Jacobsen, K. E., and Flandry, F. C.: Diagnosis of anterior knee pain. Prim. Care *15*:179–195, 1988.

Katerndahl, D. A.: Calf pain mimicking thrombophlebitis. Postgrad. Med. *68(6)*:107–115, 1980.

Lee, R. V., McComb, L. E., and Mezzadri, F. C.: Pregnant patients, painful legs: the obstetrician's dilemma. Obstet. Gynecol. Surv. *45*:290–298, 1990.

McCune, W. J., Matteson, E. L., and MacGuire, A.: Evaluation of knee pain. Prim. Care *15*:795–808, 1988.

Noble, J., and Abernathy, P. K.: The painful knee. Br. J. Hosp. Med. *22(2)*:169–176, 1979.
Polisson, R. P.: Sports medicine for the internist. Med. Clin. North Am. *70*:469–489, 1986.
Provan, J. L., Moreau, P., and MacNab I.: Pitfalls in the diagnosis of leg pain. Can. Med. Assoc. J. *121*:167–171, 1979.
Roberts, W. N., and Williams, R. R.: Hip pain. Prim. Care *15*:783–793, 1988.
Styf, J.: Diagnosis of exercise induced pain in the anterior aspect of the lower leg. Am. J. Sports Med. *16*:165–169, 1988.

Chapter 24

Pain in the Lower Extremity and Limp in Children

The physician should approach leg pain or limp in children as in adults—that is, determine whether it originates in joints or in soft tissue. The most common causes of leg pain originating in the soft tissue are unusual or strenuous *exercise* and *trauma*. Other common causes of leg pain include *growing pains, Legg-Calvé-Perthes disease, Osgood-Schlatter disease, chondromalacia patellae*, and *ossification of the Achilles insertion*.

NATURE OF PATIENT

If a limp occurs in a young child when he begins to walk, *congenital dislocation* of one or both hips should be considered. *Legg-Calvé-Perthes disease* (epiphysitis of the hip) usually occurs between ages 5 and 7. In adolescents, *slipped femoral epiphyses* and *patellar problems* are more common. In children between ages 12 and 14, pain in the heel is most often caused by a painful *bursitis* or *irregular ossification of the calcaneal apophysis*.

NATURE OF SYMPTOMS

Growing pains is a general diagnosis that is being made less frequently as physicians become more expert in making specific diagnoses. There is no doubt, however, that growing pains do exist, and they are now thought to be a form of *myalgia*. The aching pain is intermittent and usually located in the leg muscles, particularly in the front of the thigh, the calf, and the back of the knee. The pain is deep and localized to areas outside joints. It is usually bilateral and commonly occurs late in the day, although it may awaken the child from a sound sleep. Growing pains may be exacerbated by excessive running during the day, but exercise is not usually a factor. **The findings that the pain is nonarticular, bilateral, and usually unrelated to activity are essential to the accurate diagnosis of growing pains.** There are no abnormal physical findings in children with growing pains.

Most serious diseases that cause leg pain in children (except slipped capital femoral epiphyses) are usually unilateral. Pain in the hip may be due to *Legg-Calvé-Perthes disease*, a disturbance of the epiphyseal ossification of the femoral head in children ages 4 to 12 (peak age, 5 to 7 years). It often is associated with a limp. Occasionally, the pain is referred to the medial aspect of the knee.

The most common causes of knee pain in children are *acute trauma, Osgood-Schlatter disease,* and *chondromalacia patellae.* Osgood-Schlatter disease is an abnormality of the epiphyseal ossification of the tibial tubercle. It is most common in children ages 10 to 15. This condition involves painful swelling of the tibial tubercle at the insertion of the patellar tendon. Pain is worse with contraction of the quadriceps against resistance. It is exacerbated by activity and relieved by rest.

Chondromalacia patellae is an extremely common syndrome in active children and may be a precursor of adult patellofemoral arthritis. In this condition, the patellar cartilage degenerates not because of primary cartilaginous disease but because of abnormal mechanical forces acting on it. These abnormal forces may be due to direct or indirect trauma. Direct injury may occur when a force is applied to the anterior aspect of the patella; this usually results from a fall on the flexed knee. Indirect trauma is more common. This is usually the result of strenuous or repetitive quadriceps activity to which the patient is unaccustomed (e.g., hiking, jogging, calisthenics, or skiing). **The most characteristic symptom of indirect trauma is pain in the lower pole of the patella and adjacent patellar tendon that is precipitated by strenuous activity, especially running, jumping, or squatting.** After resting with the knee flexed, patients with indirect trauma experience a marked increase in pain when they initially extend the knee and begin to move around, but they usually find some relief after standing still or walking a short distance. Patients often describe a grating sensation that may be detected on physical examination when the knee is flexed and extended. The grating is noted particularly when the knee is extended against resistance. Radiographs are usually normal but may show fragmentation of the lower pole of the patella.

Chondromalacia patellae must be differentiated from *patellar osteo-chondritis, jumper's knee,* and *partial rupture of the patellar tendon.* Children with chondromalacia patellae usually have localized tenderness at the lower pole of the patella and the adjacent patellar tendon (see Fig. 23–1). Occasionally, the physician may note separation of the patellar tendon from the lower pole and a palpable defect at that point.

Other conditions that give rise to knee pain include *patellar subluxation, patellar dislocation,* and *meniscal injuries. Rheumatoid arthritis* and *popliteal cysts,* although uncommon, can occur in children.

Limping is a common complaint among children. It is never normal, although its causes are many, ranging from ill-fitting shoes to a sprained ankle to the earliest manifestation of a malignant tumor. To determine the exact cause of limping, the physician must approach the problem methodically and thoroughly, obtaining a detailed history and performing a careful examination of the child's gait.

ASSOCIATED SYMPTOMS

Although limping is often due to trauma and the most common cause of leg pain is traumatic injury to the joints or soft tissue, these facts may be misleading in some cases. **In general, when pain or limp is due to mild trauma, the symptoms should disappear within 2 to 3 weeks.** If the symptoms do not disappear, despite a report of trauma, the physician must obtain a thorough history and perform a complete physical examination to rule out more serious entities. The physician must determine whether the limp is intermittent or constant, whether it is present at the end of the day or in the morning, whether it is made worse by climbing stairs, and whether it is present only after vigorous exercise (which may be the first clue to an impending stress fracture).

The location of leg pain often provides clues to its cause, particularly in cases of referred pain. Lower back pathology most commonly refers pain to the buttocks and lateral thigh, whereas hip pathology often refers pain to the groin, medial thigh, or knee. For example, *Legg-Calvé-Perthes disease,* in which unknown factors cause infarction of the femoral head, is a common cause of knee pain and limp in children ages 4 to 12.

PHYSICAL FINDINGS

Range of motion of each joint from the hip down should be noted and compared with that of the opposite side, with careful attention given to the patellae. Leg lengths should be measured; a discrepancy of ½ inch or more can cause a *pelvic tilt* and subsequent limp.

When the patient complains of lower leg pain, particularly when

DIFFERENTIAL DIAGNOSIS OF LOWER EXTREMITY PAIN AND LIMP IN CHILDREN

CAUSE	NATURE OF PATIENT	NATURE OF SYMPTOMS	ASSOCIATED SYMPTOMS	PRECIPITATING AND AGGRAVATING FACTORS	AMELIORATING FACTORS	PHYSICAL FINDINGS	DIAGNOSTIC STUDIES
Epiphysitis of hip (Legg-Calvé-Perthes disease)	Ages 4–12 (5–7 peak incidence) Usually male Rare in blacks	Unilateral hip pain often referred to medial aspect of knee	Limp			Limitation of hip motion	Radiograph of hip Bone scintigraphy
Epiphysitis of knee (Osgood-Schlatter disease)	Ages 10–15	Painful swelling of tibial tubercle		Quadriceps contraction against resistance	Rest		Radiograph of knee
Chondromalacia patellae	Children and adolescents	Pain in lower pole of patella and adjacent patellar tendon		Running Jumping Squatting	Quiet standing or walking	Grating of knee with flexion and extension	Radiograph of knee
Trauma	History of sports participation	Joint or soft tissue			2–3 wk of rest	Local tenderness	Sonography for synovitis of hip
Growing pains		Intermittent myalgia, especially of thigh, calf, and back of knee Nonarticular and bilateral Not related to activity				No abnormal physical findings	
Slipped capital femoral epiphysis	Usually males, aged 12–15 mo More common in blacks	Hip pain Only knee pain in 25%	Limp Trendelenburg gait			Bilateral in 25%	Radiograph of hip Bone scintigraphy

there also is a limp, the gait should be examined first. Gait consists of two phases: stance and swing. In the stance phase, the foot is in contact with the floor, and one limb bears all the body weight. In the swing phase, the foot is not touching the floor. This phase begins when the toe comes off the floor and ends with heel strike. A child with a stiff hip would have a short swing phase because of limited hip joint movement. During each phase, the physician should observe one or two of the involved anatomic components: first the feet and then the knees, the pelvis, and the trunk. The sound of the walk may suggest a steppage gait, with slapping of the foot from footdrop. The shoes should be inspected for abnormal wear: Excessive wear of the toes of the shoes suggests *toe walking*, and excessive wear of the medial aspects of the shoe indicates severe *flat feet*.

If there is joint effusion, the physician must suspect an infectious process, especially if there are systemic signs. Infections may be due to gonococci, *Staphylococcus*, or *Haemophilus*.

LESS COMMON DIAGNOSTIC CONSIDERATIONS

Rheumatoid arthritis, popliteal cyst, quadriceps malalignment, supracondylar cortical avulsion, and traumatic epiphyseal injury may cause leg pain or limp, or both. Herpes zoster is relatively uncommon in children, but when it does occur, it frequently involves the lower extremity and may cause pain, burning, or itching before the typical herpetic lesion appears. Usually children with herpes zoster of the leg have only a rash and experience no pain.

Selected References

Hensinger, R. N.: Limp. Pediatr. Clin. North Am. *24(4)*:723–730, 1977.
Peterson, H.: Growing pains. Pediatr. Clin. North Am. *33*:1367–1372, 1986.
Smith, J. B.: Knee problems in children. Pediatr. Clin. North Am. *24(4)*:841–855, 1977.
Speer, D. P.: Differential diagnosis of knee pain in children. Ariz. Med. *34*:330–332, 1979.
Sty, J. R., Wells, R. G., and Smith, W. B.: The child with acute leg pain. Semin. Nucl. Med. *18*:137–158, 1988.

Chapter 25

Pain in the Upper Extremity

SHOULDER

After backache, upper extremity pain is the next most common type of musculoskeletal pain. Upper extremity pain usually occurs in the joints (shoulder, elbow, and wrist), with the shoulder being the most common site. Shoulder pain can be referred from the neck, chest, or diaphragmatic region; it usually is due to a local process. It should be remembered that the "shoulder joint" includes three large bones (the clavicle, scapula, and humerus) and four joints (sternoclavicular, acromioclavicular, glenohumeral, and thoracoscapular). For an excellent description of the anatomy of the shoulder joint and clinical entities that produce shoulder pain, the reader should refer to the 1977 article by Bland, Merrit, and Boushey and the accompanying illustrations (Figs. 25–1 to 25–3).

Several terms are used to describe painful disorders of the shoulder.

Figure 25–1. Glenohumeral, acromioclavicular, and sternoclavicular joints. The thoracoscapular joint is between the anterior scapular surface and the chest wall. (From Bland, J. H., et al.: The painful shoulder. Semin. Arthritis Rheum. 7:21–47, 1977.)

Figure 25–2. Posterior view of shoulder. *A,* Surface muscles, all groups. *B,* Rotator cuff; subscapularis not shown (medial rotator). Note that the rhomboids and levator scapulae displace the scapula medially toward the midline, whereas the scapulohumeral group rotates the humerus laterally. (From Bland, J. H., et al.: The painful shoulder. Semin. Arthritis Rheum. 7:21–47, 1977.)

These terms refer to variations of the same basic process and include *supraspinatus tendinitis, rotator cuff tendinitis, subacromial bursitis, bicipital tendinitis, painful arc syndrome, impingement syndrome, calcific tendinitis, calcific bursitis,* and *calcific bicipital tendinitis.*

Pain may originate in the bursa as well as in the shoulder joint. Many authors suggest that the only significant bursa in the shoulder is the subacromial bursa and that the subdeltoid, subcoracoid, and supraspinatus bursae are extensions of the subacromial bursa.

The initial process with shoulder pain is usually a *supraspinatus tendinitis* with extension to other muscles of the rotator cuff. With severe or continuing damage, the inflammatory process spreads first to the subacromial bursa and then to the joint capsule and intra-articular and extra-articular structures. **The greater the area of pain in the arm and shoulder and the greater the spontaneity of pain (i.e., onset without aggravating events), the greater the likelihood of an extensive lesion.**

Pain in the shoulder (as well as in the elbow and wrist) can be due

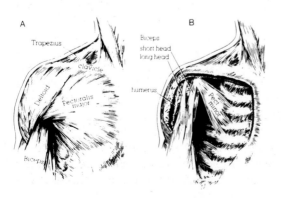

Figure 25–3. Anterior view of the shoulder. *A,* Surface muscles. *B,* Deep layer of muscles. (From Bland, J. H., et al.: The painful shoulder. Semin. Arthritis Rheum. 7:21–47, 1977.)

to *tendinitis, bursitis, trauma, arthritis,* or *referred pain.* Cartilage and bone are not very sensitive to pain. The following are listed in order of decreasing degrees of pain sensitivity: tendons, bursae, ligaments, synovial tissue, capsular reinforcements, and muscles.

Nature of Patient

Acute *subacromial bursitis,* which is painful enough to cause marked limitation of movement, is more common in younger patients. *Calcific tendinitis* is also more common in younger people and seldom is associated with tears; it is more often seen as a sequela to acute bursitis. A *supraspinatus tear,* which permits some movement, is more common in people over ages 40 to 50. *Dislocation of the shoulder* is also more common in people over age 50. With first-time dislocations after ages 40 to 50, there is a much higher incidence of a rotator cuff tear. This is a rare occurrence before age 40.

Nature of Symptoms

INVOLVEMENT OF THE SUPRASPINATUS TENDON. Shoulder pain is most commonly located in the lower part of the deltoid region; this is the referral area for pain originating in the supraspinatus tendon. When there is a dull ache in the region of the deltoid insertion that is exacerbated with abduction to 60 degrees or more (painful arc), internal rotation, reaching overhead, or putting on a coat, the physician should suspect *supraspinatus tendinitis.* Characteristically, patients report that the pain is worse at night or when they lie on the affected shoulder.

INVOLVEMENT OF THE TERES MINOR, INFRASPINATUS, AND SUBSCAPULARIS MUSCLES. If the shoulder is diffusely tender and if moving the humerus posteriorly causes pain, teres minor or infraspinatus muscle involvement should be suspected. If there is pain with resisted medial rotation, there may be subscapularis muscle involvement. In patients with teres minor, infraspinatus, and subscapularis involvement with diffuse shoulder tenderness, pain usually does not radiate into the arm or neck, and it commonly is absent or minimal when the arm is dependent.

TEARS ABD RUPTURES OF THE ROTATOR CUFF. If the patient presents with a sudden onset of shoulder pain in the deltoid area that intensifies within 6 to 12 hours after the initial trauma, a rotator cuff tear should be suspected. With this injury, there may be extreme tenderness over the greater tuberosity as well as pain and restricted motion in one plane of movement at the glenohumeral joint. Patients who present with these findings and recurrent severe pain that awakens them at night may have a rotator cuff tear, even if the arthrogram is normal. In cases of complete rotator cuff rupture, the patient has severe pain and is totally unable to abduct the arm.

CALCIFIC TENDINITIS. After a rotator cuff tear, patients may develop calcification and calcific tendinitis of the rotator cuff. Calcification has been reported in the rotator cuff in 8 per cent of the asymptomatic population over age 30. Despite the fact that 8 per cent of the asymptomatic population demonstrate calcific tendinitis, studies have shown that 35 per cent of all patients with calcific tendinitis have had symptoms at some time. If 8 per cent of the population have calcific tendinitis and 35 per cent of these people develop symptoms, about 3 per cent of patients over age 30 will eventually present with pain referable to a calcific tendinitis. Some studies have related the extent of the symptoms to the size of the calcific area. If the diameter of the calcific mass reaches 1 to 1½ cm, patients invariably develop symptoms. Patients have an abrupt onset of severe, aching pain and find all shoulder movement painful.

BICIPITAL AND TRICIPITAL TENDINITIS. When there is generalized tenderness anteriorly in the region of the long head of the biceps (the region of the anterior subacromial bursa), particularly if the pain seems to be worse at night, bicipital tendinitis should be suspected. This pain resembles that of adhesive capsulitis, except that in bicipital tendinitis, there is relative freedom of abduction and forward flexion. In patients with bicipital tendinitis, resisted forearm supination causes anterior shoulder pain. This finding is a hallmark of bicipital tendinitis. If there is pain in the triceps region with resisted extension of the elbow, tricipital tendinitis is probable.

BURSITIS. When there is point tenderness over the subacromial bursa (often associated with swelling and warmth), subacromial bursitis is probable. Pain in the acromioclavicular joint suggests that this joint is the source of pain. Patients with subacromial bursitis experience particular pain when performing activities such as lifting objects and combing their hair. Virtually all cases of subacromial bursitis are preceded by tendinitis or tenosynovitis in the rotator cuff, biceps, or biceps tendon sheath. When there is an acute onset of excruciating pain in the subdeltoid region of such severity that shoulder movement is totally limited, *calcific bursitis* is probable. Friction of an inflamed bursal surface may be detected with passive motion if the patient is unable to abduct or rotate his upper arm. This acute inflammatory process is probably secondary to calcific deposits in the coracoacromial arch, which ultimately ruptures into the bursal sac and leads to an acute bursitis.

FROZEN SHOULDER. A frozen shoulder should be suspected when there is a gradual onset of pain with limitation of motion at both the glenohumeral and scapulothoracic joint and when there is limitation of abduction, external rotation, and forward flexion. Although a frozen shoulder is most often due to inflammation of the capsule or rotator cuff, it has many other causes. The hallmark of frozen shoulder is a spontaneous onset of pain that worsens gradually and insidiously. The pain may radiate into the neck and arm, but pain below the elbow is unusual.

SUBLUXATION OR DISLOCATION. When pain in the shoulder follows severe trauma (as opposed to the minor trauma of everyday activity and routine athletic endeavors), it may be due to subluxation or dislocation of the shoulder joint. Patients may state that their shoulder "doesn't feel right," that "something popped," or that "something feels out of place." If this occurs in a child, particularly if there is other evidence of external trauma, child abuse should be considered.

IMPINGEMENT SYNDROME. An impingement syndrome secondary to sports trauma usually occurs in the vulnerable, avascular region of the supraspinatus and biceps tendon. It usually starts as an irritation in the avascular region of the supraspinatus tendon and progresses to an inflammatory response (tendinitis) that involves the biceps tendon and subacromial bursa and then the acromioclavicular joint. This inflammation may finally result in rotator cuff tears and calcification. The most reliable sign of an impingement syndrome is that the pain is reproduced when the arm is flexed forward forcibly against resistance with the elbow extended (Fig. 25–4). Magnetic resonance imaging suggests that subacromial bursitis, supraspinatus tendinitis, and impingement syndrome are variants of a single entity.

SITE OF PAIN. The location of pain is also useful in differential diagnosis. Pain in the acromioclavicular joint suggests that the source of pain is that joint. Pain that occurs in any other part of the arm, shoulder, or neck or in the C5 dermatome may be due to many other shoulder lesions. With supraspinatus tendinitis, the initial symptom frequently is pain in the deltoid insertion area that is precipitated by abduction. As the inflammation spreads to the subacromial bursa, the pain may extend to the distal arm and, occasionally, into the forearm. Pain that involves the forearm as far as the wrist suggests that the inflammatory process has spread to the capsule and has been present for 3 to 6 months. If the entire arm is painful and if there is marked limitation of motion, the inflammation has spread to involve the capsule and synovia. This condition is called frozen shoulder.

FIBROSITIS SYNDROME. Fibrositis syndrome, a form of nonarticular rheumatism, is a common cause of pain in multiple locations, including the upper extremity (Fig. 25–5). Although the existence of this syndrome is doubted by some physicians, others have demonstrated that there is exaggerated, reproducible tenderness at specific anatomic locations in patients with this condition. Even though these sites are normally somewhat tender on palpation, these patients often complain of spontaneous pain over the upper border of the trapezius, the lateral epicondyle of the humerus (the site of tennis elbow pain), and the origin of the supraspinatus muscle near the medial border of the scapula. These

Figure 25–4. Positive impingement sign. The examiner forcibly forward flexes the humerus, jamming the greater tuberosity against the anterior inferior acromial surface. The patient's facial expression on reproduction of the pain confirms the presence of impingement. This may be relieved by the injection of lidocaine directly into the subacromial bursa. (From Hawkins, R. J., and Kennedy, J. C.: Impingement syndrome in athletes. Am. J. Sports Med. 8:151–158, 1980.)

patients often complain of insomnia as well. Both the pain and the insomnia of fibrositis may respond to tricyclic antidepressants.

PAIN DUE TO VIGOROUS PHYSICAL ACTIVITY. Although the traumatic aspects of severe falls and motor vehicle accidents and the recurrent trauma of competitive sports (e.g., swimming and tennis) are recognized, the fact that trauma to the shoulder can occur as a result of ordinary, vigorous physical activity (e.g., polishing a car for a few hours) is often overlooked. Such physical exertion may cause rotator cuff

Figure 25–5. Location of 14 typical sites of deep tenderness in "fibrositis." (From Smythe, H. A., and Moldofshy, H.: Two contributions to understanding of the "fibrositis" syndrome. Bull. Rheum. Dis. *28(1)*:928, 1977–1978.)

injuries or subacromial bursitis and severe pain. At rest, pain may be poorly localized; the physician can better determine the source of pain by having the patient repeat the type of activity that apparently induced the pain.

ARTHRITIS. Arthritis of the shoulder is uncommon. When it does occur, it is usually superimposed on a previous injury. With arthritis of the acromioclavicular joint, the pain worsens with adduction of the arm across the chest or circumduction. As with other forms of degenerative arthritis, this pain is often worse in the morning and improves somewhat as the day progresses.

Nonarticular pain in the arm is most often due to *overuse syndromes.* Other common causes are *thoracic outlet syndrome, cervical disc,* and *carpal tunnel syndrome* (Table 25–1).

Associated Symptoms

Weakness and atrophy of muscles is uncommon with *supraspinatus tendinitis.* With *rotator cuff tears,* supraspinatus and infraspinatus atrophy may occur in about 3 weeks. With prolonged *frozen shoulder,* there may be atrophy of several shoulder muscles. Patients with *acute bursitis* resist any passive or active shoulder motion.

Arthritis should be suspected if other joints are involved. If paresthesia or hyperesthesia in the region of C8 or T1 is noted, especially with atrophy of the hypothenar eminence, *thoracic outlet syndrome* should be suspected. Patients with this condition also may demonstrate Raynaud's phenomenon.

TABLE 25–1. Differential Diagnosis of Thoracic Outlet, Cervical Disc, and Carpal Tunnel Syndromes

	Thoracic Outlet	Cervical Disc	Carpal Tunnel
Symptoms			
Pain	Neck, shoulder, and arm (intermittent)	Neck, shoulder, and arm (constant)	Wrist, volar forearm, fingers 1, 2, and 3 (intermittent)
Numbness	Ulnar nerve or whole hand or arm asleep	Radial nerve (dorsal web between fingers 1 and 2)	Median nerve, fingers 2, 3, and 4
Awkwardness	All fingers or 4 and 5	Thumb	Fingers 1, 2, and 3
Aggravation	Arm elevation	Neck turn or arm stretch	Sustained grasp, pinch
Color	Normal, pallid, cyanotic, or splotchy	Normal or splotchy	Normal, red, or splotchy
Edema	May be present	Absent	May be present
Signs			
Pain on percussion	Brachial plexus	Neck at disc level	Tinel sign (volar wrist)
Pain on compression	Brachial plexus	Neck and brachial plexus	Phalen sign (wrist flexion)
Symptoms reproduced	Arm elevation and brachial plexus compression	Head turn and tilt, cranial compression	Wrist and finger flexion
Nerve conduction	Positive or negative (unreliable if negative)		Positive or negative (unreliable if negative)
X-rays	Normal, long C7 process, anomalies (venoarteriogram)	Degenerative arthritis, disc space narrowed to 85% of normal on myelogram	Normal, arthritis, or old trauma

Modified from Stabile, M J., and Warfield, C. A.: Differential diagnosis of arm pain. Hosp. Pract. 25:55–58, 61, 64, 1990.

Precipitating and Aggravating Factors

Prolonged and sustained immobilization with the arm at the side may lead to a *frozen shoulder.* This immobilization may have been recommended by the physician, or the patient may have avoided movement for some other reason for a prolonged period. The *impingement syndrome* often is precipitated by repetitive use of the arm above the horizontal position (as in throwing a baseball or football, swimming, or tennis). Isolated arthritis of the sternoclavicular joint may be due to trauma or weight lifting. *Septic arthritis of the sternoclavicular joint* has been reported in heroin users and in patients with gonococcal arthritis.

Ameliorating Factors

Full trunk and hip flexion that allows the arm to hang limp or supporting the forearm in flexion may help alleviate the pain of rotator cuff tears. This finding may also help the physician establish the diagnosis.

Physical Findings

A careful physical examination with implementation of specific maneuvers is essential to effective diagnosis—and therefore management—of pain in the upper extremity. In most cases, the diagnosis can be made without radiography or arthrography. With *supraspinatus tendinitis,* there is pain on resisted abduction, limitation of joint motion (with or without disruption of the scapulohumeral rhythm), and a normal passive range of motion. Pain is absent or minimal when the arm is dependent. Pain is usually located in the deltoid region, where the supraspinatus tendon inserts.

Patients with *rotator cuff tears* usually have a full range of passive movement and experience pain at extremes of motion. They have pain and restricted movement at the glenohumeral joint and experience pain and weakness with resisted movement. These patients also may demonstrate the "drop arm" sign: weak ability to maintain abduction after passive abduction support is removed. Radiographs may show that the humeral head is high in the glenoid when the arm is in full adduction. Patients with *calcific rotator cuff tendinitis* experience pain with all movements of the shoulder. They usually have associated muscle spasm throughout the shoulder.

Patients with *bicipital tendinitis* experience exacerbation of pain on resisted forearm supination, which causes anterior shoulder pain. Likewise, there is pain with resisted flexion of the shoulder at about 80 degrees.

ELBOW

Overuse syndromes may involve the elbow. These muscle strains may be vocational or recreational due to weight lifting, throwing, or racquet sports. *Tennis elbow* is a lateral epicondylitis of the humerus that may appear in tennis players of any age or level of expertise, especially those over age 40. It also may occur in people who do not play tennis. Lateral epicondylitis is due to overexertion of the finger and wrist extensors, which originate in the region of the lateral epicondyle. There is pain and acute tenderness at the origin of the extensor muscles of the forearm, which attach just distal to the lateral epicondyle of the humerus. The pain may radiate down the back of the forearm. Patients with epicondylitis also experience pain when performing an activity such as opening a door or lifting a cup or glass.

If pain and swelling are noted in the posterior aspect of the elbow, *bursitis* should be suspected. This may occur after a forced, vigorous extension of the elbow joint. If a child develops pain in the elbow after being swung around by the hand, *radial head dislocation* is probable. *Rheumatoid arthritis* occasionally involves the elbow.

HAND AND WRIST

Pain at the base of the thumb aggravated by movement of the wrist or thumb and reproducible by flexion of the thumb is called *de Quervain's disease*. This is a *tenosynovitis* of the thumb abductors and extensors. Pain in the palm at the base of the third and fourth digits, often associated with a catching or fixation of fingers in flexion, is known as *Dupuytren's contracture*. Examination reveals a painless thickening of the palmar fascia or tendon sheath. If the pain is in the anatomic snuff box, it can be assumed to be due to *navicular bone* fracture unless another cause is determined. Pain or numbness of the fingers is seen in *Raynaud's disease* and associated conditions including *Buerger's disease, disseminated lupus,* and *scleroderma. Peripheral nerve entrapment syndromes,* such as carpal tunnel syndrome, may cause pain or numbness or both, in the wrist, hand, or forearm. Pain and swelling in the wrist *not* due to trauma are usually caused by inflammation due to *rheumatoid arthritis, gout, pseudogout,* or rarely *septic arthritis.*

Thoracic outlet syndrome (previously referred to as scalenus anticus syndrome, neurovascular compression syndrome, and hyperabduction syndrome) is most common in middle-aged women and usually occurs on the left side. This syndrome presents with intermittent pain, numbness, or weakness in the hand (occasionally the forearm) after the arm or arms have been in a hyperabducted state for a period of time. Patients often experience this discomfort after working for a long time with the arms over the head or after sleeping with the arms folded behind the neck. Physical examination is normal except when specific maneuvers are employed. For example, forcing the shoulders back and down while in forced inspiration may obliterate the radial pulse on the affected side. Likewise, the radial pulse may be obliterated by the Adson maneuver.

Degenerative arthritis usually involves the distal interphalangeal joints, whereas *rheumatoid arthritis* most often involves the proximal interphalangeal and metacarpophalangeal joints. Rheumatoid arthritis also can involve the elbow and the wrist; it seldom involves the shoulder. With active rheumatoid arthritis, there is usually joint stiffness as well as warmth, swelling, and tenderness. The pain is usually polyarticular and migratory rather than monoarticular.

DIAGNOSTIC STUDIES

Precise clinical examination is more useful than radiography in the evaluation of soft-tissue injuries. Arthroscopy and magnetic resonance imaging are useful in the diagnosis of shoulder disorders. Arthrography and CT scans are occasionally helpful. Radiographs and, occasionally, bone scans should be obtained if fracture is suspected. Electromyography and nerve conduction studies are helpful tools in the diagnosis of neural entrapment syndromes.

LESS COMMON DIAGNOSTIC CONSIDERATIONS

Less common sources of pain in the upper extremity include some types of local discomfort and referred pain. Apical lung tumors (Pancoast's tumor), cervical disc disease, and cervical spondylosis all can produce shoulder pain. Cervical spondylosis can be due to intervertebral disc protrusion or primary spondylosis. If radiculitis is present, the pain will be sharp and well localized. There may be paresthesias and numbness in the sensory distribution of the compromised nerve root. Fasciculations also may be present, and the pain may be exacerbated by movement of the cervical spine. Despite shoulder pain, a full range of motion may be possible. Cervical spondylosis often can be identified by tenderness over the motor point (where the motor nerve enters the muscle).

Sternoclavicular joint arthritis is rare but occurs in a small number of patients with rheumatic diseases as well as in weight lifters. This pain is usually an anterior chest discomfort that may radiate to the shoulder or arm. When there are significant soft-tissue swelling and warmth in a wide area around the joint, the possibility of a septic arthritis, particularly gonococcal, must be considered.

Shoulder pain can be referred from neck lesions and visceral lesions, including mediastinal disease, subphrenic abscess, and gallbladder disease. Neural entrapment syndromes (e.g., median and ulnar nerve compression) cause pain in the distribution of these nerves. Median nerve compression syndrome is due to compression of the median nerve as it passes beneath the flexor retinaculum, and its symptoms are those of carpal tunnel syndrome. This condition is most common in middle-aged and elderly women. Patients usually complain of pain and paresthesias in the thumb and in the index and middle fingers. They also may report that they feel clumsy when performing fine movements such as sewing and picking up small objects. Patients may have a sensory loss of median nerve distribution and weakness of the thenar muscles. Both the pain and the paresthesia may be worse at night and on awakening.

Cervical spine and cervical cord lesions often produce referred pain in the upper extremity. Herniation of the disc at C5–C6 or C6–C7 causes pain from the back of the neck, across the back of the shoulder, and down the arm and forearm to the wrist. Patients may have a history of recurrent stiff neck. Their pain is often aggravated by movement, particularly flexion, of the neck. They also may have paresthesias of the thumb and index finger.

Cervical spine spondylosis can cause pain and stiffness in the neck and a radicular distribution of pain in one or both arms. Compression of the cervical cord can cause weakness, wasting, and fibrillations in the upper limbs; paresthesias in the arms or legs; and, occasionally, evidence of pyramidal involvement (e.g., weakness, spasticity, increased deep tendon reflexes, and a positive Babinski sign). The combination of atrophic weakness in the arms and spastic weakness in the legs may suggest amyotrophic lateral sclerosis. Spondylosis can be distinguished from amyotrophic lateral sclerosis by a history of paresthesias and the presence of sensory impairment in the former condition.

Meningeal tumors, Pott's disease, and primary or secondary vertebral body tumors may produce upper extremity pain as a result of root compression. In elderly patients, herpes zoster may cause pain in the arm. Many of these patients have a history of an eruption and residual pigmented scars.

Angina pectoris is a common cause of pain in the arm and shoulder. This pain is most frequently located in the left upper arm and is usually associated with precordial pain. A history of pain in the arm with exertion is the major diagnostic clue for angina pectoris.

Arteritis of the great vessels, Norwegian pulseless disease, is a rare condition that can produce intermittent claudication of one or both arms. It is most common in young women and should be considered in those patients who have diminished blood pressure in one or both arms,

DIFFERENTIAL DIAGNOSIS OF UPPER EXTREMITY PAIN

CAUSE	NATURE OF PATIENT	NATURE OF SYMPTOMS	ASSOCIATED SYMPTOMS	PRECIPITATING AND AGGRAVATING FACTORS	AMELIORATING FACTORS	PHYSICAL FINDINGS
Shoulder Supraspinatus tendinitis	> Age 40	Pain in lower part of deltoid region, which is referral area for pain from supraspinatus tendon		Reaching overhead and lying on affected shoulder		Pain worse with resisted abduction Pain worse with abduction to 60 degrees and internal rotation
Subacromial bursitis	< Age 40	Severe pain with marked limitation of motion Pain may radiate to distal arm and even forearm		Lifting objects or combing hair		Point tenderness over subacromial bursa, which may be warm and swollen
Bicipital tendinitis		Generalized tenderness anteriorly in the region of long head of biceps (anterior subacromial bursa)				Resisted forearm supination causes anterior shoulder pain Free abduction and forward flexion
Calcific tendinitis	Younger adults	Usually a sequela to acute bursitis				
Rotator cuff tear	Adults	Sudden onset Pain in deltoid area that intensifies 6–12 h after initial trauma	Recurrent pain		Arm hanging limp	Restricted motion in one plane at glenohumeral joint Weakness and atrophy of supraspinatus and infraspinatus Pain over greater tuberosity
Teres minor or infraspinatus tendinitis		Diffuse shoulder pain	No pain radiation into arm or neck		Arm dependent	Pain on moving humerus posteriorly

Table continued on following page

DIFFERENTIAL DIAGNOSIS OF UPPER EXTREMITY PAIN *Continued*

CAUSE	NATURE OF PATIENT	NATURE OF SYMPTOMS	ASSOCIATED SYMPTOMS	PRECIPITATING AND AGGRAVATING FACTORS	AMELIORATING FACTORS	PHYSICAL FINDINGS
Shoulder *Continued* Subscapularis tendinitis		Diffuse shoulder pain	No pain radiation into arm or neck		Arm dependent	Pain with resisted medial rotation
Frozen shoulder		Gradual onset of pain with limitation of motion at the glenohumeral and scapulothoracic joints. Limitation of abduction, extension, rotation, and forward flexion. Pain may radiate into neck and down arm to elbow	Some atrophy of shoulder muscles	Prolonged immobilization		Marked restriction of motion of shoulder in all directions
Impingement syndrome	Athletes (e.g., participants in baseball, swimming, and tennis)	Tendinitis of the biceps and/or supraspinatus tendon progressing to subacromial bursitis and inflammation of acromioclavicular joint				Pain on forward flexion of arm with elbow extended
Fibrositis syndrome	Ages 20–60	Pain at midpoint of upper border of trapezius, origin of supraspinatus near medial border of scapula, 2–3 cm distal to lateral epicondyle of humerus	Sleep disturbance Diffuse musculoskeletal pain		Tricyclic antidepressants	Multiple tender points

Condition					
Lesion of cervical spine and cord		Referred pain to upper extremity, esp. back of neck, back of shoulder, down arm, forearm			Pain and hyperesthesia along dermatome distribution
Elbow Lateral epicondylitis	Often in tennis players, especially those > age 40 years	Pain over lateral epicondyle that may radiate down back of forearm		Resisted extension of wrist and supination of forearm	Tender to palpation over lateral epicondyle
Bursitis		Pain in back of elbow			Swelling, warmth, and tenderness over back of elbow
Radial head dislocation	Child			Swinging child around by the arms	Radial head palpable in displaced position
Hand and Wrist Tenosynovitis of abductors and extensors of wrist (de Quervain's disease)		Pain at base of thumb		Flexing thumb	
Tenosynovitis of flexors of fingers (Dupuytren's contracture)		Pain in palm at base of third and fourth digits			Catching or fixation of third or fourth digits in flexion Painless thickening of palmar fascia or tendon sheath
Thoracic outlet syndrome	More common in middle-aged women	Hand pain, weakness, or numbness (usually left) after arms are hyperabducted or on awakening	Numbness of ulnar distribution or whole hand	Prolonged hyperabduction	Decreased radial pulse with Adson's and other maneuvers
Gout and pseudogout	Adults	Wrist often involved in pseudogout			
Carpal tunnel syndrome	More common in women	Pain in wrist radiating to hand and forearm			Tinel and Phalen tests may be positive Thenar wasting

especially if they also experience transient episodes of blindness or other cerebral incidents.

Selected References

Bauze, R. J.: Orthopedic pitfalls. Austr. Fam. Phys. 7:1253–1261, 1978.

Bland, J. H., Merrit, J. A., and Boushey, D. D.: The painful shoulder. Semin. Arthritis Rheum. 7:21–47, 1977.

Gunn, C. C., and Milbrandt, W. E.: Tenderness at motor points: an aid in the diagnosis of pain in the shoulder referred from the cervical spine. J. Am. Osteopath. Assoc. 77:196–212, 1977.

Heron C. W. Imaging the painful shoulder. Clin. Radiol. 1990; 41:376–379, 1990.

Jenkins, D. G.: Clinical features of arm and neck pain. Psychotherapy 65:102–105, 1979.

Lascelles, R. G., Mohr, P. D., Neary, D., and Bloor, K.: The thoracic outlet syndrome. Braun. 100:601–612, 1977.

Matsen, F. A., and Kirby, R. M.: Office evaluation and management of shoulder pain. Orthop. Clin. North Am. 13:453–475, 1982.

Polisson, R. P.: Sports medicine for the internist. Med. Clin. North Am. 70:469–489, 1986.

Richardson, A. B., Jobe, F. W., and Collins, H. R.: The shoulder in competitive swimming. Am. J. Sports Med. 8:159–163, 1980.

Semble, E. L., and Wise, C. M.: Fibrositis. Am. Fam. Physician 38:129–139, 1988.

Smythe, H. A., and Moldofshy, H.: Two contributions to understanding of the "fibrositis" syndrome. Bull. Rheum. Dis. 28:928–931, 1977–1978.

Spiegel, T. M., and Crues, J. V.: The painful shoulder: diagnosis and treatment. Prim. Care 15:709–724, 1988.

Stabile, M. J., and Warfield, C. A.: Differential diagnosis of arm pain. Hosp. Pract. 25:55–58, 61, 64, 1990.

Wade, J. P., and Bell, J. G.: Wrist pain. Prim. Care 15:737–749, 1988.

Watrous, B. F., and Ho, G.: Elbow pain. Prim. Care 15:725–735, 1988.

Chapter 26

Palpitations

Palpitations are defined here as skipped heartbeat, irregular heartbeat, rapid or slow heartbeat, or increased awareness of the heartbeat. A patient's awareness of his heartbeat occurs most frequently at rest (e.g., while watching television or while lying in bed). In bed, the mattress serves as a resonator; this facilitates an awareness of the heartbeat, which may be fast, slow, irregular, or normal.

The most common causes of palpitations are *anxiety, stimulants* (e.g., caffeine and alcohol), *drugs* (e.g., amphetamines, cocaine, digitalis glycosides, psychotropic agents, and thyroid hormone), and *cardiac disease* (valvular disease, ischemia, myocardiopathy, and mitral valve prolapse). Other common causes include *conduction abnormalities* (e.g., *Wolff-Parkinson-White syndrome, sick sinus syndrome,* and other conduction disturbances), *hypoglycemia, reactive hypoglycemia, hyperthyroidism, hypoxia,* and *hyperventilation.* If the palpitations occur infrequently or only once, are not associated with other symptoms (e.g., chest pain, syncope, dizzy spells), and develop in an otherwise healthy patient, there is probably little need for concern or extensive workup. **If palpitations are frequent, disturbing to the patient, or associated with syncope, dizzy spells, chest pain, activity, or evidence of heart disease, further investigation is required and should include electrocardiography performed with the patient at rest, exercise electrocardiography, and often 24-hour Holter monitoring.**

NATURE OF PATIENT

In children and adolescents, the complaint of palpitations is most often a sign of *anxiety.* If a rapid arrhythmia is suspected or if the problem is recurrent, the physician should perform electrocardiographic studies and Holter monitoring to determine whether Wolff-Parkinson-White syndrome is present. The most common arrhythmias in children are supraventricular tachycardias. Children, adolescents, and young adults should be specifically questioned about the use of *stimulants* such as caffeine, alcohol, and nonprescribed illegal drugs.

In adults who have no clinical evidence of heart disease or other systemic disease, the complaint of palpitations is often only an awareness of their normal heartbeat or an occasional atrial or ventricular contraction. The patient should be questioned carefully about the excessive use of stimulants such as caffeine, alcohol, and other agents, including recreational drugs, amphetamines, psychotropic agents, over-the-counter weight-reducing agents, and thyroid replacement therapy. **With increasing age, there is often a decreasing tolerance to agents such as caffeine, alcohol, and drugs.** Although previously tolerated without symptoms, these agents may induce palpitations as the patient gets older. Occasionally, palpitations (often paroxysmal atrial fibrillation) are noted by a patient during the day after unusual but not necessarily excessive alcohol ingestion. This phenomenon has been termed the holiday heart syndrome. The most common causes of palpitations in the elderly include supraventricular and ventricular premature beats, sick sinus syndrome, and atrial fibrillation.

Patients with known cardiac disease who complain of palpitations are more likely to have serious arrhythmias, such as *atrial fibrillation, ventricular tachycardia,* and *sick sinus syndrome.* If a patient with a wide-complex tachycardia has a history of heart failure, myocardial infarction, or a recent onset of angina, the tachycardia is more likely to be ventricular in origin rather than supraventricular with aberration. Those who have poor left ventricular function are particularly prone to ventricular arrhythmias and sudden death. *Mitral valve prolapse* occurs most frequently in young women. One study revealed that the average age of patients with mitral valve prolapse is 38 and that 70 per cent of patients are women. Palpitations occur in about 44 per cent of patients with documented mitral valve prolapse. Well-conditioned athletes often have a resting bradycardia (sometimes marked). This may be associated with premature ventricular contractions, first degree atrioventricular block, and second degree atrioventricular block; these arrhythmias disappear with exercise.

NATURE OF SYMPTOMS

Patients may complain of a forceful, fast, slow, or irregular heartbeat. It is often useful to have the patient tap out what the rhythm feels like to him. If the patient cannot do this, the physician can tap out a selection of rhythms—slow and regular, slow and irregular, fast and regular, fast and irregular, and the beat of a premature contraction followed by a compensatory pause to assist patients in describing what they mean by "palpitations." Although this procedure is a useful tool, determination of the precise nature of the arrhythmia must be documented by electrocardiography or Holter monitoring.

Various types of arrhythmias are commonly found at different times in the same patient. Arrhythmias that recur in late afternoon and early evening suggest that the arrhythmias are precipitated by *reactive hypoglycemia.* For any patient with unexplained recurrent arrhythmias that occur several hours after eating, the physician should perform a 5-hour glucose tolerance test to rule out reactive hypoglycemia. These arrhythmias are usually supraventricular in origin. Arrhythmias in insulin-dependent diabetics that occur near the time of peak insulin activity are also frequently induced by hypoglycemia. Diabetics often have accelerated coronary artery disease, which is another possible cause of arrhythmias in these patients.

ASSOCIATED SYMPTOMS

Fatigue, confusion, and syncope may be noted in patients with *sick sinus syndrome,* which occurs frequently in the elderly. Sweating, tremors, and other symptoms of *hypoglycemia* suggest that hypoglycemia is contributing to the arrhythmia. Sticking chest pains that do not usually coincide with the arrhythmia should suggest *mitral valve prolapse,* a condition in which arrhythmias are common. Chest pain, congestive heart failure, syncope, and dizziness all suggest a clinically significant arrhythmia, such as *paroxysmal atrial tachycardia, sick sinus syndrome, complete heart block,* or *ventricular tachycardia.*

PRECIPITATING AND AGGRAVATING FACTORS

Although exercise may induce arrhythmias in a normal heart, arrhythmias that increase with exercise are probably due to *cardiac disease,* especially coronary artery disease, mitral valve prolapse, and cardiomyopathy—both hypertrophic and dilated forms. When premature ventricular contractions decrease with exercise (and its associated increase in sinus rate), they are probably benign. *Digitalis-induced arrhythmias* can be in the form of premature beats, tachyarrhythmias or bradyarrhythmias, supraventricular arrhythmias, supraventricular tachycardia with block, or ventricular tachycardia. Digitalis arrhythmias can be precipitated by increased digitalis dosage, hypokalemia, hypomagnesemia, or decreased renal function. *Antiarrhythmic drugs,* particularly the class I agents (quinidine sulfate, procainamide hydrochloride, lidocaine, disopyramide phosphate, and phenytoin), can both precipitate and suppress arrhythmias. Their prolongation of the Q–T interval makes the patient more vulnerable to the torsades de pointes type of ventricular tachycardia, which the patient may perceive as palpitations or dizzy spells.

Most of the beta blockers, many of the antihypertensive agents (e.g., reserpine, methyldopa, clonidine), and the calcium channel blockers cause bradycardia. Hydralazine and minoxidil can cause sinus tachycardia. Sometimes discontinuation of drugs (e.g., clonidine, phenytoin, beta blockers, and antiarrhythmics) is associated with the development of palpitations.

AMELIORATING FACTORS

If the palpitations abate with cessation of stimulants or other drugs, it is most likely that the arrhythmias were caused by the agent or agents that were discontinued. Some patients find that performing Valsalva's maneuver, pressing on their carotid sinus, or gagging themselves to induce vomiting terminates the arrhythmias. In these cases, the arrhythmias are probably supraventricular in origin.

PHYSICAL FINDINGS

Auscultation of a midsystolic click or late systolic murmur is found in patients with *mitral valve prolapse* (balloon mitral valve, click-murmur syndrome, and Barlow's syndrome). Premature atrial or ventricular contractions occur most commonly in patients with mitral valve prolapse; supraventricular tachycardia or ventricular tachycardia occurs in about 12 per cent of these patients.

There are many clinical maneuvers (well documented in cardiology texts) that may help the physician determine the nature of arrhythmias. **Precise diagnosis requires electrocardiographic documentation.** In anxious patients who complain of palpitations, the arrhythmias may be precipitated by *hyperventilation*. If this is suspected, the physician can instruct the patient to hyperventilate forcibly for 3 or 4 minutes to determine whether this activity induces an arrhythmia that should be recorded.

DIAGNOSTIC STUDIES

If arrhythmias cannot be documented clinically or electrocardiographically, and if they are frequent or associated with dizziness, syncope, or other cardiac symptomatology, Holter monitoring must be performed. Several studies of 24-hour Holter moni-

DIFFERENTIAL DIAGNOSIS OF PALPITATIONS

CAUSE	NATURE OF PATIENT	NATURE OF SYMPTOMS	ASSOCIATED SYMPTOMS	PRECIPITATING AND AGGRAVATING FACTORS	PHYSICAL FINDINGS*	DIAGNOSTIC STUDIES†
Anxiety	Most common cause of palpitations in children and adolescents		Sweaty palms	Hyperventilation	Have patient hyperventilate for 3–4 min to see whether arrhythmias can be induced	
Ingestion of stimulants or drugs (caffeine, alcohol, amphetamines, cocaine)	Patients have decreased tolerance to these agents with increased age		Nervousness Tremor	Caffeine Alcohol Drugs (amphetamines, psychotropic agents, thyroid hormone)	Premature ventricular contractions Tachycardia	Toxicology screening tests
Digitalis glycosides			Nausea Anorexia	Increased digitalis dose Hypokalemia Hypomagnesemia Decreased renal function	Premature ventricular contractions Tachyarrhythmias Bradyarrhythmias Second- or third- degree heartblock Bradycardia	Serum digitalis levels Electrocardiography Holter monitoring Serum potassium Serum magnesium Creatinine
Beta blockers Antihypertensives Calcium channel blockers Hydralazine Minoxidil	Patients with angina or hypertension				Sinus tachycardia	
Hypoglycemia	Insulin-dependent diabetics	Arrhythmias occur near the time of peak insulin activity	Sweating Headache Tremor Weakness	Increased insulin Decreased carbohydrate	Premature ventricular contractions Tachycardia	Blood sugar

*Arrhythmias are often absent.
†All arrhythmias should be documented by electrocardiography or Holter monitoring.

Table continued on following page

DIFFERENTIAL DIAGNOSIS OF PALPITATIONS *Continued*

CAUSE	NATURE OF PATIENT	NATURE OF SYMPTOMS	ASSOCIATED SYMPTOMS	PRECIPITATING AND AGGRAVATING FACTORS	PHYSICAL FINDINGS*	DIAGNOSTIC STUDIES†
Hyperthyroidism	More common in older men	Atrial premature contractions May be silent	Nervousness Tremors Weight loss	Heart disease	Atrial fibrillation Premature contractions Tachycardias	Thyroid function tests
Exercise	Normal More frequent in patients with coronary heart disease, hypertension, mitral valve prolapse, and cardiomyopathy			Exercise		
Reactive hypoglycemia		Recurrent arrhythmias in late afternoon and early evening Arrhythmias occur several hours after ingestion of carbohydrates	Sweating Tremors Headache	Anxiety		5-hour glucose tolerance test

Cardiac Disease

Mitral valve prolapse	Most common in young women (average age, 38 years)		Sticking chest pain	Exercise	Midsystolic click Late systolic murmur Premature ventricular contractions or premature atrial contractions Tachycardia	Echocardiography
Wolff-Parkinson-White syndrome	Often detected in children and adolescents	Recurrent palpitations Frequent paroxysmal tachycardia		Exercise Digitalis	Paroxysmal tachycardia	Electrocardiography Holter monitoring
Sick sinus syndrome	Older patients	Bradyarrhythmia Tachyarrhythmia	Chest pain Syncope Congestive heart failure Dizziness	Exercise Digoxin Beta blockers Calcium channel blockers	Bradyarrhythmia Tachyarrhythmia	Electrocardiography Holter monitoring Electrophysiologic studies
Coronary artery disease	Older patients	Palpitations	Angina pectoris Congestive heart failure		Premature ventricular contractions Paroxysmal atrial fibrillation	Exercise electrocardiography Holter monitoring

toring have shown that a significant number of patients note palpitations when there is no abnormality detected on their Holter tape and, conversely, that many patients demonstrate arrhythmias on their Holter tape but are unaware of palpitations at that time.

Other studies that may help the physician determine the cause of palpitations include thyroid function tests, the 5-hour glucose tolerance test, drug screens, determination of serum digitalis and arterial blood gas levels, echocardiography, invasive cardiac electrophysiologic tests, and, rarely, coronary arteriography.

LESS COMMON DIAGNOSTIC CONSIDERATIONS

Less common causes of palpitations include infiltrative diseases of the myocardium, such as amyloidosis, sarcoidosis, and tumors. Hypothyroidism can cause sinus bradycardia; hyperthyroidism can cause sinus tachycardia, paroxysmal atrial tachycardia, and paroxysmal atrial fibrillation.

Selected References

Chung, E. K.: Wolff-Parkinson-White syndrome—current views. Am. J. Med. *62*:252–266, 1977.

Goldberg, A. D., et al.: Ambulatory electrocardiographic records in patients with transient cerebral attacks or palpitations. Br. Med. J. *4*:569–571, 1975.

Kung, G., et al.: What does the symptom "palpitation" mean? Correlation between symptoms and the presence of cardiac arrhythmias in the ambulatory EKG. Z. Kardiol. *66*:138–141, 1977.

Ladenson, P. W.: Recognition and management of cardiovascular disease related to thyroid dysfunction. Am. J. Med. *88:*638–641, 1990.

Marcus, F. I., Ruskin, J. N., and Surawicz, B.: Cardiovascular disease in the elderly. Arrhythmias. J. Am. Coll. Cardiol. *10(2 Suppl. A):*66A–72A, 1987.

Rodriguez, R. D., and Schocken, D. D.: Update on sick sinus syndrome; a cardiac disorder of aging. Geriatrics *45:*26–30, 33–36, 1990.

Swartz, M. H., et al.: Mitral valve prolapse: a review of associated arrhythmias. Am. J. Med. *62*:377–389, 1977.

Toff, W. D., Joy, M., and Comm, A. J.: Exercise-induced arrhythmias. Eur. Heart J. *9(Suppl. G):*119–126, 1988.

Zeldis, S. M., et al.: Correlation with cardiac arrhythmias on 24-hour electrocardiographic monitoring. Chest *78*:456–461, 1980.

Chapter 27

Shortness of Breath

Dyspnea or breathlessness has been defined as patient awareness of respiratory discomfort, unpleasant sensation of labored breathing, or shortness of breath. Dyspnea can be caused by increased rigidity of lung tissue, increased airway resistance, enhanced ventilation during exercise, or any combination of these factors. Some investigators have suggested that determining the cause of dyspnea is often facilitated by first classifying it into different types, such as wheezing dyspnea, dyspnea on exertion, paroxysmal nocturnal dyspnea, hyperventilation, and dyspnea of cerebral origin. Perhaps a simple classification is acute, chronic, or recurrent. The common causes of dyspnea include *chronic obstructive pulmonary disease (COPD), asthma, congestive heart failure, anxiety, obesity,* and *poor physical condition.*

NATURE OF PATIENT

Acute dyspnea in children is most frequently due to *asthma, bronchiolitis, croup,* and *epiglottitis.* Rarely, it may be due to *foreign body aspiration.* An acute onset of dyspnea in a woman who is pregnant or who is taking oral contraceptives suggests *pulmonary embolism.* Pulmonary embolism should also be suspected if dyspnea occurs in patients who are in the postoperative period, in people who have had prolonged recumbency, and in patients who have a history of phlebitis or cardiac arrythmias.

The most common cause of chronic and recurrent shortness of breath in children is asthma. In elderly patients, chronic dyspnea is frequently due to COPD or heart failure, which are rare conditions in patients under age 30. Chronic dyspnea is more common in people who are heavy smokers because smoking is one of the most important factors in the development of *emphysema, chronic bronchitis,* and *COPD. Obese* and *physically inactive* patients frequently complain of recurrent dyspnea on minimal exertion because of their poor cardio-pulmonary reserve.

NATURE OF SYMPTOMS

ACUTE DYSPNEA. In patients with acute dyspnea, the physician should consider the possibility of *pulmonary embolus, asthma, upper airway obstruction, foreign body aspiration, panic disorder, hyperventilation, pneumonia, pneumothorax, pulmonary edema,* and occasionally *respiratory failure.* Asthma is usually episodic and often is precipitated by allergens, exercise, or infections. It is characterized by bilateral wheezing and a decreased respiratory flow rate.

Upper airway obstruction can be caused by *aspiration, vocal cord paralysis, tumors,* and *epiglottic* and *laryngeal edema.* In cases of *foreign body aspiration* (more common in children), the onset of respiratory difficulty is acute. When acute respiratory difficulty occurs during eating, especially in the intoxicated or semiconscious patient, foreign body aspiration is probable. When complete respiratory obstruction occurs, severe respiratory distress, cyanosis, gasping, and loss of consciousness occur quickly. Incomplete respiratory obstruction causes tachypnea, inspiratory stridor, and localized wheezing.

Patients with acute dyspnea due to *hyperventilation* are usually anxious. They often complain of numbness and tingling in the perioral region and the extremities. These patients also often complain of light-headedness, sighing respiration, and an inability to "get enough air in."

A gradual onset of shortness of breath occurs in patients with *congestive heart failure, anemia, lung tumors,* and *parenchymatous lung disease.*

CHRONIC DYSPNEA. Chronic dyspnea in adults is most often due to *chronic pulmonary disease, chronic congestive heart failure,* and *obesity.* It also may be seen with *severe anemia* and *infiltrative pulmonary carcinomatosis.*

ASSOCIATED SYMPTOMS

DYSPNEA IN CHILDREN. When dyspnea occurs in young children, especially when it is associated with coughing and expectoration, *cystic fibrosis* and *bronchiectasis* should be considered.

ACUTE DYSPNEA. When chest pain accompanies acute dyspnea, *spontaneous pneumothorax, pulmonary embolism, chest trauma,* and *myocardial infarction* should be suspected. *Pulmonary embolism* is a common cause of acute dyspnea in adults. Patients usually appear severely ill and may complain of chest pain, faintness, and, occasionally, loss of consciousness. Peripheral cyanosis, low blood pressure, and rales may be present. When acute dyspnea is due to severe *anemia* of acute onset, there are usually symptoms of dizziness, weakness, and sweating. There may be signs of hemorrhage (e.g., hypotension, tachycardia, and rapid, shallow respirations). When acute dyspnea is a manifestation of *anxiety neurosis* or *panic disorder,* the patient usually also complains of dizziness, lightheadedness, palpitations, and paresthesias. The patients do not appear dyspneic and often complain of "not being able to take in enough air." Patients who complain of dyspnea at rest have either a severe physiologic impairment or anxiety hyperventilation.

CHRONIC DYSPNEA. The most common causes of chronic dyspnea on exertion are *cardiac* and *pulmonary.* **Although paroxysmal nocturnal dyspnea is most frequently due to cardiac pathology, it should be noted that some asthmatics develop symptoms primarily when recumbent, usually at night.** Associated findings are often helpful in differentiating pulmonary from cardiac causes of dyspnea. When dyspnea is primarily due to lung disease, the dyspnea is intensified by effort, there is a daily productive cough, the respirations are shallow and rapid, and postural changes have little or no effect. When dyspnea is of cardiac cause, it is intensified by recumbency, and the respirations are shallow but not necessarily rapid.

Other clues also help differentiate pulmonary from cardiac causes of dyspnea on exertion. When the cause is pulmonary, the rate of recovery to normal respiration is fast, and dyspnea abates a few minutes after cessation of exercise. Patients with dyspnea due to cardiac causes, however, remain dyspneic much longer after cessation of exercise. Likewise, in these patients the heart rate also takes longer to return to preexercise levels. Patients with pulmonary dyspnea do not usually have dyspnea at rest. Patients with severe cardiac dyspnea demonstrate a volume of respiration that is greater than normal at all levels of exercise; they also experience dyspnea sooner after the onset of exertion.

PRECIPITATING AND AGGRAVATING FACTORS

Smoking is the most frequent precipitating and aggravating factor of chronic pulmonary dyspnea. When *exercise* precipitates wheezing or dyspnea, *bronchial asthma* or *congestive heart failure* may be the diagnosis. *Exposure to cold* often precipitates wheezing and shortness of breath in asthmatics. Bronchial asthma is also probable when *air-borne allergens, noxious fumes,* or *respiratory infections* precipitate dyspnea, cough, or wheezing. *Drugs* (e.g., beta blockers) may precipitate wheezing or dyspnea in asthmatics. Beta blockers and calcium channel blockers may exacerbate dyspnea in cardiac patients. Less common precipitating and aggravating factors include trauma, shock, hemorrhage, and gaseous anesthesia.

AMELIORATING FACTORS OTHER THAN MEDICAL THERAPY

Some patients with severe chronic obstructive lung disease obtain relief by leaning forward while seated or by lying supine with their heads down. These positions increase the efficiency of diaphragmatic movement and facilitate the use of the accessory muscles of respiration. Performance of the Heimlich maneuver (abdominal thrust) may dislodge a foreign body from the upper airway.

PHYSICAL FINDINGS

Patients with *upper airway obstruction* have coarse sonorous rhonchi and impaired inspiration. Stridor as well as suprasternal retraction may be noted with inspiration. Sibilant, whistling expiratory sounds are usually heard in asthmatics. Expiration appears to be prolonged in asthmatics, whereas inspiration seems to be prolonged in patients with upper airway obstruction. The trachea may be shifted to the opposite side in patients with *pneumothorax* or a *large pleural effusion*.

Wheezing dyspnea at rest associated with rhonchi and a productive cough suggests *asthmatic bronchitis*. In contrast, patients with a history of progressive dyspnea that precedes the development of cough or sputum production often have *emphysema*. The physical findings are a hyperinflated lung, decreased breath sounds, decreased diaphragmatic movement, increased anteroposterior chest diameter, and hyperresonance to percussion. Classically, emphysematous patients have been described as "pink puffers"; patients with chronic bronchitis are called "blue bloaters."

Bilateral wheezing usually is heard when acute dyspnea is due to *asthma*. Bilateral wheezing also may occur with *pulmonary edema*. Wheezing frequently may be heard before the auscultation of rales at the bases and other more classic signs of congestive heart failure. Bilateral wheezing also may be heard in patients with *pulmonary emboli*, but more frequently the wheezing is limited to the side of the pulmonary embolus. Unilateral wheezing may also indicate a *bronchial obstruction* by a foreign body, polyp, or mucous plug. Other causes of dyspneic wheezing include *upper airway obstruction, localized bronchial obstruction,* and *hypersensitivity pneumonitis*.

DIAGNOSTIC STUDIES

Although there are many clinical findings that help the physician differentiate the causes of dyspnea, pulmonary function tests are most helpful and frequently can be performed in an outpatient setting. **Pulmonary function tests should be an integral part of the clinical evaluation of all patients with dyspnea.** Patients with *simple acute bronchitis* may have a persistent productive cough but demonstrate no signs of airway narrowing on spirometry. In patients with *chronic bronchitis* and a persistent cough, spirometry may indicate widespread narrowing of the airways, but dyspnea may not be present. *Chronic obstructive lung disease* may be diagnosed with simple spirometry. Occasionally, patients with obstructive lung disease demonstrate airway narrowing on spirometry without any other symptoms except cough.

Pulmonary function tests do not provide a specific diagnosis; rather, they demonstrate a pattern of the physiologic abnormality. Typical, but not exclusive, patterns of physiologic abnormalities are seen in most patients with chronic pulmonary diseases, in most people with diseases of pulmonary circulation, and in patients with mild cardiac or valvular disease. Pulmonary function tests may help the physician differentiate dyspnea due to hyperventilation or psychologic factors from pulmonary dysfunction.

Pulmonary function tests demonstrate increased obstruction to inspiration when there are extrathoracic (upper airway) obstructive lesions and increased obstruction to expiration when there are intrathoracic obstructive lesions. Expiratory airway obstruction is indicated by decreased airflow rates, decreased forced expiratory volume in 1 second (FEV_1), decreased peak flow rate (PFR), decreased maximum midexpiratory flow rate (FEF 25–75 per cent), decreased maximum voluntary ventilation (MVV), increased tidal volume, and increased residual volume. These findings are often observed in patients with *asthma, bronchitis, emphysema,* and *bronchial adenoma.* The abnormal findings of bronchospasm can usually be transiently reversed with the inhalation of a bronchodilator drug. Lung volume restriction is indicated by a decreased total lung capacity (TLC), increased respiratory minute volume (VE), and decreased compliance. Decreased compliance is found in patients with *fibrosis, sarcoidosis, pneumoconiosis, pulmonary edema, pneumonia, pleural effusion, kyphoscoliosis, obesity,* and *ascites.* Pulmonary vascular disease is evidenced by increased ventilation (VE) and increased dead space (VD). Ventilation and perfusion scanning and digital subtraction angiography are useful in the diagnosis of pulmonary embolism. An electrocardiogram may show P pulmonale and right ventricular strain.

Chest radiographs may show pulmonary parenchymal disease, pleural effusions, tumors, or signs of congestive heart failure.

Text continued on page 306

DIFFERENTIAL DIAGNOSIS OF SHORTNESS OF BREATH

CAUSE	NATURE OF PATIENT	NATURE OF SYMPTOMS	ASSOCIATED SYMPTOMS	PRECIPITATING AND AGGRAVATING FACTORS	AMELIORATING FACTORS	PHYSICAL FINDINGS	DIAGNOSTIC STUDIES
Acute or Recurrent Dyspnea Asthma	Most common cause of recurrent dyspnea in children	Acute dyspnea Episodic May rarely be dyspneic only at night	Cough (indicates asthmatic bronchitis)	Allergens Exercise Noxious fumes Respiratory tract infections Recumbency Exposure to cold or beta blockers		Bilateral wheezing Sibilant, whistling sounds Prolonged expiration	Pulmonary function tests: Decreased respiratory flow rates Decreased maximum voluntary ventilation Increased tidal volume Pre- and post-bronchodilator evidence for reversible airway obstruction ($>10\%$)
Pulmonary emboli	Women using birth control pills Patients in postoperative period Long-term recumbent patients Patients with phlebitis Patients in postpartum period	Acute onset of dyspnea	Chest pain Faintness Loss of consciousness	Oral contraceptives Prolonged recumbency		Tachypnea Peripheral cyanosis Low blood pressure Rales Wheezing (usually only on side of emboli) Pleural friction later with pulmonary infarction	Ventilation and perfusion studies Digital subtraction angiography Electrocardiography indicates acute right ventricular strain Pulmonary infarction or effusion on x-ray

Hyperventilation and anxiety	Usually anxious	Acute dyspnea "Sighing" respirations	Lightheadedness Palpitations Paresthesias (especially in perioral region and extremities)	Stress Panic	Signs of anxiety but no signs of dyspnea	Pulmonary function tests are usually normal
Poor physical conditioning	Obese Physically inactive	Dyspnea on minimal exertion			Obesity After exercise pulse slows very gradually	Pulmonary function tests: Decreased total lung capacity Increased respiratory minute volume Decreased compliance
Foreign body aspiration	Most common in children May occur in intoxicated or semiconscious people during eating	Acute dyspnea		Removal of foreign body Heimlich maneuver	Tachypnea Inspiratory stridor Localized wheezing Suprasternal retraction with respiration May be unilateral wheezing	Chest radiograph may show atelectasis or the foreign body

Table continued on following page

DIFFERENTIAL DIAGNOSIS OF SHORTNESS OF BREATH *Continued*

CAUSE	NATURE OF PATIENT	NATURE OF SYMPTOMS	ASSOCIATED SYMPTOMS	PRECIPITATING AND AGGRAVATING FACTORS	AMELIORATING FACTORS	PHYSICAL FINDINGS	DIAGNOSTIC STUDIES
Pulmonary edema		Acute onset Episodic	Dyspnea on exertion Orthopnea Paroxysmal nocturnal dyspnea			Gallop rhythm Rales at bases	Decreased ejection fraction Chest radiograph shows cardiomegaly with upper lobe redistribution or Kerley's B lines
Pneumothorax	Often a prior history of similar episode May be familial	Acute onset		Cystic fibrosis Chronic obstructive pulmonary disease		Decreased or absent breath sounds Tracheal shift	Chest radiograph shows pneumothorax
Chronic Dyspnea Chronic obstructive pulmonary disease	Older adults Rarely patients under age 30 Most often smokers	Chronic dyspnea Dyspnea with exertion	Fast rate of recovery to normal respiration after stopping exercise Leaning forward while seated or supine with head down History of smoking	Smoking Exertion Postural changes have little or no effect	With severe disease patients may obtain some symptomatic relief by leaning forward while sitting	Rapid and shallow respirations	Pulmonary function tests: Spirometry

Disease	Patients	Symptoms		Physical findings	Diagnostic findings
Emphysema		Progressive dyspnea precedes onset of cough Usually no dyspnea at rest		"Pink puffers" Hyperventilated lungs Decreased breath sounds Decreased diaphragmatic movement Increased anteroposterior chest diameter Hyperresonance	Decreased respiratory flow rate Increased tidal volume Decreased maximum voluntary volume Increased residual volume
Chronic bronchitis		Persistent, minimally productive cough Dyspnea not necessarily presenting symptom Cough precedes dyspnea		"Blue bloaters" Rhonchi	Same as with emphysema Spirometry shows widespread airway narrowing
Congestive heart failure	Older patients	Edema Chronic dyspnea with gradual onset Paroxysmal nocturnal dyspnea Dyspnea remains long after stopping exercise	Exercise Beta blockers Calcium channel blockers Recumbency Trauma Shock Hemorrhage Anesthesia	Nocturnal dyspnea may be relieved by sitting Shallow respirations (not necessarily rapid) Edema Hepatomegaly Jugular venous distention Third heart sound Basilar rales	Spirometry Respiratory volume is greater than normal at all exercise levels Pulmonary congestion and cardiomegaly on radiograph

LESS COMMON DIAGNOSTIC CONSIDERATIONS

Dyspnea is occasionally the presenting symptom in patients with hyperthyroidism. Pregnant patients may complain of dyspnea. Patients with idiopathic pulmonary hemosiderosis may present with dyspnea on exertion, chronic cough, hemoptysis, and recurrent epistaxis. People who work in grain elevators or with hay also may have severe wheezing and dyspnea. Progressive dyspnea and a nonproductive cough may be the presenting symptoms of patients with interstitial pulmonary fibrosis, which may result from drugs (e.g., phenytoin) and from sarcoidosis and other granulomatous diseases. Patients with recurrent pulmonary emboli may present with recurrent episodes of dyspnea. Patients with interstitial pulmonary diseases (e.g., pulmonary fibrosis and pneumoconiosis), as well as those with constrictive cardiomyopathy and constrictive pericarditis, may present with dyspnea on exertion, chronic cough, and paroxysmal nocturnal dyspnea.

Selected References

Andrews, J. L.: The clinical roles of pulmonary function testing. Med. Clin. North Am. *63(2)*:355–377, 1979.

Angelillo, V. A.: Evaluation of dyspnea: is it really present and, if so, why? Postgrad. Med. *73(2)*:336–345, 1983.

Campbell, E.J.M., and Howard, J.B.L.: The sensation of breathlessness. Br. Med. Bull. *19*:36–40, 1963.

Golish, J. H., Ahmad, M., and Yarnal, J. R.: Chronic upper airway obstruction; methods of detection and recognition. Cleve. Clin. Q. *47*:9–15, 1980.

Gulsvik, A.: Prevalence of and manifestations of obstructive lung disease in the city of Oslo. Scand. J. Respir. Dis. *60*:286–296, 1979.

Mahler, D. A.: Dyspnea: diagnosis and management. Clin. Chest Med. *8*:215–230, 1987.

Neff, T. A.: The diagnosis and management of chronic obstructive lung disease. Cleve. Clin. Q. *47*:17–24, 1980.

Schmitt, B. P., Kushner, M. S., and Weiner, S. L.: The diagnostic usefulness of the history of the patient with dyspnea. J. Gen. Intern. Med. *1*:386–393, 1986.

Spiro, G.: Exercise testing in the assessment of respiratory disease. Can. Med. Assoc. J. *122*:890–896, 1980.

Williams, M. H.: Expiratory flow rates: their role in asthma therapy. Hosp. Pract. October, 1982, pp. 95–105.

Chapter **28**

Skin Problems

Skin problems are one of the most common reasons for which patients seek medical attention. The ten most common skin problems for which patients consult dermatologists are *acne, fungal infections, seborrheic dermatitis, atopic* or *eczematous dermatitis, warts,* benign and malignant *skin tumors, psoriasis, hair disorders, vitiligo,* and *herpes simplex. Occupational dermatoses* most commonly appear as an eczematous *contact dermatitis,* although they occasionally present as skin cancers, vitiligo, or infectious lesions. Other common lesions include infestations such as *scabies* and *pediculosis, contact dermatitis, pityriasis rosea, herpes zoster,* and *seborrheic keratoses.* These are not necessarily the most common skin problems; some of the most prevalent are handled by physicians other than dermatologists. About one-third of all patients with a primary dermatologic complaint consult a general physician.

In this chapter, the most common dermatologic problems are presented in tabular form. Because dermatologic diagnosis is based on the type of lesion, its configuration, and the distribution of the lesions, the summary table is organized accordingly. Because most of the pediatric exanthems such as measles (rubeola), German measles (rubella), and chicken pox (varicella) are easily diagnosed, they are not discussed in this chapter, and the reader therefore should consult pediatric textbooks for their description.

Skin tumors are most common later in life. The most common malignant lesions are *basal cell epithelioma* and *squamous epithelioma.* **If there is any uncertainty about whether a skin lesion is malignant, it should be biopsied.** For the differential diagnosis of benign and malignant skin tumors, the reader is referred to several excellent texts and articles (see Selected References).

Figure 28–1. Comedones and lesions. Patient posing in front of mirror reveals comedones, papular lesions, and small superficial pustules on both sides of face. (From Chalker, D. K., and Smith, J. G.: Acne vulgaris: causes and preferred regimens. Medical Times, June 1977, p. 57.)

Figure 28–2. Impetigo. This starts with mild discomfort and is followed in a few hours by serous exudation and crusting. The condition is contagious and can be spread both to other people and to different parts of the body. Culture may grow either *Staphylococcus aureus* or, less commonly, *Streptococcus hemolyticus*. (From Vickers, H. R.: Problems of dermatological diagnoses. Br. J. Clin. Pract. *32*:159–166, 1978.)

Figure 28–3. Impetigo circinata. Occasionally, the center of an impetiginous lesion heals, leaving a ringed, crusted edge culture from which the diagnosis can be established. (From Vickers, H. R.: Problems of dermatological diagnoses. Br. J. Clin. Pract. *32*:159–166, 1978.)

Figure 28–4. Lichenified pruritic areas in flexural regions and on the face are typical locations for adult atopic dermatitis. (From Lamberg, S. I.: Common problems of the skin. *In* Barker, L. R., Binton, J. R., and Zieve, P. D. [Eds.]: Principles of Ambulatory Medicine. Baltimore, Williams & Wilkins, 1982.)

Figure 28–5. Atopic dermatitis. Characteristic facial appearance, chronic excoriated dermatitis, and "sad" and "strained" look. (From Huff, J. C., and Weston, W. L.: Eczematous dermatitis. Maj. Probl. Clin. Pediatr. *19*:86–122, 1978.)

Figure 28–6. Atopic dermatitis—characteristic lesions. *A,* Sharply marginated excoriated lesions of popliteal spaces. *B,* Lichenification and thickening—antecubital fossa. (From Huff, J. C., and Weston, W. L.: Eczematous dermatitis. Maj. Probl. Clin. Pediatr. *19*:86–122, 1978.)

Figure 28–7. Nummular eczema. (From Welton, W.: Dermatology and syphilology. *In* Rakel, R. E., and Conn, H. F. [Eds.]: Family Practice. 2nd ed. Philadelphia, W. B. Saunders Co., 1978.)

Common site for herald patch

Figure 28–8. Pityriasis rosea typically starts with a "herald patch" followed by oval patches in a fernlike pattern. (From Lamberg, S. I.: Common problems of the skin. *In* Barker, Z. R., Binton, J. R., and Zieve, P. D. [Eds.]: Principles of Ambulatory Medicine. Baltimore, Williams & Wilkins, 1982.)

Figure 28–9. Pityriasis rosea. Trunk with central distribution. Discrete papulosquamous lesions. Larger initial plaque ("herald patch"). (From Gilbert, R., and Rosenthal, D.: Dermatology. *In* Rakel, R. E.: Textbook of Family Practice. 3rd ed. Philadelphia, W. B. Saunders Co., 1984.)

Figure 28–10. Pityriasis rosea with herald patch. (From Welton, W.: Dermatology and syphilology. *In* Rakel, R. E., and Conn, H. F. [Eds.]: Family Practice. 2nd ed. Philadelphia, W. B. Saunders Co., 1978.)

Figure 28–11. Psoriasis tends to be found on extensor surfaces and areas of repeated trauma, such as the waistline. (From Lamberg, S. I.: Common problems of the skin. *In* Barker, L. R., Binton, J. R., and Zieve, P. D. [Eds.]: Principles of Ambulatory Medicine. Baltimore, Williams & Wilkins, 1982.)

Figure 28–12. Minute pits are commonly seen on the surface of nails in patients with psoriasis. (From Lamberg, S. I.: Common problems of the skin. *In* Barker, L. R., Binton, J. R., and Zieve, P. D. [Eds.]: Principles of Ambulatory Medicine. Baltimore, Williams & Wilkins, 1982.)

Figure 28–13. Psoriasis of the toes with marked thickening, yellow discoloration, and crumbling of all toenails. (From Loeffel, E. D.: The true heartbreaks of psoriasis. Medical Times, June 1977, p. 51.)

Figure 28–14. Psoriasis. White scale and palm lesions. (From Welton, W.: Dermatology and syphilology. *In* Rakel, R. E., and Conn, H. F. [Eds.]: Family Practice. 2nd ed. Philadelphia, W. B. Saunders Co., 1978.)

Figure 28–15. Usual location of erythema and scale in seborrheic dermatitis. (From Lamberg, S. I.: Common problems of the skin. *In* Barker, L. R., Binton, J. R., and Zieve, P. D. [Eds.]: Principles of Ambulatory Medicine. Baltimore, Williams & Wilkins, 1982.)

Figure 28–16. Seborrheic dermatitis. Erythema and scaling on ears and scalp is typical of this condition. (From Medical Times, June 1977, p. 67.)

Figure 28–17. Pruritic papules are most prevalent about the waist, pelvis, elbows, hands, and feet in scabies. (From Lamberg, S. I.: Common problems of the skin. *In* Barker, L. R., Binton, J. R., and Zieve, P. D. [Eds.]: Principles of Ambulatory Medicine. Baltimore, Williams & Wilkins, 1982.)

Figure 28–18. Insect bites (clustered itching papules). (From Vickers, H. R.: Problems of dermatological diagnoses. Br. J. Clin. Pract. *32*:159–166, 1978.)

Figure 28–19. Tinea versicolor in varying stages of pigmentation and depigmentation. (From Welton, W.: Dermatology and syphilology. *In* Rakel, R. E., and Conn, H. F. [Eds.]: Family Practice. 2nd ed. Philadelphia, W. B. Saunders Co., 1978.)

Figure 28–20. Short hyphae and spores of *Malassezia furfur* seen in tinea versicolor (KOH preparation, ×400). (From Lamberg, S. I.: Common problems of the skin. *In* Barker, L. R., Binton, J. R., and Zieve, P. D. [Eds.]: Principles of Ambulatory Medicine. Baltimore, Williams & Wilkins, 1982.)

Figure 28–21. Contact dermatitis caused by laundry detergent. Note sparing of the folds. (From Jacob, A. H.: Eruptions in the diaper area. Pediatr. Clin. North Am. *25*:209, 1978.)

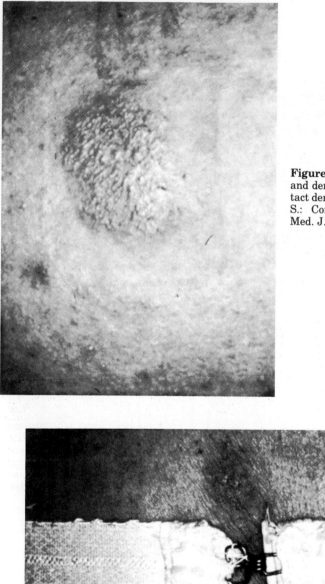

Figure 28–22. Microvesicles and dermal edema in acute contact dermatitis. (From Basler, R. S.: Contact dermatitis. Nebr. Med. J. *65*:296–299, 1980.)

Figure 28–23. Chronic contact dermatitis. (From Basler, R. S.: Contact dermatitis. Nebr. Med. J. *65*:296–299, 1980.)

Figure 28–24. Ringworm of scalp *(Trichophyton tonsurans).* (From Vickers, H. R.: Problems of dermatological diagnosis. Br. J. Clin. Pract. *32*:159–166, 1978.)

Figure 28–25. Tinea capitis round areas of broken hairs and some scale. (From Welton, W.: Dermatology and syphilology. *In* Rakel, R. E., and Conn, H. F. [Eds.]: Family Practice. 2nd ed. Philadelphia, W. B. Saunders Co., 1978.)

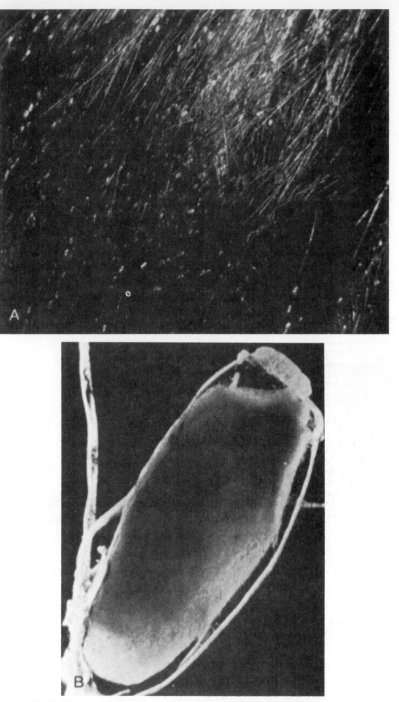

Figure 28–26. Pediculus humanus var. capitis (head louse). *A,* Gross appearance of nits on the hair shaft. *B,* Microscopic appearance (× 100; photograph *B* courtesy of Reed & Carnrick, Kenilworth, N. J.). (From Lamberg, S. I.: Common problems of the skin. *In* Barker, L. R., Binton, J. R., and Zieve, P. D. [Eds.]: Principles of Ambulatory Medicine. Baltimore, Williams & Wilkins, 1982.)

Figure 28–27. *A*, Hyphae of tinea (KOH preparation. × 400). *B*, Pseudohyphae of *Candida* (KOH preparation, × 400; photograph *B* courtesy of William G. Merz, Ph.D.). (From Lamberg, S. I.: Common problems of the skin. *In* Barker, L. R., Binton, J. R., and Zieve, P. D. [Eds.]: Principles of Ambulatory Medicine. Baltimore, Williams & Wilkins, 1982.)

Figure 28–28. Candidiasis (moniliasis). Groin with intense erythema with satellite papules and pustules. Requires blood sugar determination in adult. (From Gilbert, R., and Rosenthal, D.: Dermatology. *In* Rakel, R. E. [Ed.]: Textbook of Family Practice. 3rd ed. Philadelphia, W. B. Saunders Co., 1984.)

Figure 28–29. Candidiasis. (From Welton, W.: Dermatology and syphilology. *In* Rakel, R. E., and Conn, H. F. [Eds.]: Family Practice. 2nd ed. Philadelphia, W. B. Saunders Co., 1978.)

Figure 28–30. Tinea cruris. (From Welton, W.: Dermatology and syphilology. *In* Rakel, R. E., and Conn, H. F. [Eds.]: Family Practice. 2nd ed. Philadelphia, W. B. Saunders Co., 1978.)

Figure 28–31. Tinea pedis, macerated acute type. (From Welton, W.: Dermatology and syphilology. *In* Rakel, R. E., and Conn, H. F. [Eds.]: Family Practice. 2nd ed. Philadelphia, W. B. Saunders Co., 1978.)

Figure 28–32. Tinea pedis, chronic rubrum type. Nails also are involved. (From Welton, W.: Dermatology and syphilology. *In* Rakel, R. E., and Conn, H. F. [Eds.]: Family Practice. 2nd ed. Philadelphia, W. B. Saunders Co., 1978.)

TABLE 28–1. Common Areas of Involvement and Causes of Allergic Contact Dermatitis

Area	Causes
Earlobes	Earrings (nickel)
Postauricular area	Hair dye (paraphenylenediamine) Shampoos (formalin) Hearing aids or glasses (nickel or plastic)
Ear canal	Medications
Face	Hair dye (paraphenylenediamine) Poison ivy Cosmetics Sprays or any airborne contactant
Eyelids	Sprays or any airborne contactant Cosmetics Eyelash curlers (rubber accelerators or nickel) Any contactant on the hands (topical medications, formalin in nail polish)
Perioral area	Lipstick Toothpaste
Neck	Jewelry (nickel) Perfumes Sprays or other airborne contactants
Axilla	Deodorants Clothing (formalin)
Chest	Brassieres (rubber accelerators) Metal objects carried in pockets (nickel)
Back	Metal fasteners (nickel)
Waist	Belt buckles or snaps (nickel) Waist bands or girdles (rubber accelerators)
Extremities	Poison ivy Airborne contactants
Wrists	Jewelry (nickel)
Hands	Rings (nickel) Gloves (rubber accelerators)
Feet	Components of shoes (rubber accelerators, dichromates in leather)
Scrotum	Any contactant on the hands or agent applied in the groin (topical medications)

From Huff, J. C., and Weston, W. L.: Eczematous dermatitis. Maj. Probl. Clin. Pediatr. *19*:86–122, 1978.

DIFFERENTIAL DIAGNOSIS OF SKIN PROBLEMS

NATURE OF LESION	DISTRIBUTION OF LESION	ASSOCIATED FINDINGS	NATURE OF PATIENT	LESIONS WITH SIMILAR APPEARANCE	DIAGNOSIS
Papules and pustules	Face, back, and chest (Fig. 28–1)	Comedones	Start at puberty and last several years		Acne
Papules, vesicles, and pustules	Face, head, and neck Occasionally diaper area in infants	Oozing, honeycomb-colored crusting	Mostly children		Impetigo (Figs. 28–2 and 28–3)
Scaling and lichenification	Face, extensor surfaces, and exposed areas in children Flexural folds (antecubital, popliteal), wrists, neck, upper arms, and thighs in adults Symmetrical (Fig. 28–4)	Often family history of hay fever or asthma Itching, erythema, often lichenification In blacks, the rash tends to be more papular 10% of general population have atopic dermatitis Erythematous or with plaques Rash in adults is usually localized, dry, excoriated, or lichenified	Often begin in infancy at age 5 mo Often clear spontaneously at age 5 yr Rare in elderly people	Seborrheic dermatitis (different location and yellow scales) Psoriasis (typical locations and silvery scales) Contact dermatitis is usually asymmetrical	Atopic dermatitis or eczema (Figs. 28–4 and 28–6)
Scaling plaques	Mostly extensor surface of extremities, back, buttocks, and hands, but can occur anywhere	Coin-shaped lesions Itching Oozing	Children and adults	Ringworm (positive KOH) Contact dermatitis (exposed areas) Psoriasis (elbows and knees)	Nummular eczema or nummular dermatitis (Fig. 28–7)
Scaling plaques or patches	Trunk and proximal extremities (Fig. 28–8)	Herald patch (2 × 6 cm), usually on trunk, precedes generalized lesion More common in winter Salmon-colored May itch Oval patches (1 × 2 cm) with long axis along skin lines giving a Christmas tree pattern Collarette scaling	Children Young adults	Fungus, psoriasis, secondary syphilis, and drug eruptions	Pityriasis rosea (Figs. 28–9 and 28–10)

Plaques	Usually on the covered parts of body and face Often multiple	Irregular greasy surface Superficial—on top of skin ("stuck to the skin") Yellow, tan, dark brown, or, rarely, black Sharply defined edges	Adults (mostly elderly people)	Actinic keratoses occur in sun-exposed areas and are smaller	Seborrheic keratoses
Erythematous plaques	Extensor surfaces, esp. knees and elbows Scalp Coccygeal region Nails Rare on face (Fig. 28–11)	Silvery, loosely adherent scales Occasional itching Arthritis, especially in distal interphalangeal joints Sharp margins Scalp lesions usually stop at hairline	Adults Rare in young children	Seborrheic dermatitis can involve scalp but doesn't stop at hairline Nummular eczema	Psoriasis (Figs. 28–12 to 28–14)
Scaling patches	Scalp Eyebrows Nasolabial fold Midchest Umbilicus (Fig. 28–15)	Yellow, greasy scaling Greasy scaling with poor margin Some erythema Cradle cap in infants	More common in adults	Dandruff with little erythema and no other areas involved (Fig. 28–16) Psoriasis involves extensor surfaces Psoriasis of scalp usually stops at hairline with well-defined plaques	Seborrheic dermatitis
Papules inflamed with excoriation and crusting Linear burrows not always seen	Fingerwebs Wrists Antecubital Elbows Areolar Umbilicus Lower abdomen Genitalia Gluteal cleft	Itching (worse at night) Excoriation Weeping Other in household may have same problem	Adults and children	Pediculosis pubis (nits attached to hair; lice often seen on skin)	Scabies (Fig. 28–17)

Table continued on following page

DIFFERENTIAL DIAGNOSIS OF SKIN PROBLEMS *Continued*

NATURE OF LESION	DISTRIBUTION OF LESION	ASSOCIATED FINDINGS	NATURE OF PATIENT	LESIONS WITH SIMILAR APPEARANCE	DIAGNOSIS
Papules inflamed	Usually on trunk Grouped	Itching; flea bites often grouped	Sand flies and fleas in adults on lower legs Flea bites in children can be anywhere	Scabies Drug eruptions Lymphoma	Insect bites (Fig. 28–18)
Depigmentation	Orifices Eyes Extensor surfaces Areas of trauma	Positive Wood's light (bright white) Increased familial incidence	Familial Thyroid disease Addison's disease	Postinflammatory hypopigmentation Tinea versicolor alba Exposure to phenolic compounds	Vitiligo
Depigmentation and pink-red-brown macules	Mainly trunk Upper arms (Fig. 28–19)	Positive Wood's light (pale yellow) Pink-red-brown macules Scaling Positive KOH Mild itching	Young adults	Postinflammatory hypopigmentation as seen with seborrheic dermatitis and pityriasis rosea, especially in blacks Other fungi	Tinea versicolor (Figs. 28–19 and 28–20)
Depigmentation	Exposed areas, especially hands and arms		Janitors Chemical workers	Vitiligo	Exposure to phenolic compounds
Vesicles	Anywhere (often asymmetrical exposed areas)	Itching, oozing May occur hours to a few days after exposure	Adults and children	Allergy to systemic medications Atopic dermatitis	Contact dermatitis (Table 28–1)
	Hands				Detergents Chemicals (Fig. 28–21)
	Axilla				Deodorant

Vesicles on erythematous areas	Exposed areas (especially extremities)	Lesions often in streaks Itching	Adults and children		Plants (ivy, oak, sumac) (Fig. 28–22)
	Near hands, zippers, jewelry (e.g., wrist or earlobe)	Itching			Nickel (Fig. 28–23)
	Where medication is applied (e.g., eye, hair, face, neck)			Eczema	Medications, hair preparations, cosmetics
	Hands and other exposed areas Genital region Buttocks				Industrial agents
Vesicles with erythematous base	Genital area	Pain, not itch Positive Tzanck's test	Adults		Herpes (genitalia) simplex II
	Cold sore (rarely in genital area)	Pain Systemic symptoms Positive Tzanck's test	Neonates	Acute contact dermatitis Erythema multiforme	Herpes simplex I
Vesicles	Dermatome distribution	Tingling Occasional itch Pain Vesicles	Adults and children	Contact dermatitis (usually itches) Cellulitis	Herpes zoster
	Leg most common site in children	In children, not usually painful Often sciatic distribution			
Patchy alopecia	Scalp	Hairs broken and short Positive KOH *Trichophyton tonsurans* is the most common fungal scalp infection	Preadolescents	Alopecia areata	Fungal infections mostly *Trichophyton tonsurans* (Figs. 28–24 and 28–25)

Table continued on following page

DIFFERENTIAL DIAGNOSIS OF SKIN PROBLEMS *Continued*

NATURE OF LESION	DISTRIBUTION OF LESION	ASSOCIATED FINDINGS	NATURE OF PATIENT	LESIONS WITH SIMILAR APPEARANCE	DIAGNOSIS
		Does not fluoresce Culture in dermatology test medium (DTM) *Microsporum audouini* and *canis* give apple-green Wood's light			
Patchy alopecia (possibly scarring)	Scalp	Pustular lesion Boggy scalp Culture in DTM	Most common in children	Fungal infection	Bacterial infection
	Scalp	Pinhead-sized nits on hair shaft May be superimposed bacterial infection Itching	More common in children but can occur in adults	Seborrheic dermatitis Bacterial infection	Pediculosis capitis (Fig. 28–26)
Erythematous Some scaling Occasional maceration and oozing	Groin (Figs. 28–28 and 28–29) Under breasts	Border not sharp; pustules at edge Positive KOH Moist	Children Diabetics	May all look similar (KOH required for differentiation) (Fig 28–27)	Candidiasis
	Groin	Border sharp and accentuated Itch No pustular edge Positive KOH	Often complicates simple herpes rash More common in males Not seen in children		Tinea cruris (Fig. 28–30)
	Groin Groin	Moist Border sharp Positive Wood's light (coral-red) Reddish brown macules	Obese adults Adults		Seborrheic intertrigo Erythrasma (*Corynebacterium*)
Scaling, vesicles	Feet (soles)	Scaling Itch (worse in summer) Positive KOH	Adults and children	May coexist*	Tinea pedis (dyshidrotic form) (Figs. 28–31 and 28–32)
Vesicles	Feet (soles, sides, dorsum)	Negative KOH Often associated with similar process in hands	Adults	May coexist*	Dyshidrotic eczema

				May coexist*	
Maceration	Feet (between toes, mainly 4th and 3rd spaces)	Itch (worse in summer) Positive KOH	Adults and children		Tinea pedis (intertriginous form)
Scaling	Face or feet (soles)	Erythema and fissuring Negative KOH, spares toewebs	Children		Juvenile plantar dermatosis
Erythema scaling	Feet (dorsum and toes; toewebs and soles not involved)	Negative KOH	Adults and children	Tinea pedis	Contact dermatitis
Tumor	Most common on face and other sun-exposed areas	Smooth surface Atrophic center Pearly edge Roundish shape Tannish brown Telangiectasia on border	Elderly people Those often exposed to sun	Squamous cell cancer Melanoma Sebaceous nevi	Basal cell carcinoma
Tumor	Most common on sun-exposed areas (especially hands, face, and ears)	Smooth or irregular surface Firm Irregular edge May be scaling Tannish brown	Elderly people Those often exposed to sun	Basal cell cancer Warts Actinic keratoses	Squamous cell carcinoma
Tumor	Men: mostly on trunk (47%) Women: mostly on legs (39%)	Pigmented, often with different colors in same lesion (blue, purple, white, tan) Irregular border Change in size Satellites	Adults	Mole (melanocytic nevus) Pigmented lesions Seborrheic keratosis Dermatofibroma Angiokeratoma Lentigo	Malignant melanoma

*Different forms of tinea pedis may coexist with each other as well as with dyshidrotic eczema.

Selected References

August, P. J.: Iatrogenic skin disease. Practitioner *224*:471–478, 1980.

Basler, R. S.: Contact dermatitis. Nebr. Med. J. *65*:296–299, 1980.

Berger, T. G., Obuch, M. L., and Goldschmidt, R. H.: Dermatologic manifestations of HIV infection. Am. Fam. Physician *41*:1729–1743, 1990.

Cripps, D. J.: Skin care and problems in the aged. Hosp. Pract. *12*:119–127, 1977.

Epstein, E.: Common skin disorders. Oradell, N.J., Medical Economics Co., 1979.

Feigold, D. S., and Bachta, M.: Common skin diseases seen by the internist. DM *25(8)*:1–39, 1979.

Hanifin, J. M.: Eczematous conditions in the elderly: common and curable. Geriatrics *34*:29–38, 1979.

Huff, J. C., and Weston, W. L.: Eczematous dermatitis. Maj. Probl. Clin. Pediatr. *19*:86–122, 1978.

Lamberg, S. I.: Common problems of the skin. *In* Barker, L. R., Binton, J. R., and Zieve, P. D. (Eds.): Principles of Ambulatory Medicine. Baltimore, Williams & Wilkins, 1982.

McLauria, C. I.: Unusual patterns of common dermatoses in blacks. Cutis *32(4)*:352–355, 358–360, 1983.

Scott, D. A.: Disorders of the hair and scalp in blacks. Dermatol. Clin. *6*:387–395, 1988.

Stevenson, C. J.: Occupational skin disease. Postgrad. Med. J. *65*:374–386, 1989.

Symposium on Pediatric Dermatology. Pediatr. Clin. North Am. *25(2)*:189–389, 1978.

Verou, J. L.: Skin problems in children. Practitioner *217*:403–415, 1976.

Vickers, H. R.: Problems of dermatological diagnoses. Br. J. Clin. Pract. *32*:159–166, 1978.

White, J. E.: Skin cancer. Practitioner *224*:501–503, 1980.

Chapter 29

Sore Throat

In this chapter, sore throat is defined as pain in the throat at rest that often worsens with swallowing. The most common causes of sore throat without pharyngeal ulcers include *viral pharyngitis, bacterial pharyngitis* and *tonsillitis, allergic pharyngitis, pharyngitis secondary to sinusitis,* and *infectious mononucleosis.* Common causes of sore throat with pharyngeal ulceration include *herpangina, herpes simplex, fusospirochetal infection, candidiasis, herpes zoster,* and *chicken pox* (varicella). The less common primary and secondary syphilitic ulcerations are usually not painful.

Pharyngitis is a vexing problem because it is extremely prevalent and it is difficult to establish a precise diagnosis. The annual cost of laboratory tests and medications ordered for patients with sore throats is about $300 million. Despite the fact that streptococcal and viral pharyngitis (including infectious mononucleosis) are the most common causes of sore throat, studies have shown that even with careful diagnostic techniques, a precise cause can be determined only in about 50 per cent of patients.

Prompt diagnosis and treatment of *streptococcal pharyngitis* are essential to reduction of spread to close contacts; treatment also prevents acute rheumatic fever. Prompt antibiotic therapy also shortens the clinical course and decreases morbidity. Rapid screening tests for streptococcal antigens are useful in selected cases. For a precise diagnosis of streptococcal pharyngitis, there must be a positive culture for group A streptococci and a fourfold rise in the antistreptolysin (ASO) titer. The carrier state exists when there is a positive culture without antibody response. According to one large study in which these criteria were used, most patients were found to be carriers. Because the ASO titer does not rise until 1 to 6 months after an acute streptococcal infection, the ASO titer in the acute serum is of no value in the diagnosis of a current infection. The foregoing information does not mean that throat cultures are of no value, but it does reinforce the need for sound clinical judgment in the diagnosis and treatment of patients with sore throats (Table 29–1).

NATURE OF PATIENT

Streptococcal pharyngitis is most prevalent in patients under age 25, particularly those between ages 6 and 12. Likewise, *herpangina, herpes simplex, fusospirochetal infections*, and *candidiasis* are more common in children. As a cause of pharyngitis, *infectious mononucleosis* is most prevalent in adolescents and young adults. It does occur, although less frequently, in patients over age 60. It is particularly notable that 70 per cent of elderly patients with infectious mononucleosis do not develop pharyngitis, adenopathy, or splenomegaly.

Neisseria gonorrhoeae presenting with oropharyngeal symptoms is becoming more common as a cause of pharyngitis, yet it is often unrecognized. It has been cultured from the throat in 10 per cent of patients with anogenital gonorrhea. Of those with positive cultures, most do not have pharyngeal symptoms. It is more common in people who engage in orogenital sex. Male homosexuals have a higher incidence of oropharyngeal gonorrheal infections than other groups do.

Common ulcerative and vesicular pharyngeal lesions include *recurrent aphthous stomatitis, herpes zoster, herpes simplex, fusospirochetal infections*, and *candidiasis* (particularly if the patient is immunosuppressed or taking antibiotics; see Table 29–2). The last three, although common causes of ulcerative pharyngeal lesions in adults, are somewhat more prevalent in children. Although rare, primary and secondary syphilitic lesions occasionally are seen in adults. They should be suspected if the lesion is not painful and if there is an absence of the usual accompanying symptoms of upper respiratory infection.

NATURE OF SYMPTOMS

Marked pain in the throat (frequently associated with dysphagia), an oral temperature exceeding 100° to 101°F, and a rapid onset of symptoms suggest the probability of a *streptococcal* or *viral pharyngitis*. A low-grade temperature, gradual onset of pharyngeal symptoms, and systemic symptoms that are more persistent suggest *infectious mononucleosis*. In reality, it is difficult for the physician to determine the cause of pharyngitis on the basis of the nature of the chief complaint; predisposing factors and physical examination are frequently more useful indicators.

TABLE 29–1. Probabilities of Streptococcal Isolation in Four Series* with Different Clinical Predictors*

	Present Series (n = 693) (%)	Walsh et al. (n = 418) (%)	Crawford et al. (n = 472) (%)	Centor et al. (n = 234) (%)
Tonsillar exudate	25.4	19.9	18.5	18.9
Anterior cervical adenopathy	13.8	12.6	15.3	16.5
Temperature >100°F	22.2	14.3	NR†	NR
Temperature >101°F	26.1	23.9	25.0	19.5
History of recent exposure to streptococcus	11.1	18.8	20.0	NR
No cough	15.0	14.8	14.7	19.3
No rhinorrhea	14.8	13.4	NR	11.9
"High risk" according to Walsh algorithm‡	26.4	19.0	22.7	NR

*Probabilities in all series adjusted to an assumed prevalence rate of 10%, using Bayes' theorem.
†NR = not reported.
‡"High-risk" patients are those with enlarged or tender cervical nodes *and* pharyngeal exudate *or* history of recent exposure to someone with diagnosed streptococcal infection.
From Komaroff, A., et al.: The prediction of streptococcal pharyngitis in adults. J. Gen. Intern. Med. *1*:1–7, 1986.

TABLE 29–2. Common Infections Causing Oropharyngeal Ulceration

Disease	Location	Vesiculation	Pain	Size of Lesion (mm)	Diagnostic Criteria
Local herpangina	Tonsils, pillars, uvula	Yes	Yes	1–2	Characteristic clinical presentation, coxsackievirus in culture of lesion exudate, positive serologic test
Herpes simplex	Lips, gingivae, buccal mucosa, tongue	Yes	Yes	1–2	Multinuclear giant cells with ballooning degeneration in Tzanck smear of ulcer-crater exudate
Fusospirochetal infection	Gingivae, may spread diffusely	No	Yes	2–30	Characteristic lesions, foul breath, anaerobic forms and spirochetes in smear of lesion exudate
Candidiasis	All parts of oropharynx	No	Yes	3–10	*Candida albicans* in Gram-stained smear and culture of scrapings
Primary syphilis	Lips, tonsils, tongue	No	No	5–15	Indurated "heaped-up" lesion, positive serologic test (periodic evaluation necessary)
Herpes zoster	Unilateral involvement of tongue, lip, buccal mucosa	Yes	Yes	2–4	Unilateral involvement, painful prodromes, giant cells in Tzanck smear of lesion exudate
Systemic hand-foot-and-mouth disease	All parts of oropharynx	Yes	Yes	1–10	Exanthem on hands and feet, coxsackievirus in culture of lesion exudate, positive serologic test
Varicella	All parts of oropharynx	Yes	No	2–4	Characteristic exanthem
Secondary syphilis	Symmetrical involvement of all parts of mouth and oropharynx	No	No	2–10	Other evidence of secondary syphilis, positive serologic test, spirochetes visible on darkfield microscopy

From Brown, R. B., and Clinton, D.: Vesicular and ulcerative infections of the mouth and oropharynx. Postgrad. Med. 67(2):107–116, 1980.

PREDISPOSING FACTORS

Herpangina, herpes simplex, and *candidiasis* are most common in immunosuppressed patients. *Candidiasis* also is most prevalent in diabetic patients and in those taking broad-spectrum antibiotics. *Herpangina* is most common in children and shows a strong seasonal propensity for summer and autumn, whereas *streptococcal pharyngitis* is most prevalent in fall and winter.

PHYSICAL FINDINGS

Marked erythema and swelling of the throat (often associated with an exudative pharyngitis or tonsillitis), temperature greater than 101°F, tachycardia, and occurrence between September and April all strongly indicate *streptococcal pharyngitis*. Likewise, a history of streptococcal exposure within the family during the past week, prior history of acute rheumatic fever, diabetes, tender anterior cervical nodes, or a scarlatiniform rash increases the likelihood that streptococcal pharyngitis is the correct diagnosis. As mentioned previously, streptococcal pharyngitis is rare after age 30 and is most common between ages 6 to 12.

Although many authors stress an association between tonsillopharyngeal exudate and *streptococcal pharyngitis*, it is important to note that only 50 per cent of the patients with proven streptococcal pharyngitis have an exudate, and only 50 per cent of all patients with a pharyngeal exudate have streptococcal pharyngitis. Despite this, many physicians presume a streptococcal cause if a tonsillar exudate is present and if one or more of the following signs also are demonstrated: temperature greater than 101°F, tender anterior cervical nodes, or duration of sore throat greater than 6 days, particularly if there is no cough (see Table 29–2).

Viral pharyngitis is the most common cause of pharyngitis and, unlike streptococcal pharyngitis, has no particular distribution with regard to age or time of year, although it is slightly more frequent in the winter months. Patients with viral pharyngitis usually have less severe pharyngeal symptoms and severer systemic symptoms. These patients are less likely to have an exudate or marked erythema of the pharynx. The pharynx is usually slightly injected but also may appear swollen, boggy, or pale. There is usually no exudate or follicular tonsillitis present, but systemic symptoms (malaise, fever, cough, headache, and fatigue) are more prominent than with streptococcal pharyngitis.

Patients with the pharyngitis of *infectious mononucleosis* may present with an exudate, although most do not. The enanthem of infectious mononucleosis, palatine petechiae, is almost diagnostic. They resemble small, red, raised grains of sand surrounded by 0.5-mm pale bases. The pharyngitis of infectious mononucleosis is almost invariably (i.e., in 90 per cent of cases) accompanied by posterior cervical adenopathy. Some authors are reluctant to diagnose infectious mononucleosis in the absence of posterior cervical adenopathy.

Epiglottitis, which is not uncommon in children but is rare in adults, is usually caused by a Haemophilus *infection.* When epiglottitis is suspected, appropriate cultures should be performed, and antibiotics should be administered promptly. *Gingivitis* is most often seen in patients with poor oral hygiene. In some cases, it can involve the entire oropharynx. The most common presentation of *ulcerative gingivitis (trench mouth)* is an acute onset of painful bloody gums, foul breath, and a grayish exudate covering the interdental papillae. Ulcerative gingivitis is a *fusospirochetal* infection and responds well to improved oral hygiene and appropriate antibiotics. Pharyngeal involvement with fusospirochetal organisms *(Vincent's angina)* may occur primarily or secondary to a spread of fusospirochetal infection from anterior sites. In patients with this infection, sore throat is the most common complaint, and there may be necrotic, gray, ulcerative lesions about the tonsillar pillars. If the "pseudomembrane" is removed, there is usually bleeding of the undersurface. Although in most cases involvement is initially unilateral, it often spreads and becomes bilateral.

Patients who have frequent sore throats, without evidence of pharyngitis or fever, may have an *allergic pharyngitis.* This is often associated with an intermittent postnasal drip that leads to minor irritation and inflammation of the posterior pharynx. Some patients with recurrent or chronic low-grade *sinusitis* may present with a sore throat induced by a postnasal drip from the affected sinuses. **It is particularly important to note that when a patient complains of a sore throat that becomes worse with swallowing, and when the physical examination of the oropharynx is negative, the physician should suspect thyroiditis and palpate the thyroid for swelling or pain on palpation.** This is a common way by which the uncommon illness of thyroiditis presents.

Retropharyngeal abscess is most common in infants and young children, but it does occur infrequently in adults. There may be an unexplained fever, an upper respiratory tract infection, loss of appetite, difficulty in swallowing, and stridor. The last sign is particularly common in children. Retropharyngeal abscess is a medical emergency and should be evaluated promptly. The study of choice is a CT scan. Some investigators believe that earlier treatment with antibiotics reduces the incidence of this complication and the need for surgical intervention.

The presence of oropharyngeal ulcerations, with or without vesiculation, is often helpful in differential diagnosis. In patients with *herpangina*, usually children, the painful ulcerations measure 1 to 2 mm and occur on the tonsils, pillars, and the uvula. The pharyngeal ulcers (2 to 30 mm) due to *fusospirochetal infections* are usually present on the gingivae, but they may spread diffusely throughout the oropharynx. These lesions are usually painful, but there is no associated vesiculation. In adults and children with *herpes simplex*, the painful ulcers measure 1 to 2 mm and can occur on the lips, gingivae, buccal mucosa, or rarely tongue. The painful ulcerations of *herpes zoster* usually are unilateral and involve the tongue, lip, or buccal mucosa. These lesions are usually 2 to 4 mm and associated with vesiculation. In infants and adults with *candidiasis*, the ulcerations measure 3 to 11 mm and can involve any part of the oropharynx. Vesiculation does not occur with candidiasis.

DIAGNOSTIC STUDIES

Tests that are often helpful in the differential diagnosis of sore throat are a complete blood count with differential, throat cultures, rapid screening tests for streptococcal antigens, Gram staining, Monospot test, and antistreptolysin titers. Komaroff (1978) developed a decision table that recommends culture if any one of the following is present: age less than 25 years, definite streptococcal exposure during the previous week, history of acute rheumatic fever, diabetes, known epidemic of streptococcal pharyngitis, oral temperature greater than 37.7°C, exudate, tender anterior cervical nodes, or scarlatiniform rash. Difficulty with follow-up, a known epidemic of nephritogenic streptococcal infections, or presence of a scarlatiniform rash is an indication for both throat culture and treatment with penicillin. In addition, if there is a history of rheumatic fever or if diabetes is present, treatment with penicillin is indicated despite the clinical picture. A patient with a temperature greater than 37.7°C, tonsillar exudate, and tender anterior cervical nodes probably has a *streptococcal pharyngitis*, and immediate treatment is justified. A complete blood count with a lymphocytosis of greater than 50 per cent or an absolute lymphocytosis of greater than 4500 lymphocytes per mm³ with more than 10 per cent atypical lymphocytes suggests *infectious mononucleosis*. This is confirmed by a positive Monospot test. **There are virtually no false-negative Monospot tests, although some studies have shown 10 per cent false-positive results**. Most of these characteristic hematologic and serologic abnormalities occur within 1 week from onset of symptoms in 80 per cent of patients.

LESS COMMON DIAGNOSTIC CONSIDERATIONS

Patients with thyroiditis may present with a sore throat or dysphagia or both. In a patient complaining of a sore throat whose throat examination is negative, the thyroid gland should be palpated. If it is tender, thyroiditis should be suspected. Patients with hypothyroidism

DIFFERENTIAL DIAGNOSIS OF SORE THROAT

TYPE OF PHARYNGITIS	NATURE OF PATIENT	NATURE OF SYMPTOMS	PREDISPOSING FACTORS	PHYSICAL FINDINGS	DIAGNOSTIC STUDIES
Without Pharyngeal Ulcers					
Viral	All ages	Pain in the throat Rapid onset Systemic symptoms		Exudate less likely than with streptococcal infections	
Infectious mononucleosis	Adolescents and young adults Uncommon in elderly	Gradual onset		Low-grade temperature Occasional exudate Enanthem Posterior cervical adenopathy Hepatosplenomegaly	Monospot test
Streptococcal pharyngitis	Patients younger than age 25, especially those between ages 6 and 12	Pain in throat Rapid onset Few systemic symptoms	Fall and winter Streptococcal infection in family Diabetes	Marked erythema and throat swelling Temperature > 101°F Tachycardia Tender anterior cervical nodes Scarlatiniform rash Exudate more likely than with viral infection	Culture Increased antistreptolysin titer
Gonococcal pharyngitis	Most common in male homosexuals and those with anogenital gonorrhea	Often no symptoms	Orogenital sex		Culture

Sinusitis with postnasal drip	Adults	Mild throat soreness Symptoms often worse with recumbency		Evidence of sinusitis Postnasal drip	Sinus radiographs
Allergic pharyngitis			Seasonal allergies	No fever Intermittent postnasal drip Swollen pharynx with minimal injection	Eosinophils in nasal secretions
With Pharyngeal Ulcers Herpangina	More common in children	Painful ulcers on tonsils, pillars, or uvula	Immunosuppression Summer and autumn	Vesicles 1–2-mm ulcers	Serologic tests
Fusospirochetal infection (Vincent's angina)	Children and those with poor oral hygiene	Painful ulcers Bleeding gums Foul breath		No vesicles Ulcerative gingivitis Gray necrotic ulcers 2–30-mm ulcers Pseudomembrane	Spirochetes on Gram stain
Candidiasis	Children and those who are immuno-suppressed or taking antibiotics		Immunosuppression Antibiotics	3–11-mm ulcers No vesicles	KOH smear shows *Candida* Culture
Herpes simplex	Most common in children	Not usually a cause of sore throat	Immunosuppression	1–2-mm painful ulcers Vesicles present on lips, gingivae, buccal mucosa, or tongue	Tzanck smear shows multinucleated giant cells

may complain of a sore throat or hoarseness, regardless of whether a goiter is present. Some patients with seasonal allergy present with a sore throat. In most instances, there is minimal pharyngeal swelling. Occasionally, a postnasal drip is seen, and other allergic symptoms usually can be elicited as well. Patients who have swallowed a coarse foreign body such as a bone, rough vegetable, or piece of meat may complain of a sore throat with or without dysphagia, even if they have successfully swallowed the object. If this complaint persists or is severe, the possibility that a foreign body is lodged in the posterior pharynx or proximal esophagus should be considered. Patients with leukemia, agranulocytosis, or diphtheria also may present with a sore throat.

Selected References

Balciunos, B. A., and Overholser, C. D.: Diagnosis and management of common oral lesions. Am. Fam. Physician *35*:206–220, 1987.

Brown, R. B., and Clinton, D.: Vesicular and ulcerative infections of the mouth and oropharynx. Postgrad. Med. *67(2)*:107–116, 1980.

Everett, M. T.: The uninflamed sore throat. Practitioner *222*:835–838, 1979.

Komaroff, A. L.: A management strategy for sore throat. J.A.M.A. *239*:1429–1432, 1978.

Komaroff, A. L., Pass, T. M., Aronson, M. D., et al.: The prediction of streptococcal pharyngitis in adults. J. Gen. Intern. Med. *1*:1–7, 1986.

Sloan, P. D.: Sore throats. Consultant *22(5)*:110–127, 1982.

Todd, J. K.: The sore throat: pharyngitis and epiglottitis. Infect. Dis. Clin. North Am. *2*:149–162, 1988.

Chapter 30

Swelling of Legs

Swelling of one or both legs is a frequent presenting complaint. Common causes include systemic edema states such as *heart failure, nephrotic syndrome, cirrhosis, acute and chronic thrombophlebitis, chronic venous insufficiency, cellulitis, lymphedema, salt-retaining drugs,* and mechanical factors such as *dependency* and *constricting garters* or *pantyhose.* Although the causes are numerous and the pathophysiology complex, diagnosis is simplified by determining whether one or both legs are involved, whether onset is sudden or gradual, whether pain is present, and other associated symptoms. **Certainly the most common cause of unilateral leg edema is chronic venous insufficiency, and the most common causes of bilateral leg edema are the systemic edema states, salt-retaining drugs, dependency, and primary lymphedema.**

NATURE OF PATIENT

Primary lymphedema is an inherited defect in the lymphatic system caused by hypoplasia, aplasia, or digitation of the lymphatic vessels. In the neonate, unilateral edema of a leg is termed *congenital lymphedema* and is due to a form of primary lymphedema. If the swelling of the leg becomes apparent around age 10, it is called *lymphedema praecox.* Traumatic thrombophlebitis, cellulitis, and *compartment syndromes* also cause unilateral leg edema in children. In children, bilateral leg edema usually is due to a systemic illness, such as acute glomerulonephritis, nephrotic syndrome, hypoproteinemia, and primary lymphedema. Unilateral or bilateral edema in teenagers or older women may be due to constricting garments such as tight jeans, pantyhose, or, rarely, garters. In a runner, sudden onset of painful calf swelling suggests *rupture of the medial head of the gastrocnemius,* whereas intermittent pain and swelling of the upper or lower leg suggests a compartment syndrome.

343

In obese women, the development of bilateral leg swelling that spares the feet suggests *lipedema*. Lipedema occurs exclusively in obese women and is a bilateral and symmetrical deposition of fat in the lower extremities. Lipedema can be differentiated from lymphedema, since the foot is not involved in the former, whereas in the latter, the swelling starts in the most distal part of the foot.

In a chronic alcoholic, bilateral edema of the leg suggests edema caused by cirrhosis, with or without ascites. In a diabetic, unilateral and occasional bilateral swelling of the legs suggests cellulitis, especially if it is accompanied by warmth and tenderness. Leg swelling due to venous insufficiency is more common in women, and frequently there is a history of varicose veins in female relatives. In patients with heart failure or cirrhosis, bilateral leg edema is usually a manifestation of their systemic disease. In patients with *rheumatoid arthritis,* a painful unilateral swelling of the calf may be due to a ruptured Baker's cyst, sometimes referred to as pseudophlebitis. A localized, pretibial swelling in a patient with tachycardia, exophthalmos, or other signs or symptoms of hyperthyroidism suggests *pretibial myxedema,* which is a rare finding in hyperthyroidism.

NATURE OF SYMPTOMS

Unilateral swelling of the lower or upper leg suggests *local* mechanical or inflammatory processes. These include *lymphedema, venous insufficiency* (the most common cause of unilateral leg edema), *thrombophlebitis, cellulitis, ruptured gastrocnemius muscle, compartment syndrome, ruptured Baker's cyst,* and, rarely, an acquired or inherited *arteriovenous fistula.* Bilateral leg swelling is most often due to systemic conditions, including *congestive heart failure, nephrotic syndrome, cirrhosis, acute glomerulonephritis, salt-retaining drugs, constricting garments,* or *prolonged dependency* of the legs. Less common causes of bilateral leg swelling include *idiopathic edema, lipedema, primary lymphedema,* and exposure to *extremes of temperature.*

A sudden onset of calf swelling suggests a ruptured Baker's cyst, ruptured gastrocnemius, arterial occlusion, thrombophlebitis, cellulitis, or a compartment syndrome. Chronic bilateral swelling of the legs occurs in the aforementioned systemic illnesses as well as lymphedema, lipedema, lymphatic obstruction, chronic venous insufficiency, and cellulitis, which may be secondary to bilateral venous stasis dermatitis. The gradual onset of edema that starts in the distal part of the foot and involves the dorsum of the foot and ankle suggests lymphedema. **Painless unilateral leg edema in a woman over age 40 should make the physician suspicious of a gynecologic cancer with obstruction of the lymphatics, causing secondary lymphedema.**

ASSOCIATED SYMPTOMS

When warmth, redness, moderate pain, and tenderness to palpation is associated with calf swelling, cellulitis or thrombophlebitis is probable. The absence of pain does not eliminate the diagnosis of thrombophlebitis. When pain is associated with calf swelling, thrombophlebitis, compartment syndrome, arterial thrombosis, ruptured Baker's cyst, or ruptured medial head of the gastrocnemius should be suspected. Dyspnea on exertion, orthopnea, or paroxysmal nocturnal dyspnea suggests heart failure as the cause of leg edema. If spider angiomas, palmar erythema, hepatomegaly, or jaundice is present in a patient with swollen legs, cirrhosis should be suspected. Patients with nephrotic syndrome often have generalized edema and swelling of the eyelids, which is particularly noticeable after prolonged recumbency. If leg swelling is absent or minimal after recumbency but develops as the day progresses, venous insufficiency is most likely.

PRECIPITATING AND AGGRAVATING FACTORS

Prolonged sitting or standing may cause swelling of the lower extremities, particularly in patients with venous insufficiency. Garments such as jeans or pantyhose tight enough to impede venous return may also cause swelling of the legs. Patients may gain weight gradually so that their thighs are fatter yet are not recognized as such by the patient. The garments that previously fit adequately now impede venous return. Trauma to a vein causing thrombophlebitis may cause unilateral, painful swelling of the leg. Conditions such as pregnancy and large uterine fibroids that increase intra-abdominal pressure may mechanically impede venous return and cause painless unilateral or bilateral swelling of the legs. Fluid-retaining drugs such as estrogens, oral contraceptives, nonsteroidal anti-inflammatory agents, psychotropic agents (lithium and tricyclic antidepressants), and vasodilators (calcium channel blockers, nitrates, prazosin, and minoxidil) can cause fluid retention with minimal to moderate painless swelling of both legs. Other drugs that may give rise to bilateral gradual leg swelling include corticosteroids, progesterone, testosterone, methyldopa, hydralazine, and diazoxide.

AMELIORATING FACTORS

Cessation of salt-retaining and vasodilating drugs will alleviate edema if these drugs were causal. Marked weight loss alleviates some of the swelling of lipedema. Support hose alleviate the edema of venous insufficiency. Muscle activity of the lower legs alleviates the edema of

DIFFERENTIAL DIAGNOSIS OF SWELLING OF LEGS

CAUSE	NATURE OF PATIENT	NATURE OF SYMPTOMS	ASSOCIATED SYMPTOMS	PRECIPITAT-ING AND AGGRAVAT-ING FAC-TORS	AMELIO-RATING FACTORS	PHYSICAL EXAMINA-TION	DIAGNOSTIC STUDIES
Systemic Heart failure	Hypertension or coronary artery disease	Bilateral	Dyspnea on exertion Orthopnea Paroxysmal nocturnal dyspnea	Myocardial infarction		Pulmonary rales, distended neck veins, tachycardia, cardiac enlargement, gallop	Chest radiograph Echocardiogram
Cirrhosis	Alcoholic	Bilateral	Ascites Jaundice Abdominal swelling			Hepatomegaly, jaundice, ascites, gynecomastia	Abnormal liver function tests Liver biopsy
Nephrotic syndrome	Often children	Bilateral	Polyuria Eyelid swelling			Edema of eyelids, hypertension	Albuminuria Hypercholes-terolemia
Hypoproteinemia	Malnourished	Bilateral					Serum protein Electrophoresis
Venous insufficiency	Usually female	Often unilateral	Minimal on arising		Recumbency	Varicose veins	
Thrombophlebitis		Usually unilateral, sudden onset of swelling with redness and pain	Pain, warmth, and redness	Trauma, immobilization, childbirth, drugs (estrogen), birth control pills		Tender cord Positive Homans' sign Warmth, low-grade fever	Duplex ultrasonography Venogram Doppler ultrasonography Computed tomography

Mechanical—							
Ruptured gastrocnemius	Runners	Sudden onset	Pain			Ecchymoses of ankle	Computed tomography
Baker's cyst	Rheumatoid arthritis		Arthritis				Arthrogram
Constrictive garments	Usually female		Painless	Weight gain	Weight loss	Fat thighs	
Dependency	Post stroke		Impaired mobility	Venous insufficiency	Muscle activity of legs		
Lymphatic							
Congenital	Neonate	Unilateral					
Secondary Lymphedema	> Age 40, usually female			Pelvic cancer Radiation		Peau d'orange skin, involves foot, dorsal hump	Lymphangiography
Lipedema	Obese, female	Bilateral	Obesity	Weight gain	Weight loss	Spares foot	
Salt-retaining drugs		Bilateral		Estrogen, oral contraceptives, NSAIDs, lithium, vasodilators			

dependency. Edema due to a ruptured gastrocnemius or a ruptured Baker's cyst gradually subsides, as does the edema from thrombophlebitis and cellulitis. Diuretics and aldosterone blocking agents often assist in the mobilization of edema in patients with cirrhosis, nephrosis, and heart failure.

PHYSICAL EXAMINATION

Physical examination of the legs should include inspection and palpation. The patient should be examined to determine the area of the swelling, which may be in the knee, the anserine bursa, or Cooperman's fat pad, none of which causes true edema of the lower extremity. Lipedema excludes the foot and is a deposition of fat in the leg, whereas lymphedema begins at the distal area of the foot and involves the dorsum of the foot with a so-called "hump." The character of the skin in the area of edema is also diagnostically helpful. Thick, taut, and fibrotic skin suggests that the causative process is chronic rather than acute. Redness or lymphangitic streaks suggests a cellulitis. Ecchymoses in the dependent part of the ankle associated with mid-calf pain suggests a tear of the gastrocnemius muscle. Tenderness to palpation over the vein, warmth, low-grade fever, and a positive Homans' sign suggest thrombophlebitis. Painful swelling of one calf in a patient with the stigmata of rheumatoid arthritis and popliteal cyst on the opposite side suggests pseudophlebitis, a ruptured Baker's cyst. Physical findings of systemic illnesses associated with swelling of the legs include pulmonary rales, distended neck veins, tachycardia, gallop rhythm, cardiac enlargement, heart failure, hepatomegaly, jaundice, ascites, palmar erythema gynecomastia, spider angiomas, cirrhosis, hypertension, periorbital edema, nephrotic syndrome, peau d'orange (skin of the orange) skin, and lymphatic obstruction.

DIAGNOSTIC STUDIES

Although venography is the gold standard for the diagnosis of deep vein thrombosis, it is not necessary or advisable in all instances. Duplex ultrasonography or, if not available, Doppler ultrasonography can be used to confirm the diagnosis of venous thrombosis when invasive or radiographic procedures are contraindicated.

A computed tomographic scan can be used to determine the distribution of edema in instances of leg swelling: venous obstruction exhibits an increased cross-sectional area of muscle tissue and edema in the muscular and interstitial compartment; obesity and lipedema exhibit increased subcutaneous fat; lymphedema exhibits increased fluid in the interstitial space with a honeycombed pattern when the condition is chronic; popliteal cysts exhibit an extension of fluid from the joint space to between the muscle planes. Direct and indirect lymphangiography is used to visualize lymphatics, which are dilated in instances of congenital and acquired lymphatic obstruction.

LESS COMMON DIAGNOSTIC CONSIDERATIONS

Lipedema is a bilateral, symmetrical deposition of fat in the lower extremities that spares the foot. Spontaneous venous thrombosis occurs more frequently during pregnancy, parturition, surgical trauma, severe illness, polycythemia, malignant disease, and dehydration. Retroperitoneal fibrosis (most commonly induced by the antimigraine drug methysergide) can cause obstruction of lymphatic or venous drainage. The swelling may be unilateral or bilateral. Pretibial myxedema, a localized edema in the pretibial area, occurs in patients with hyperthyroidism. Thrombosis of the iliac vein, or compression of the iliac vein by a distended bladder, is another rare cause of unilateral edema of the leg. Cyclic or idiopathic edema occurs mostly in obese women and is usually bilateral. These patients can develop fluid retention of several pounds in a few days.

Selected References

Ruschhaupt, W. F.: Differential diagnosis of edema of the lower extremities. Cardiovasc. Clin. *13*:307–320, 1983.

Ruschhaupt, W. F., and Graor, R. A.: Evaluation of the patient with leg edema. Postgrad. Med. *78*:132–139, 1985.

Sachs, M. K.: The optimum use of needle aspiration in the bacteriologic diagnosis of cellulitis in adult. Arch. Intern. Med. *150*:1907–1912, 1990.

Satiani, B., Rustin, R., Biggers, K., and Bordner, L.: Noninvasive diagnosis of deep venous thrombosis. Am. Fam. Physician *44*:569–574, 1991.

Vaughan, B. F.: CT of swollen legs. Clin. Radiol. *41*:24–30, 1990.

Young, J. R.: The swollen leg. Am. Fam. Physician *15*:163–173, 1977.

31

Urethral Discharge and Dysuria

Dysuria denotes burning or pain associated with urination and can have several causes. Frequency, hesitancy, urgency, and strangury (slow, painful urination) are other symptoms commonly associated with micturition disorders. Urinary urgency occurs as a result of *trigonal* or *posterior urethral irritation* produced by inflammation, stones, or tumor; it most commonly occurs with *cystitis*. Acute inflammatory processes of the bladder cause pain or urgency when only a small quantity of urine is present in the bladder. Frequency of urination, when due to bladder problems, occurs with either a decreased bladder capacity or with pain on bladder distention. Frequency is caused most commonly by lesions of the bladder or urethra, although diseases of the nervous system involving the bladder's nerve supply (either centrally as in tabes and multiple sclerosis or peripherally as in diabetic neuropathy) may produce bladder decompensation with voiding abnormalities. Urinary frequency may also be a manifestation of overflow incontinence; this can occur with either *prostatic hypertrophy* or *neurologic bladder disorders*.

Inflammatory lesions of the prostate, bladder, and urethra are the most common cause of dysuria and frequency and include *prostatitis* in men, *urethrotrigonitis* in women, and *bladder* and *urethral infections* in men and women. Both men and women may have *chronic inflammation of the posterior urethra*. In the United States, women with symptoms of lower urinary tract infections account for more than 5 million office visits per year; only 50 per cent of these women, however, have classic cystitis with urine culture bacteria concentrations greater than 10^5 organisms per milliliter. **Several studies indicate that symptomatic women with urinary bacteria counts less than 10^5 organisms per milliliter (female urethral syndrome) should be considered to have an infectious cause and be treated accordingly.**

About 2 million cases of urethritis (men and women) occur annually in the United States; about 50 per cent of cases are nongonorrheal. There is increasing evidence that *Chlamydia,* which causes nongonorrheal urethritis, is a major cause of sexually transmitted disease in the United States. Because of the frequency of complaints of dysuria and urethral discharge, the associated public health problem, and the ease of treatment, it is essential that physicians be expert in recognizing the causes of these symptoms.

NATURE OF PATIENT

In children, *meatal stenosis* may cause recurrent lower urinary tract infections. Up to 20 per cent of children with urinary complaints may have some degree of meatal stenosis. Dysuria and urethral discharge are uncommon in children. When these symptoms occur in young girls, they frequently are due to a *chemical vaginitis* or a *mechanical urethritis.* When these findings are seen in young boys, they are often secondary to a mechanical urethritis, which can result from continued jarring of the perineum from bicycle riding, horseback riding, a foreign body, or masturbation. *Sexually transmitted diseases* must be considered in instances of urethritis or vaginitis that occurs in boys or girls. If discovered in young children, child abuse is usually the cause.

Bacteriuria is rare in school-age boys and occurs in only 0.1 per cent of men. The incidence of bacteriuria increases in men at age 50 and rises to about 1 per cent at age 60 and to between 4 and 15 per cent in later years, coinciding with the onset of prostatic disease. Among women under age 18, there is a 5 per cent incidence of asymptomatic bacteriuria. Women between ages 15 and 34 account for most of the patients who present with symptoms of urinary tract infections. A study in Great Britain showed that 20 per cent of women in this age group developed dysuria and frequency. Dysuria in women is most frequently caused by *cystitis, vaginitis, female urethral syndrome,* and *mechanical irritation of the urethra.* Dysuria in men is most commonly caused by *urethritis, prostatitis, cystitis,* and *mechanical irritation of the urethra.* Urethral discharge, which is essentially limited to men, is usually caused by *gonorrheal* or *nongonorrheal urethritis (Chlamydia or Trichomonas).*

NATURE OF SYMPTOMS

CYSTITIS. In women who complain of frequency and dysuria without clinical evidence of an upper urinary tract infection, *bacterial cystitis* is usually suspected. Several studies, however, have shown that 30 to 50 per cent of women complaining of these symptoms do not have a positive urine culture according to traditional criteria (isolation of a pathogen in concentrations greater than 10^5 bacteria per milliliter of urine in a clean-voided specimen). There are several possible reasons for this. First, dysuria often represents a vaginal rather than a urinary tract infection. When carefully questioned, women with dysuria due to cystitis usually describe an internal discomfort, whereas women with dysuria due to vaginitis usually describe a more external discomfort; their burning sensation appears to be in the vagina or the labia and is due to urine flow over an inflamed vaginal mucosa. **All women with dysuria should be questioned about an associated vaginal discharge or irritation.** Second, many women who present with symptoms due to bacterial cystitis (i.e., dysuria and frequency) have colony counts less than 10^5 bacteria per milliliter of urine. Various studies have shown that if pathogens are found in a concentration less than 10^5 per milliliter in symptomatic women, there is probably a significant bacterial infection. Third, *Chlamydia trachomatis* is frequently the causative agent. Patients who are infected with this organism have symptoms and pyuria but a negative routine urine culture. Chlamydial infections of the bladder and urethra in women are somewhat analogous to nongonorrheal urethritis in men; in both, there is pyuria but no growth on routine culture. Although rare, *urinary tract tuberculosis* also may present with pyuria and a negative routine culture.

It is important that the physician inquire about the duration and onset of symptoms. Longer duration and gradual onset of symptoms suggest a chlamydial infection, whereas a history of hematuria and sudden onset of symptoms indicate a bacterial infection. Dysuria that is more severe at the end of the stream, particularly if associated with hematuria, suggests *cystitis;* dysuria that is worse at the beginning of the stream is a sign of *urethritis.* Patients with the *female urethral syndrome* often have dysuria, frequency, suprapubic pain, onset of symptoms over 2 to 7 days, and some pyuria. Besides having dysuria, frequency, and suprapubic pain, patients with *cystitis* demonstrate symptoms that develop quickly—pyuria, bacteriuria, and positive urine cultures (Table 31–1). Fever, nausea, back pain, and leukocytosis are not common findings in either female urethral syndrome or cystitis.

URETHRITIS. Urethral discharge in male patients is accepted as objective evidence of *urethritis,* but patients may have urethritis without a significant urethral discharge. **If the patient has dysuria and more than four polymorphonuclear cells per high-powered field in a urethral smear, urethritis is probable.** Nongonorrheal urethritis is defined to include inflammations in men who have negative urethral cultures for *Neisseria gonorrhoeae* and a urethral discharge or more than four polymorphonuclear cells per high-powered field in the urethral smear. *Chlamydia trachomatis* is the most common isolate from patients with nongonorrheal urethritis (Table 31–2). Other causative organisms may include *Mycoplasma,* group D streptococci, *Trichomonas,* and,

TABLE 31–1. Clinical Features of Female Urethral Syndrome and Cystitis

Clinical Features	Female Urethral Syndrome	Cystitis
Dysuria, frequency, suprapubic pain	+	+
Fever, nausea, back pain, other systemic signs	–	–
Duration of symptoms (days)	2–7	1–2
Leukocytosis	–	–
Urinalysis:		
Pyuria	+ or –	+
Bacteriuria	–	+
Hematuria	–	+ or –
White blood cell casts	–	–
Urine cultures	–	+
Blood cultures	–	–

From Meadows, J. C.: The acute urethral syndrome: diagnosis, management, and prophylaxis. Continuing Education, December 1983, pp. 112–120.

rarely, *Candida albicans.* Although a significant number of patients with nongonorrheal urethritis are asymptomatic, most have mild dysuria and a minimal or absent urethral discharge. When a discharge does appear, it is usually clear or whitish. In contrast, about 80 per cent of patients with gonorrheal urethritis have a moderate to heavy urethral discharge that is usually purulent. Dysuria with a mucoid or mucopurulent urethral discharge usually develops 1 to 3 weeks after coitus with an infected partner.

Urethral discharges are usually observed on awakening, after a long period without urination, or after penile stripping. Other symptoms include urgency, frequency, and meatal or urethral irritation. The usual presentation of nongonorrheal urethritis is a low-grade inflammation; the symptoms of gonorrheal urethritis tend to be more acute and severer and include a urethral discharge that is purulent, spontaneous, and greater in volume. **It is important to recognize that a patient may have gonorrheal as well as nongonorrheal urethritis at the same time.** Both may be contracted simultaneously from the same contact.

ASSOCIATED SYMPTOMS

When hematuria accompanies dysuria, *cystitis* is most probable, although the possibility of a *tumor* or *stone* should be considered. If dysuria and frequency are associated with a high fever or chills, an upper urinary tract infection such as *pyelonephritis* may be present. When frequency and dysuria are associated with backache or costovertebral angle tenderness, *pyelonephritis* or *prostatitis* should be suspected.

TABLE 31–2. Comparison Between *Chlamydia trachomatis* and *Neisseria gonorrhoeae* as Venereal Disease Agents

Subject	*C. trachomatis*	*N. gonorrhoeae*
Organism	Obligate intracellular parasite	Gram-negative diplococcus often found within cells (as leukocytes on Gram's stain)
Transmission	Venereal	Venereal
Incubation period	8–21 days	2–6 days (can be longer, up to 10–16 days in rare cases)
Major infection	Urethritis (men); cervicitis (women)	Urethritis (men); cervicitis (women)
Local complications	Yes: epididymitis, bartholinitis, urethral syndrome, salpingitis, others	Yes: same, and others, including prostatitis
Systemic complications	Possibly: arthritis, perihepatitis, peritonitis, and endocarditis reported	Well known: gonococcal septicemia, with resultant arthritis, dermatitis, endocarditis, and meningitis; perihepatitis and peritonitis also reported
Pharyngitis	Yes	Yes
Conjunctivitis	Yes	Yes
Proctitis	Cultured from the rectum	Yes: common venereal infection in homosexuals
Maternal infection with effect on neonate or infant	Well known: inclusion conjunctivitis and pneumonia	Less well established
Carrier state	Recognized, especially in women; can last for months	Recognized, especially in women; can last for months
Reservoir	Cervix (male urethra a minor role)	Cervix (male urethra a minor role)
Treatment	Tetracycline (antibiotic of choice) Erythromycin, sulfonamides, streptomycin, and tri-methoprim-sulfamethoxazole also effective Regimen of 14 days often used	Current Centers for Disease Control recommendation involves procaine penicillin, ampicillin, amoxicillin, tetracycline, or specti-nomycin; probenecid used; shorter treatment regimen
Treatment of sexual contacts	Yes	Yes

From Greydanus, D. E., and McAnarney, E. R.: *Chlamydia trachomatis:* an important sexually transmitted disease in adolescents and young adults. J. Fam. Pract. *10*:611–615, 1980.

Patients who have prostatitis often present with an unexplained backache, with or without fever. The physician should perform a gentle rectal examination of any man who complains of frequency, dysuria, and fever to determine whether the prostate is tender to palpation. Pyelonephritis should be suspected if nausea and vomiting accompany dysuria. Patients who demonstrate prostatic enlargement or experience severe pain on micturition that causes them to resist voiding have outflow obstruction. This causes bladder distention, which may also induce nausea, vomiting, or mild ileus, resulting in abdominal distention.

Frequency of urination without discomfort on voiding may be due to a *diminished bladder capacity, overflow incontinence, or habit* in patients with a normal bladder. It also is observed in patients who pass a large volume of urine owing to diabetes, hypercalcemia, hypokalemia, congestive heart failure, loss of renal concentrating capacity, or the use of diuretics. The absence of nocturia in a patient with urinary frequency suggests that the increased frequency of urination may be of psychogenic origin. Rarely, this may be due to a polyp or irritative lesion in the posterior urethra that is relieved by recumbency.

PRECIPITATING AND AGGRAVATING FACTORS

Patients who have multiple sexual contacts are more likely to develop a sexually transmitted disease such as *gonorrheal* or *nongonorrheal urethritis* or *cervicitis.* An abrupt alteration in the frequency of ejaculation may result in symptoms of *prostatitis.* This often occurs on the patient's return from a vacation during which the frequency of intercourse and subsequent ejaculation were increased. The use of vaginal sprays, douches, and bubble baths (particularly in children) may induce a *chemical vaginitis* that may present with dysuria. It is important for the physician to ask women who complain of dysuria whether a vaginal discharge is present because, in the absence of a recognizable discharge, *vaginitis* is an unlikely cause of dysuria.

AMELIORATING FACTORS

Some patients with *cystitis* believe that they can alleviate their pain by avoiding urination; they actually mean that the pain is made worse with micturition, particularly at the end of urination, when the inflamed bladder walls become apposed. Some symptoms of cystitis are ameliorated by warm tub baths. Patients who complain of persistent frequency, nocturia, terminal hematuria, and suprapubic pain relieved by voiding may have *chronic interstitial cystitis,* a condition that is most common in middle-aged women.

If *Neisseria gonorrhoeae* is the offending organism, the symptoms of urethritis occasionally abate without treatment after a few months. In contrast, the symptoms of nongonorrheal urethritis, although low-grade, usually persist if not treated appropriately.

PHYSICAL FINDINGS

The physical findings of gonorrheal urethritis in men include a spontaneous urethral discharge or one that can be elicited by penile stripping. The most common physical finding in patients with dysuria due to cystitis is suprapubic tenderness to palpation or percussion. When dysuria is due to vaginitis, a vaginal discharge is apparent on pelvic examination.

DIAGNOSTIC STUDIES

In men, *urethritis* is present if a urethral smear shows more than four polymorphonuclear cells per high-power field. All urethral discharges should be examined by Gram stain and culture. A culture should be obtained for *Neisseria gonorrhoeae* and, when indicated, *Chlamydia*. Urine cultures should be obtained for all patients with symptoms of cystitis. In uncomplicated cases, some physicians use only reagent test strips, including the leukocyte esterase test strips, before beginning empiric antibiotic therapy. When sterile pyuria is demonstrated on routine culture, the urine should be cultured for *Chlamydia* and tuberculosis-causing species of *Mycobacterium*.

Laboratory tests are required to distinguish gonorrheal from nongonorrheal urethritis. Because it is frequently difficult to culture *Chlamydia,* physicians often diagnose nongonorrheal urethritis by establishing the presence of urethritis and then excluding gonorrheal infection by smear and culture. *Trichomonas vaginalis* and *Candida albicans* are uncommon causes of urethritis and need not be considered at the initial visit. A Gram smear or a KOH preparation may help identify patients with candidal urethritis, and a saline wet-mount should be examined if trichomonal urethritis is suspected.

The following are considered indications for urologic evaluation: an initial urinary infection in a child, initial urinary tract infection in men, urinary infections in pregnant women, recurrent urinary tract infections (three per year) in women, severe acute urinary tract infections suggesting upper tract involvement, and painless hematuria.

DIFFERENTIAL DIAGNOSIS OF URETHRAL DISCHARGE AND DYSURIA

CAUSE	NATURE OF PATIENT	NATURE OF SYMPTOMS	ASSOCIATED SYMPTOMS	AMELIORATING FACTORS	PRECIPITATING AND AGGRAVATING FACTORS	PHYSICAL FINDINGS	DIAGNOSTIC STUDIES
Cystitis	Most common in women aged 15–34	Dysuria (worse at end of flow) Urgency Frequency "Internal" discomfort Acute onset of symptoms with bacterial infection	Hematuria Nocturia Fever	Avoidance of urinating Warm baths	Meatal stenosis may cause recurrent UTI in children	Suprapubic tenderness to palpation or percussion Fever	Urine culture positive Cystoscopy Special test for *Chlamydia* Pyuria by urinalysis or leukocyte esterase test
Female Urethral Syndrome		Dysuria Urgency Frequency Gradual onset of symptoms over 2–7 days	Suprapubic pain			Suprapubic pain No fever	Minimal pyuria Urine culture usually negative
Vaginitis (see Chapter 32)	Candidiasis more common in diabetics	Dysuria "External burning"	Vaginal itching			Vaginal discharge on pelvic exam	KOH and saline wet-mounts for *Candida* and *Trichomonas* Gram stain and culture for gonococci
Chemical vaginitis	Common cause of dysuria and urethral discharge in young girls	Dysuria "External burning" Urethral discharge (minimal)			Bubble baths Vaginal sprays and douches	Vaginitis	
Prostatitis	Men over age 50	Dysuria Frequency	Backache Fever Decreased or intermittent stream		Abrupt change in frequency of ejaculation (e.g., after a vacation)	May be costovertebral tenderness Prostate tender to palpation on rectal examination	Examination and culture of prostatic secretions

Meatal Stenosis	Children	Dysuria Recurrent urinary tract infection symptoms		
Urethritis				
Gonorrheal	Most common in men	Sexually transmitted Urethral discharge is moderate to large, purulent, mucoid, or mucopurulent and develops 1–3 wk after coitus with infected partner Dysuria (worse at beginning of urine flow)	Sexual contact	Urethral discharge is spontaneous or elicited by penile stripping Gram's stain and culture of urethral smear
Nongonorrheal (chlamydial or trichomonal)	Most common in men	Sexually transmitted Symptoms usually minimal or absent Discharge (if present) is observed on awakening and is thin and clear or whitish Dysuria (ranges in severity) Urgency Frequency	Multiple sexual partners Meatal or urethral irritation	Thin, scanty, and whitish Urethral discharge appears on penile stripping Gram's stain and culture of urethral smear Special test for *Chlamydia* Saline wet-mount for *Trichomonas*
Mechanical	Most common in young boys and girls	Dysuria Minimal urethral discharge	Horseback or bike riding Masturbation Foreign body	

LESS COMMON DIAGNOSTIC CONSIDERATIONS

Less common causes of dysuria and urinary frequency include genital herpes simplex virus, *Trichomonas,* and *Candida* urethritis. Rarely, frequency is an early symptom of a bladder tumor or carcinoma in situ of the bladder.

Relatively uncommon causes of urethritis include infections with *Mycoplasma hominis.* Urethritis secondary to *Mycoplasma* is most common in lower socioeconomic groups and in men and women who have multiple sexual partners. Another uncommon cause of urethritis is Reiter's syndrome, which frequently begins with a urethritis after sexual contact and is followed in a few days by conjunctivitis, mucocutaneous lesions (including balanitis), and arthritis. This type of urethritis is characterized by mucopurulent discharge and dysuria, but it may be asymptomatic. Sometimes Reiter's syndrome may be initiated by a gonorrheal urethritis. In such cases, the urethritis responds to penicillin so that the purulent discharge disappears and is replaced by the less purulent, mucoid discharge of nonspecific urethritis.

Selected References

Bodner, D. R.: The urethral syndrome. Urol. Clin. North Am. *15*:699–703, 1988.

Greydanus, D. E., and McAnarney, E. R.: *Chlamydia trachomatis:* an important sexually transmitted disease in adolescents and young adults. J. Fam. Pract. *10*:611–615, 1980.

Kiel, D. P., and Moshowitz, M. A.: The urinalysis: a critical appraisal. Med. Clin. North Am. *71*:607–624, 1987.

Komaroff, A. L.: Acute dysuria in women. N. Engl. J. Med. *310(6):*368–374, 1984.

Komaroff, A. L.: Urinalysis and urine culture in women with dysuria. Ann. Intern. Med. *107*:212–218, 1986.

Lipsky, B. A.: Urinary tract infections in men. Epidemiology, pathophysiology, diagnosis, and treatment. Ann. Intern. Med. *110*:138–150, 1989.

Martin, D. H., Pollock, S., Kuo, C. C., et al.: *Chlamydia trachomatis* infections in men with Reiter's syndrome. Ann. Intern. Med. 100:207–213, 1984.

Meadows, J. C.: The acute urethral syndrome: diagnosis, management, and prophylaxis. Continuing Education, December 1983, pp. 1112–1129.

Parrott, T. S.: Cystitis and urethritis. Pediatr. Rev. *10*:217–222, 1989.

Chapter 32

Vaginal Discharge and Itching

Vaginal discharge, which may be accompanied by vulvar itching or burning, is one of the most common problems seen in the physician's office. Usually, these symptoms indicate *moniliasis (Candida albicans), trichomoniasis (Trichomonas),* or *Gardnerella vaginalis (Haemophilus vaginalis).* Other common causes of vaginal discharge include *acute cervicitis, gonorrhea,* and *herpes genitalis.* Many discussions of vaginitis emphasize a "typical" appearance of the discharge: cheesy, frothy, or mucoid. Appearances, however, may be misleading. **In addition, 15 to 20 per cent of patients in one series had two coexistent infections.** Other studies of patients with vaginitis have shown that 35 per cent had a *Gardnerella vaginalis,* 25 per cent had moniliasis, and 20 per cent had trichomoniasis. The remaining 20 per cent had less common types of vaginitis.

Vaginitis, in contrast to cervicitis, is an inflammatory change of the vaginal mucosa in the absence of profuse discharge from the cervix. A vaginal discharge can be produced by cervicitis without a significant vaginal infection, as can be the case with *gonorrhea. Chlamydia* also causes a mucopurulent cervicitis.

NATURE OF PATIENT

PREPUBERTAL PATIENTS. Prepubertal girls may develop a vaginal discharge in association with *vulvovaginitis* or an *exocervicitis.* These young girls are particularly susceptible to vulvovaginitis because of the

361

anterior location of the vagina, the proximity of the vagina to the anus, the lack of labial fat pads, a neutral to alkaline vaginal pH, a thin, atrophic vaginal wall, and, occasionally, poor hygiene. *Trichomonas vaginitis* is rare in children and in women over age 60 but does occur in neonates of infected mothers. Conversely, *monilial vaginitis* can occur at any age. It is a common cause of vulvovaginitis in children. In prepubertal girls, vulvovaginitis is more common than vaginitis. Vulvovaginitis can be caused by *bubble baths, other chemical irritants, tight nylon panties, mixed bacterial infections,* and *foreign bodies. Gardnerella* infections are rare in premenarchal girls. **Gonorrheal infections in premenarchal children are rare but do occur. In such cases, sexual abuse must be suspected.** Although a girl may be asymptomatic when a gonococcal infection is present, vulvovaginitis and exocervicitis are usually present.

ADOLESCENTS. After puberty, a vaginal discharge may be due to physiologic factors, cervicitis, or vaginitis. Although *trichomonas vaginitis* and *monilial vaginitis* may occur in adolescents, the most common cause of vaginitis with discharge in adolescent girls is *Gardnerella.* Adolescents are especially susceptible to *Gardnerella* because the changes in vaginal secretions at menarche provide a favorable environment for the *Gardnerella vaginalis* bacillus to grow. *Monilia* is the second most common cause of specific leukorrhea in adolescents. There is a high and increasing incidence of *gonorrhea* among postpubertal women. Among young mothers, the growing prevalence of gonorrhea may increase the incidence of this infection among neonates and some children. It is important to question the patient about genital or urinary infections in other family members (male or female) or sexual partners (male or female).

It must be remembered that a *physiologic leukorrhea* may occur in menarchal girls. This is not usually profuse or associated with itching. Although these girls may be concerned about a vaginal discharge, they may not present with it as a chief complaint. Therefore, the physician should provide reassurance concerning this and other normal changes that may occur with menarche. The discharge that occurs just before and after menarche is often thick, grayish white, and odorless and has a pH of 4.5 to 6.0. There are no signs of inflammation because this discharge is a physiologic reaction to the initial phase of cyclic estrogen production.

ADULTS. In adult women of reproductive age, the common causes of vaginitis are *Candida, Gardnerella,* and *Trichomonas,* in decreasing order of frequency. The three most common causes of cervicitis are *Chlamydia trachomatis, Neisseria gonorrhoeae,* and *herpes simplex virus.* In elderly, postmenopausal women, *senile atrophic vaginitis* often causes a discharge, as do other specific forms of vaginitis.

NATURE OF SYMPTOMS

Vulvovaginitis in premenarchal girls usually causes only minor discomfort, which may include perineal pruritus, burning, and a discharge that may be profuse or scanty.

The duration and type of symptoms do not consistently distinguish the common infectious causes of vaginitis. Certain symptoms and findings, however, strongly suggest the diagnosis. For instance, although an acute onset of vaginal discharge or vulvar irritation indicates that a yeast infection is the probable cause, these symptoms are often unreliable. Likewise, a curdlike discharge (resembling cottage cheese) strongly suggests a yeast vaginitis; **however, the gross appearance is less sensitive and less specific in establishing the diagnosis than is a microscopic examination of the vaginal discharge.** A curdlike appearance virtually eliminates the possibility of a trichomonas vaginitis, which usually produces a profuse, frothy, white or grayish green, malodorous discharge. The discharge in *trichomonas vaginitis* is typically described as frothy, whereas the discharge in *Gardnerella vaginalis (Haemophilus)* may also be frothy in 15 per cent of cases.

Because itching and burning may occur with virtually all forms of vaginitis, these symptoms are not particularly helpful in the differentiation of the cause. Itching is most prominent in *monilial vaginitis* and least prominent in *Gardnerella*. Itching and burning are uncommon with *gonococcal* infections, but a significant percentage of patients with a gonococcal infection have a combined infection. They may have gonorrhea with their itching caused by *Trichomonas* or *monilia*.

If a vaginal discharge is sticky, brown, or yellowish and occurs in an elderly woman, an *atrophic vaginitis* should be suspected.

ASSOCIATED SYMPTOMS

Dysuria may be a symptom of both a vaginal infection and a urinary tract infection. **Therefore, all women who complain of dysuria should be asked about the presence of a vaginal discharge or irritation or both.** About 30 per cent of patients who have vaginitis but no evidence of urinary tract infection complain of dysuria. Usually, these patients complain of "external" dysuria (pain felt in the inflamed vaginal labia as the urinary stream passes) rather than "internal" dysuria (felt inside the body). Internal dysuria seems to correlate with urinary tract infections, whereas external dysuria usually corresponds to vaginal infections.

Dyspareunia usually indicates vulvar disease rather than vaginitis. When dyspareunia is associated with a purulent discharge, *acute cervi-*

citis should be suspected. *Trichomonas vaginitis* is often associated with gonococcal or *Bacteroides* cervicitis. *Trichomonas* and *Chlamydia* may produce a vaginitis as well as a coexisting urethritis that causes dysuria and frequency. If dysuria, rectal infections, or pain on walking or climbing stairs is present, *gonorrhea* should be suspected.

If there are symptoms of diabetes or ingestion of birth control pills or antibiotics, a *monilial vaginitis* is probable. Refractory fungal vulvo-vaginitis may be secondary to undiagnosed diabetes.

PRECIPITATING AND AGGRAVATING FACTORS

Oral contraceptives, antibiotics, and pregnancy predispose the patient to a *Candida vaginitis*. Uncontrolled diabetes and long-term use of tetracycline for acne increase the intestinal reservoir of *Candida*, which predisposes the patient to recurrent monilial vaginitis. *Gardnerella* vaginitis is common and increasing in incidence. It is most frequently spread through venereal contacts. *Trichomonas vaginitis* is usually transmitted by sexual intercourse; in children, however, it may be spread by direct nonsexual contact. The increasing incidence of venereal diseases such as gonorrhea, *Gardnerella,* and trichomoniasis is due to earlier sexual activity, multiple partners, and failure to use protective barrier contraceptives (e.g., diaphragms and condoms).

In young children and in some adults, inappropriate genital hygiene (i.e., wiping the perineal region from back to front) may increase the incidence of recurrent vaginal infections. *Chemical vaginitis* is precipitated by douches, bubble baths, and vaginal sprays. It may be aggravated by powders and panties made of synthetic fibers.

PHYSICAL FINDINGS

Physical examination should include thorough evaluation of the genital and pelvic areas. The appearance of the labia, vulva, entire vagina, and cervix should be noted, and the vaginal discharge should be inspected. Nonspecific vaginitis, which occurs particularly in premenarchal girls, usually does not extend above the lower one-third of the vagina. Atrophic vaginitis can occur in premenarchal girls, as can infections due to insertion of foreign bodies into the vagina. When atrophic vaginitis occurs in postmenopausal women, there is often a sticky, brownish vaginal discharge, and the vaginal mucosa is usually thick, pale, and smooth, demonstrating loss of normal rugosal folds. The pelvic examination should include adnexal palpation and cervical manipulation so that the physician can determine whether there are any masses or points of tenderness. Adnexal tenderness and pain on motion of the cervix ("chandelier sign") suggest *pelvic inflammatory disease*—not merely cervicitis. When these findings occur in conjunction with a vaginal discharge, a *gonococcal* infection is probable. In such cases, if smear and culture are negative for gonorrhea, *Chlamydia* should be suspected and appropriately treated.

DIAGNOSTIC STUDIES

Ninety per cent of patients with vaginitis can be classified into one of four major clinical categories on the basis of symptomatology, vaginal pH, and wet-smear findings; the importance of vaginal pH and wet-smear findings, therefore, is readily apparent (Table 32–1).

In patients whose only symptom of vaginitis is vaginal discharge, a Gram stain is not indicated because it is not specific. However, if a patient has a purulent discharge from the cervical os and a Gram stain that reveals more than three polymorphonuclear leukocytes per high-power field, a chlamydial or gonococcal infection is likely. Intracellular gram-negative diplococci on the Gram stain is highly specific for a gonococcal infection. False-positive results are rare. A Gram stain is recommended whenever there is a purulent discharge from the cervical or urethral os. **Simultaneous chlamydial infections are present in 30 to 50 per cent with cervical gonococcal infections.**

In some populations in which there is a high prevalence of asymptomatic gonococcal carriers, a cervical culture for *Neisseria gonorrhoeae* on Thayer-Martin medium is considered appropriate whenever a patient has a pelvic examination. It certainly should be performed in any woman with a purulent discharge from the cervical os or urethra.

In all patients with a vaginal discharge, saline and KOH wet-mounts should be examined. The saline mount should be inspected for "clue cells" (epithelial cells with bacilli adherent to their surface), which are virtually pathognomonic of *Gardnerella vaginalis*. *Gardnerella vaginalis* may also be diagnosed on the basis of a positive culture in Casman's broth or blood agar. These cultures must be done promptly because the organisms are susceptible to drying and alkaline pH. The

TABLE 32–1. Classification of Vaginitis

Type of Vaginitis	Symptom	pH	Wet Smear Findings
Candidiasis (moniliasis)	Pruritus	4.2–4.9	Hyphae or spores
Gardnerella vaginitis	Malodorous	5.6–6.3	"Clue" cells
Trichomoniasis	Profuse discharge	4.9–5.6	Protozoa and white blood cells
Atrophic vaginitis	Discharge	7	Parabasal cells

pH range of secretions in patients with *Gardnerella* infection is usually greater than 4.5. A positive "sniff test" (presence of a fishy or amine odor when 10 per cent KOH is added to a sample of the discharge) also indicates *Gardnerella* vaginitis.

The saline wet-mount is the most reliable laboratory test for confirmation of the motile protozoan *Trichomonas*. It should be done as soon as possible after the specimen is obtained. The pH of the vaginal secretions in patients with *Trichomonas* infection ranges from 4.9 to 5.6.

The best test for detection of *monilial* vaginitis is microscopic examination of the discharge in a KOH preparation; this will show the *Candida* mycelia. The pH in patients with monilial vaginitis ranges from 4.2 to 4.9. Cultures, though most sensitive, should be reserved for certain circumstances because 15 to 20 per cent will be positive in asymptomatic healthy women.

LESS COMMON DIAGNOSTIC CONSIDERATIONS

Increased physiologic leukorrhea has a pH of 3.8 to 4.2, an absence of yeast and *Trichomonas,* and a culture with a preponderance of *Lactobacillus.* Dermatoses (e.g., psoriasis and seborrheic dermatitis) and infestations with parasites (e.g., amebiasis, pinworms, and lice) can cause vaginal discharge in rare cases. Allergy to nylon underwear and feminine deodorants, sprays, and douches may cause a vulvovaginitis leading to vaginal discharge or itching. Vaginal and cervical neoplasms can cause a serosanguineous discharge. Poor anal and vulvar hygiene also may produce vaginal discharge and itching. Tuberculosis is a rare cause of vulvovaginitis. In premenarchal girls, particularly young children, coliform bacterial infections may produce vaginitis. This is usually a low-grade, somewhat chronic infection and may be associated with pinworm infestation or insertion of foreign body into the vagina. Retained tampons and other foreign objects may be found occasionally in adults.

Herpes simplex type II, herpes genitalis, is a relatively uncommon cause of vaginal discharge (although a common cause of cervicitis), but it is increasing in frequency. It is certainly receiving much attention from the media and the public. It is most common in adolescents and appears less frequently in patients over age 35. Herpetic lesions, which can be excruciating, affect not only the vulva but also adjacent areas (thighs, buttocks, vagina, and cervix). The lesions begin as vesicles that progress in 5 to 10 days to shallow, exquisitely painful ulcerations with a clear, watery discharge. The ulcers last for 3 to 10 days and are prone to secondary infections, especially with *Streptococcus* and *Candida.* Unfortunately, genital herpes is often recurrent; some patients experience repeated flare-ups for many years. The presenting symptoms may

DIFFERENTIAL DIAGNOSIS OF VAGINAL DISCHARGE AND ITCHING

CAUSE	NATURE OF PATIENT	NATURE OF SYMPTOMS	ASSOCIATED SYMPTOMS	PRECIPITATING AND AGGRAVATING FACTORS	PHYSICAL FINDINGS	DIAGNOSTIC STUDIES
Vulvovaginitis due to: *Candida* Chemical irritants Douches Vaginal sprays Bubble baths Bacteria Foreign bodies	Most common cause of vaginal discharge in prepubertal girls	Variable discharge (scanty to profuse) Perineal pruritus Burning	May be "internal" dysuria		Vulvovaginitis does not usually extend above lower third of vagina Thin atrophic vaginal wall	
Physiologic discharge	Menarchal girls	Discharge is thick, grayish white, odorless, but not profuse No pruritus		Beginning estrogen effect occurs just before or after menarche	No signs of inflammation	pH of discharge is 4.5–6.0
Moniliasis (candidiasis)	Any age Common cause of vulvovaginitis in children Common during reproductive years	Acute onset of discharge or vulvar irritation Discharge is often curdlike (resembles cottage cheese) Pruritus is prominent	May be "external" dysuria	Diabetes Antibiotics Birth control pills Pregnancy	Vaginitis	Saline or KOH wet-mount shows hyphae or spores Vaginal pH is 4.2–4.9

Table continued on following page

367

DIFFERENTIAL DIAGNOSIS OF VAGINAL DISCHARGE AND ITCHING *Continued*

CAUSE	NATURE OF PATIENT	NATURE OF SYMPTOMS	ASSOCIATED SYMPTOMS	PRECIPITATING AND AGGRAVATING FACTORS	PHYSICAL FINDINGS	DIAGNOSTIC STUDIES
Trichomoniasis	Common cause of vaginal discharge in women of child-bearing age Rare in children Rare in women over age 60 May occur in neonates of infected mothers	Discharge is usually profuse, frothy, gray-greenish and malodorous Varying degrees of pruritus	May be associated with gonococcal or *Bacteroides* infection Urethritis may cause dysuria and frequency	Often sexually transmitted Multiple sex partners	Vaginitis Vaginal petechiae Mucosal inflammation	Vaginal pH is 4.9–5.6 Saline wet-mount shows white blood cells and motile protozoa
Bacterial vaginosis (*Gardnerella vaginalis* and other anaerobes)	Most common cause of vaginitis in adolescents Common during reproductive years Rare in premenarchal girls	Discharge is malodorous but not usually frothy Pruritus not prominent	Urethritis may cause dysuria and frequency	Change in vaginal secretions at menarche Sexually transmitted Multiple sex partners	Vaginitis	Saline wet-mount shows "clue" cells Vaginal pH is 5.6–6.3
Gonorrhea	Increased incidence in neonates of infected mothers Rare in premenarchal girls (if present, sexual abuse must be suspected)	Itching and burning uncommon Purulent cervical discharge Pelvic pain Fever	Dysuria Rectal infection (often asymptomatic) Pain on walking or climbing stairs	Symptoms often worse near time of menstrual period Sexually transmitted	Cervicitis and cervical discharge Pain with cervical manipulation Adnexal tenderness	Gram stain of discharge reveals intracellular gram-negative diplococci Positive culture Chlamydial infections common
Chlamydia			Dysuria	Sexually transmitted	Cervicitis and cervical discharge Pain with cervical manipulation	Tests for chlamydia Often coexists with cervical gonococcal infections

Herpes genitalis	Most commonly sexually active adolescents Less frequently patients over age 35 years	Pain can be excruciating Vulvar pruritus uncommon Burning Vulvar tenderness	Dyspareunia Dysuria	Secondary *Streptococcus* or *Candida* infection	Cervicitis Widespread clusters of vesicles over vulvar and perineal areas, vagina, and cervix Herpetic lesions: Affect vulva and adjacent areas Begin as vesicles Progress in 5–10 days to shallow, painful ulcers Ulcers last 3–10 days Recurrent Does not usually produce vaginitis	Tzanck smear
Senile atrophic vaginitis	Elderly women	Discharge is sticky, brown, or yellowish		Loss of estrogen effect	Vaginal mucosa is thin, pale, and smooth (owing to loss of rugosal folds)	Vaginal pH is 7.0 Parabasal cells

include pain, vulvar pruritus, burning, and frequently extreme vulvar tenderness that makes intercourse unbearable. Micturition also may be excruciating. Examination reveals widespread clusters of vesicles that may involve the vulvar and perineal areas as well as the vagina and cervix. It is important for the physician to remember that herpes does not usually produce vaginitis, although it may infect the vagina and cervix. A Tzanck smear of the base of the vesicle is a simple, definitive diagnostic test.

Selected References

Adler, M. W.: ABC of sexually transmitted diseases. Vaginal discharge: diagnosis. Br. Med. J. 287(6404):1529–1531, 1983.

Berg, A. O., and Soman, M. P.: Lower genitourinary infections in women. J. Fam. Pract. 23:61–67, 1986.

Eschenbach, D. A., and Hillier, S. L.: Advances in diagnostic testing for vaginitis and cervicitis. J. Reprod. Med. 34(8 Suppl):555–564, 1989.

Hammill, H. A.: Unusual causes of vaginitis (excluding trichomonas, bacterial vaginosis and Candida albicans). Obstet. Gynecol. Clin. North Am. 16:337–345, 1989.

Quan, M.: Diagnosis and management of infectious vaginitis. J. Am. Board Fam. Pract. 3:195–205, 1990.

Schneider, G. T.: Vaginal infections. How to identify and treat them. Postgrad. Med. 73:255–262, 1983.

Singleton, A. E.: Vaginal discharge in children and adolescents—evolution and management: a review. Clin. Pediatr. 19:799–804, 1980.

Weaver, C. H., and Mengel, M. B.: Bacterial vaginoses. J. Fam. Pract. 27:207–215, 1988.

Woodruff, J. D.: Vulvar disease: a spectrum of clinical pictures. Postgrad. Med. 73:232–245, 1983.

Chapter 33

Voiding Disorders and Incontinence

Voiding disorders and incontinence are common disorders of micturition that present to the physician. They occur more frequently in the elderly. Currently 12 per cent of Americans are over age 65, and by the year 2000, 15 per cent of Americans will be over 65. **Voiding dysfunction is the rule rather than the exception in elderly men.** Signs and symptoms of *benign prostatic hypertrophy* have been found in about 70 per cent of elderly men. **Incontinence is so frequent in women that many patients consider it normal.** Decreased bladder capacity and involuntary bladder contractions have been found in as many as 20 per cent of continent elderly. About 10 to 20 per cent of community-dwelling elderly patients have *urinary incontinence* severe enough to be considered a social or health problem. Large-scale studies have reported that one-third of people over age 60 occasionally experience an involuntary loss of urine. An even larger percentage of hospitalized and institutionalized elderly patients are troubled with incontinence.

Childhood enuresis (bed-wetting), whether primary or secondary, should be considered a symptom by the physician rather than a specific diagnosis. Most cases of *enuresis* represent *primary enuresis,* a maturational delay that occasionally is familial. Secondary enuresis is when a child who has been continent develops enuresis. *Secondary enuresis* may be due to emotional stress (birth of a sibling, beginning school) or urinary tract infection. In these children, bacteriuria may cause uninhibited bladder contractions. Most children with nocturnal or daytime incontinence (99 per cent) do not have an anatomic abnormality; rather, there is a disturbance in urodynamics, such as bladder instability.

NATURE OF PATIENT

Enuresis is common until about ages 4 to 5. **Most children with voiding disturbances do not have anatomic or neurologic disease**

causing their enuresis. Voiding dysfunction is common in elderly men. The amount of prostatic enlargement does not necessarily correlate with the symptoms of prostatism. Some young men without prostatic enlargement on rectal examination have symptoms of prostatism—the so-called trapped prostate. Incontinence is more common in women than in men. It occurs more frequently in multiparous and menopausal women. Age-related changes in bladder function include decreased capacity, increased residual urine, increased involuntary bladder contractions (detrusor muscle instability), and increased nocturnal urine production. **Incontinence has been reported in 26 per cent of women during their reproductive years, but in the postmenopausal years, the incidence is 30 to 40 per cent.**

NATURE OF SYMPTOMS

The symptoms of prostatism can be divided into two categories: obstructive symptoms, including weak stream, abdominal straining, hesitancy, intermittency of stream, incomplete emptying, and terminal dribbling, and irritative symptoms, including frequency, nocturia, and urgency. Some patients have symptoms of prostatic enlargement and also have symptoms related to unstable detrusor muscle contractions. The symptoms of benign prostatic hypertrophy often wax and wane spontaneously probably because of changes in dynamic factors, which include bladder tone, bladder neck obstruction, and tone in the prostate and prostatic capsule.

An abrupt onset of symptoms of stress incontinence or urge incontinence suggests an infectious cause. The gradual onset of symptoms of stress incontinence, particularly after menopause or oophorectomy, suggests that the symptoms are related to estrogen deficiency. When the amount of urine leakage is small to moderate and coincides with instances of increased abdominal pressure, stress incontinence is probable. Large amounts of urine incontinence suggest detrusor muscle instability, as does incontinence associated with the sensation of a full bladder. A precipitous loss of large quantities of urine unrelated to increased abdominal pressure suggests involuntary detrusor contractions, as does incontinence associated with an extreme desire to void because of pain, inflammation, or a sense of impending micturition. Moderate dripping suggests a partially incompetent outlet, overflow, or congenital or acquired anomalies.

ASSOCIATED SYMPTOMS

Microscopic or gross hematuria, from rupture of blood vessels coursing over an enlarged prostate, often occurs in patients with prostatic hypertrophy. In these instances, cystoscopy or intravenous pyelography is indicated to rule out a stone or cancer. *Infection, neurologic disease,* and *bladder carcinoma* may produce hematuria and other symptoms similar to those of benign prostatic hypertrophy. In addition, gradual obstruction from prostatic enlargement or carcinoma may lead to a large, distended bladder with overflow incontinence. Urinary retention is more common when symptoms of prostatism develop in less than 3 months or when secondary to drugs. Urinary retention is less common when symptoms develop gradually. Recurrent cystitis occurs more frequently in patients with persistent residual urine due to an atonic bladder, cystocele, prostatic hypertrophy, or diabetes mellitus.

Table 33–1 shows some of the factors that help in differentiating unstable bladder contractions from stress incontinence. Nocturia is rare in stress incontinence but occurs frequently with detrusor instability. Urgency and frequency occasionally occur in patients with stress incontinence but is the rule in patients with detrusor instability. Voluntary inhibition of incontinence is frequently present in patients with stress incontinence but is less probable in patients with detrusor muscle instability.

PRECIPITATING AND AGGRAVATING FACTORS

Stress incontinence may be precipitated or aggravated by coughing, lifting, exercising, and change in position. Incontinence caused by detrusor muscle instability may be precipitated or aggravated by the urge to void, a full bladder, or position change. Detrusor muscle instability is aggravated by bladder wall inflammation and estrogen deficiency. Drugs that may precipitate or aggravate stress incontinence include methyldopa, prazosin, phenothiazines, diazepam, and diuretics. Drugs that may

TABLE 33–1. Comparison of Presenting Symptoms in Patients with Genuine Stress Incontinence and Detrusor Instability

Symptoms	Genuine stress incontinence	Detrusor instability
Precipitating factor	Cough, lifting, exercise, position change	Preceding urge, position change
Timing of leakage	Immediate	Delayed
Amount of leakage	Small → large	Large
Voluntary inhibition	Frequently	Possibly
Urgency, frequency	Occasionally	Yes
Nocturia	Rarely	Yes
Spontaneous remission	No	Occasionally

From Horbach, N. S.: Problems in the clinical diagnosis of stress incontinence. J. Reprod. Med. *35*:751–756, 1990.

DIFFERENTIAL DIAGNOSIS OF VOIDING PROBLEMS AND INCONTINENCE

CONDITION	NATURE OF PATIENT	NATURE OF SYMPTOMS	ASSOCIATED SYMPTOMS	PRECIPITATING AND AGGRAVATING FACTORS	AMELIORATING FACTORS	PHYSICAL EXAMINATION	DIAGNOSTIC STUDIES
Benign prostatic hypertrophy	Common in older men	Nocturia, dribbling, hesitancy, decreased force of stream, incomplete emptying	Hematuria	Prostatitis, residual urine, drugs: alcohol, anticholinergics, decongestants, sympathomimetics, antidepressants	Occasional spontaneous remission of symptoms	Enlarged prostate, distended bladder	Ultrasound for prostate size and residual volume, Intravenous urography, Cystoscopy, Urinalysis, Creatinine level
Incontinence stress	Multiparous and menopausal women, Postprostatectomy men	Small-quantity incontinence with cough, sneezing, laughing, and running	Recurrent cystitis	Cystitis, laughing, coughing, and upper respiratory infections		Weakness or laxity of pelvic floor or urethral sphincter, Atrophic vagina in elderly women	Urinalysis, Residual volume, Creatinine level
Urge (unstable detrusor contractions)	Elderly men more than women, Poststroke, Dementia	Uncontrolled urge to void, Large-quantity incontinence	Unable to delay voiding long enough to reach toilet	Cystitis, urethritis, bladder calculi, alcohol, diuretics			In selected cases: cystometry, urodynamics, uroflowometry, or video-urodynamics

Type	Causes	Symptoms		Contributing Factors	Course/Management	Physical Findings	Workup
Overflow	Multiple sclerosis Severe benign prostatic hypertrophy Atonic bladder Diabetic neuropathy Tabes dorsalis	Small-quantity incontinence, nearly continuous dribbling		Medications, including anticholinergics and sympathomimetics Prostatitis in patients with severe benign prostatic hypertrophy		Distended bladder, anatomic bladder obstruction from benign prostatic hypertrophy or stricture, evidence of spinal cord disease or diabetic neuropathy	
Functional	Impaired mobility or mental status Dementia	Can void normally with assistance		Deterioration in mental or physical status	Toilet training	Severe mental or physical disability preventing normal toilet habits Lower urinary tract function is normal	
Enuresis	Children older than age 5, generally not significant if <4½ years	Bed-wetting while sleeping	Very sound sleep	Emotional stress Urinary tract infections	Usually spontaneous improvement as child grows older (> age 5)	Usually normal	Urinalysis and culture Rarely: ultrasound for hydroureteronephrosis or residual urine Urodynamics

precipitate urinary retention include alpha-adrenergic agents, androgens, and sympathomimetic agents such as ephedrine and pseudoephedrine. Psychotropic and sedative agents may diminish alertness and facilitate or precipitate urinary incontinence. Some autonomic agents precipitate incontinence, whereas others precipitate urinary retention.

AMELIORATING FACTORS

The symptoms of prostatism may spontaneously diminish without appreciable change in the size of the prostate. The symptoms and degree of obstruction vary over time despite the absence of change in prostatic size. Cessation of drugs that aggravate urinary retention or incontinence alleviates symptoms. Systemic and local estrogens often improve the symptoms of stress incontinence, although they may not have been administered for that reason. Antibiotics may improve cystitis, and thereby reduce detrusor instability. Improvement in mental status or mobility of the patient often ameliorates the symptoms of incontinence.

PHYSICAL EXAMINATION

Examination of patients with voiding disorders or incontinence must include assessment of their mental and neurologic status, mobility, and general health. Prostatic enlargement may be detected by rectal examination, although symptoms of bladder outlet obstruction may occur without prostatic enlargement being appreciated. In these instances, a so-called trapped prostate or median bar obstruction may only be detected by cystoscopic examination. Neurologic examination may provide clues to sensory or motor dysfunction of the bladder, which is under the control of S2, S3, and S4. Flexion and extension of the ankle, knee, and hip against resistance, as well as assessment of rectal sphincter tone, should be performed to assess whether S2–S4 are intact. Pelvic examination should be performed to assess the patient's estrogen status as well as the presence of a cystocele. The urethra, trigone, and vaginal area are all estrogen-dependent. The presence of a large, distended bladder may be detected on physical examination, although more sophisticated tests are needed to assess the amount of residual urine.

DIAGNOSTIC STUDIES

Patients with voiding disturbances or incontinence may have increased residual urine. Postvoid residual urine can be assessed by abdominal ultrasonography. This technique permits serial, noninvasive measurements of residual urine. Likewise, postvoid residual urine can be determined by catheterization, transabdominal ultrasonography, and postvoid films taken after intravenous pyelography. The Q-tip test is also useful in the evaluation of stress incontinence. This test provides information on the mobility of the urethrovesical junction. It is positive if the Q-tip inserted in the urethra moves 30 degrees or more from the horizontal with coughing or straining. Incontinent patients should have a urinalysis to rule out infection or hematuria. The stress test (in which the patient, with a full bladder, coughs in both the erect and the recumbent position) is also useful in the evaluation of stress incontinence.

Cystoscopy allows visualization of the bladder wall and determination of the degree of urethral obstruction. Trabeculation of the bladder wall suggests chronic obstruction. Urodynamic studies assess urine flow and force of the stream. Cystometry measures filling pressures and detrusor tone to evaluate bladder function. Videourodynamics combines video of voiding with the simultaneous measurement of intravesicular, perivesicular, and rectal pressure. Transrectal prostatic ultrasonography can be used to determine prostate size as well as the presence of prostatic nodules. It can be used to guide prostatic biopsies. Prostatic specific antigen is helpful in screening for prostatic cancer.

LESS COMMON DIAGNOSTIC CONSIDERATIONS

Multiple sclerosis, spinal cord disease, tumors, trauma, syphilis, and diabetic neuropathy can all cause voiding disorders as well as incontinence, usually overflow incontinence. Urethral stricture, dyssynergic bladder neck contracture, prostate cancer, chronic prostatitis, and bladder cancer may cause symptoms similar to those of benign prostatic hypertrophy. Ureterovaginal prolapse or prolapse of a large cystocele may cause urethral obstruction.

Selected References

Bowen, L. W.: Voiding dysfunction. Obstet. Gynecol. Clin. North Am. *16*:869–882, 1989.

Christensen, M. M., and Bruskewitz, R. C.: Clinical manifestations of benign prostatic hyperplasia and indications for therapeutic interaction. Urol. Clin. North Am. *17*:509–516, 1990.

Horbach, N. S.: Problems in the clinical diagnosis of stress incontinence. J. Reprod. Med. *35*:751–757, 1990.

Koff, S. A.: Evaluation and management of voiding disorders in children. Urol. Clin. North Am. *15*:769–775, 1988.

McLorie, F. A., and Husmann, D. A.: Incontinence and enuresis. Pediatr. Clin. North Am. *34*:1159–1174, 1987.

Ouslander, J. G., and Bruskewitz, R.: Disorders of micturition in the aging patient. Adv. Intern. Med. *34*:165–190, 1989.

Parulkar, B. G., and Barrett, D. M.: Urinary incontinence in adults. Surg. Clin. North Am. 68:945–963, 1988.
Ruff, C. C., and Reaves, E. L.: Diagnosing urinary incontinence in adults. Nurse Pract. 14:8–10, 12–14, 16–18, 1989.
Saxton, H. M.: Urodynamics: the appropriate modality for the investigation of frequency, urgency, incontinence and voiding difficulties. Radiology 175:307–316, 1990.
Smith, R. A., Wake, R., and Soloway, M. S.: Benign prostatic hyperplasia. Postgrad. Med. 83:79–85, 1988.
Weiss, B. D.: Nonpharmacologic treatment of urinary incontinence. Am. Fam. Physician 44:579–586, 1991.

Chapter 34

Weight Gain and Weight Loss

WEIGHT GAIN

Without doubt, the most common cause of weight gain is *increased caloric intake,* regardless of what the patient states. Recent studies have investigated causes of obesity other than excessive caloric intake. Rather than defining obesity simply as excessive weight for height and build (greater than 30 kg/m^2), it is better defined as an abnormally high deposition of fat. This is best measured with calipers and a body-mass index. Weight gain due to *fluid retention* occurs in patients with the nephrotic syndrome, congestive heart failure, or cirrhosis with ascites; in these patients, there are clear signs of edema. *Hypothyroidism* can lead to decreased metabolic needs and to weight gain, but for significant weight gain to occur, hypothyroidism must be pronounced, and it is usually clinically apparent. *Physiologic weight gain* occurs as a result of pregnancy and premenstrual fluid retention. Commonly prescribed *drugs* (e.g., steroids and antidepressants) can cause weight gain by promoting salt and water retention or by stimulating appetite.

Nature of Patient

Although the most common type of obesity in children is *exogenous,* this diagnosis requires that endocrine and genetic causes of obesity be considered. Children with exogenous obesity often show accelerated or at least normal linear growth and may reach puberty early. **Most children with endogenous obesity are short for their age and have other associated abnormalities. All obese children with short stature should be evaluated promptly and carefully.**

There are no particularly distinguishing characteristics of patients who are obese other than excessive weight. Although it is said that fat people are jolly, they may experience *depression,* which can be either the result of their being overweight or the cause of their overeating. Some patients with mild depression due to seasonal affective disorder have a carbohydrate craving. Their mood improves after carbohydrate ingestion. There are rare instances of *familial obesity;* in most instances, this probably represents an acquired propensity to overeat. In cases of familial obesity, various members of the family are short and obese. Their obesity tends to be proximal but can have a generalized distribution.

Weight increase in patients with *edema syndromes* (cirrhosis, nephrosis, and congestive heart failure) usually is accompanied by symptoms that suggest a deteriorating clinical status.

Nature of Symptoms

Patients may present complaining of weight gain, uncontrollable appetite, inability to diet, or too-tight garments. The weight gain associated with fluid retention in the *premenstrual period* usually is described as bloating and often is accompanied by breast tenderness, breast swelling, or finger swelling. Some patients with *hypothyroidism* comment that their skin seems puffy or that they are unable to lose weight on diets that previously had resulted in weight loss.

Associated Symptoms and Ameliorating Factors

Sudden, marked changes in weight that occur over 1 to 2 days usually are related to changes in fluid balance. Changes may range from a few pounds gained because of *premenstrual edema* or *salt-retaining drugs* to many pounds added as the result of *cyclic edema.* The weight gain of premenstrual edema usually dissipates after menstruation. Patients usually can alleviate fluid retention that occurs with *cyclic edema* by maintaining a recumbent posture for 48 to 72 hours. The weight gain caused by salt-retaining *drugs* is not continuously progressive; it levels off after a weight increase of several pounds. When weight gain is progressive and the patient appears to be obese without evidence of edema, it is reasonably certain that the patient's weight gain is due to *overeating.*

Precipitating and Aggravating Factors

Weight gain results from ingestion of more calories than are metabolized. Thus, although weight gain usually is related to increased caloric intake, it also can be produced by reduction of either physical activity or metabolic rate. These weight changes occur gradually.

Although most people eat less when they are tense or upset, 15 to 25 per cent respond to stress with increased caloric intake, or *reactive hyperphagia*. These patients often are overweight. They eat excessively when they are depressed or anxious and likewise celebrate good times with elaborate meals.

Drug ingestion is an important factor in weight gain. Steroids, nonsteroidal anti-inflammatory agents, phenylbutazone, and lithium all may cause fluid retention and produce a weight gain of several pounds. Birth control pills increase weight by causing fluid retention, increasing appetite, and creating an anabolic effect. Psychotropic agents (e.g., tricyclic antidepressants, some phenothiazines, and some other antipsychotics) may produce a carbohydrate craving in patients taking these drugs. In addition, when antidepressant drugs alleviate the anorexia of depression, a pronounced weight gain may occur. Propranolol may cause weight gain through its induction of hypoglycemia.

Physical Findings

In obese patients, adipose tissue usually is generally distributed, but it occasionally is proximally concentrated in the extremities. Proximal obesity associated with a "buffalo hump," hirsutism, hypertension, or diabetes suggests *Cushing's disease*. Marked weight gain due to *edema* usually is associated with pitting edema of the legs, ascites, gallop rhythm, or, in the nephrotic syndrome, swelling of the eyelids and facial edema. The physical findings of *hypothyroidism* may include somewhat coarse, dry skin; coarse hair; loss of the outer third of the eyebrows; a low, hoarse voice; an enlarged thyroid; and "hung-up" ankle jerks (delayed contraction and relaxation phase of deep tendon reflexes). The hung-up ankle jerk is often more readily detected when the patient kneels on a bed, chair, or examining table with his feet extended over the edge. Tapping the Achilles tendon with a reflex hammer may show a prompt contraction phase but a more readily perceived slowed relaxation phase.

Diagnostic Studies

Although hypothyroidism is an uncommon cause of obesity, it is readily diagnosed by thyroid function tests.

Less Common Diagnostic Considerations

Endogenous causes of obesity are rare but usually can be diagnosed by other associated findings. Several causes are associated with short

Text continued on page 386

DIFFERENTIAL DIAGNOSIS OF WEIGHT GAIN

CAUSE	NATURE OF PATIENT	NATURE OF SYMPTOMS	ASSOCIATED SYMPTOMS	PRECIPITAT-ING FACTORS	AMELIORAT-ING FACTORS	PHYSICAL FINDINGS
Physiologic Factors Pregnancy	Females of reproductive age	Amenorrhea				Enlarged uterus
Premenstrual fluid retention	Menstruating females	Premenstrual weight gain	Breast tenderness and breast swelling Finger swelling	End of menstrual cycle	End of menstruation	Swelling of extremities Tender, swollen breasts
Excessive Ca-loric Intake (most common cause of weight gain)	Patients who over-eat	Gradual, pro-gressive weight in-crease	Children Show normal linear growth May reach pu-berty early Adults Show depression or psychologic dependency on food	Increased stress ("reactive hy-perphagia")	Decreased caloric intake and/or in-creased caloric needs	No evidence of edema Obesity is gener-ally distributed (may have proxi-mal concentra-tion)
Drugs	Users of: Steroids Nonsteroidal anti-inflam-matory agents				Cessation of drug	

Phenylbutazone Lithium Antipsychotics Antidepressants Propranolol Birth control pills			
Edema Syndromes Nephrotic syndrome Congestive heart failure Cirrhosis (with ascites)	Weight increase may be sudden and rapid (over 24–48 hours)	Edema Signs of deteriorating clinical status Signs of primary condition	Depends on primary disease Edema (may be pitting in legs) Periorbital edema Gallop rhythm Ascites
Metabolic Causes Hypothyroidism	Patient unable to lose weight on previously successful plan	Constipation Intolerance of cold weather Skin is puffy, coarse, and dry	Enlarged thyroid "Hung-up" ankle jerk Coarse hair Loss of outer one-third of eyebrows Low, hoarse voice
Cushing's disease	Proximal obesity	Diabetes Proximal obesity	"Buffalo hump" Hirsutism Hypertension

DIFFERENTIAL DIAGNOSIS OF WEIGHT LOSS

CAUSE	NATURE OF PATIENT	NATURE OF SYMPTOMS	ASSOCIATED SYMPTOMS	PRECIPITAT-ING FACTORS	AMELIORAT-ING FACTORS	PHYSICAL FINDINGS
Aging	Elderly people	Anorexia	Occasional dyspepsia	Poverty Depression Drugs Inadequate caloric intake	Increased caloric intake	Decreased lean body mass
Depression	All ages, especially elderly people	Dysphoria Anorexia	Insomnia Fatigue Decreased libido Sleep disorders	Loss of any type	Antidepressants Improved social situation	Depressed affect
Systemic diseases, especially cardiopulmonary, infectious, metabolic		Those of underlying disease	Dyspnea Edema Fatigue Fever	Deterioration of underlying disease		Those of underlying disease

Medications	Drug administration and/or increased dosage	Cessation of drug administration
Users of: Sedatives Antidepressants Clonidine Diuretics NSAIDs Theophylline Digoxin ACE inhibitors Antibiotics Thyroid supplements Levodopa Chemotherapeutic agents	Drowsiness Dry mouth Drowsiness Cramps Indigestion Nausea Nausea Distortion of taste Nervousness Nausea and vomiting	
Cancer	Anorexia Those of the cancer	Those of underlying disease
AIDS	More common in young men Recurrent infections	Adenopathy

stature. Pseudohypoparathyroidism is characterized by short stature, short metacarpals, hypocalcemia, and occasionally mental retardation. The Prader-Willi syndrome is characterized by short stature, mental retardation, and hypogenitalism. The Laurence-Moon-Biedl syndrome is characterized by short stature, mental retardation, hypogonadism, and retinal pigmentation.

Other rare causes of obesity that are not particularly associated with short stature include Cushing's syndrome and insulinomas. Patients with insulinomas invariably have symptoms of hypoglycemia. Patients with hypothalamic tumors may present with obesity, but there usually are other findings suggestive of an intracranial tumor. Cyclic edema is more common in women than in men. Postencephalitic obesity, tumors of the third ventricle, obesity that develops after cerebral trauma, and certain brain tumors (e.g., chromophobe adenomas and craniopharyngiomas) are other rare causes of hyperphagia.

WEIGHT LOSS

Unexplained weight loss of greater than 5 per cent within 6 to 12 months suggests underlying pathology. It is important to differentiate anorexia (loss of the desire to eat) from true weight loss, although true weight loss results from anorexia when caloric intake is substantially reduced. Significant weight loss may occur in patients with anorexia secondary to psychological, cardiac, pulmonary, hepatic, renal, and metabolic diseases as well as drug ingestion. Weight loss is often the presenting symptom in patients with cancer and chronic infectious processes. Weight loss with anorexia occurs often in patients with depression, anxiety, anorexia nervosa and gastrointestinal disorders, including malabsorption, regional enteritis, granulomatous colitis, ulcerative colitis, chronic liver disease, and carcinoma of the stomach and pancreas.

Weight loss may occur with a normal appetite and adequate intake in patients with diabetes mellitus, acquired immunodeficiency syndrome (AIDS), hyperthyroidism, and decreased intestinal absorption (sprue, short bowel syndrome, parasitic infestation, and inflammatory bowel disease). Athletes in their zest to decrease fatness may develop food aversion and experience weight loss.

Anorexia and weight loss are frequent in elderly people. The causes are numerous, and range from loose dentures and poverty to drug ingestion, metabolic disease, and cancer cachexia. Robbins (1989) described the "nine d's" of weight loss in the elderly: dentition, dysgeusia, dysphagia, diarrhea, disease (chronic), depression, dementia, dysfunction, and drugs. The most common causes are psychiatric, cancer, drugs, and benign upper gastrointestinal disease.

Selected References

Ackerman, S.: The management of obesity. Hosp. Pract. March 1983, pp. 117–139.

Alemany, M.: The etiologic basis for the classification of obesity. Prog. Food Nutr. Sci. *13*:45–66, 1989.

Kalucy, R. S.: Drug induced weight gain. Drugs *19*:278–288, 1980.

Morley, J. E., Silver, A. J., Miller, D. K., and Rubenstein, L. Z.: The anorexia of the elderly. Ann. N.Y. Acad. Sci. *575*:50–59, 1989.

Olsen-Noll, C. G., and Bosworth, M. F.: Anorexia and weight loss in the elderly. Causes range from loose dentures to debilitating illness. Postgrad. Med. *85*:140–144, 1989.

Richmond, D. A., Blyer, E. M., and Linscheid, T. R.: The obese child. Am. Fam. Physician *28*:129–134, 1983.

Robbins, L. J.: Evaluation of weight loss in the elderly. Geriatrics *44*:31–34, 37, 1989.

Wurtman, J. J.: Disorders of food intake. Excessive carbohydrate snack intake among a class of obese people. Ann. N.Y. Acad. Sci. *499*:197–202, 1987.

INDEX

Note: Page numbers followed by an i indicate illustrations; those followed by a t indicate tables.

Abdomen, acute, 1
Abdominal pain, 1–17
  associated symptoms with, 9
  children with, 19–28
    appendicitis and, 20
    associated symptoms in, 22
    characteristics of, 19–20
    diagnostic studies for, 24–25
    differential diagnosis in, 26t–27t
    physical findings in, 22–23
    surgery for, 19
    symptoms in, 20–21
  diagnostic studies for, 12–13
  differential diagnosis of, 14t–16t
  in elderly, 2–3
  factors in, 8–9
  laparotomy for, 12
  location of, 5–8, 21–22
  nature of, 4–5, 20–21
  patient characteristics and, 2–4
  peritonitis with, 10
  physical findings with, 10
  rarer causes of, 13–17, 25–28
  surgery for, 2–4
  vomiting with, 9
Abortion, spontaneous, 221t
Abruptio placentae, 213
Abscess, dental, 138, 147t, 162
Abuse, child, 352, 362
  substance. See Substance abuse.
Achalasia, 239t
Achilles tendinitis, 243–244, 249t
Acidosis, diabetic, 21–22, 24
Acne, 307–308, 326t. See also Skin
    problems.
Acoustic neuroma. See Neuroma, acoustic.
Acquired immunodeficiency syndrome
    (AIDS), 76, 385t, 386
Adenoids, enlarged, cough with, 96
Adenoma, bronchial, 301
Aerophagia. See Belching.
AIDS. See Acquired immunodeficiency
    syndrome (AIDS).
Alcohol, abuse of. See Substance abuse.
  palpitations and, 289–290, 293t

Allergies, 95, 97, 100t. See also specific
    types, e.g., Dermatitis, contact.
Alopecia, patchy, 329t–330t
Amebiasis, abdominal pain from, 13
Amenorrhea, 215–223. See also
    Dysmenorrhea and Menstruation.
  drug-induced, 216t
  primary, 215–217
  rarer causes of, 217–223
  secondary, 215, 216t, 217, 218t
Ampulla of Vater, cancer of, 9
Amyloidosis, palpitations and, 296
Anal fissure, 84, 89t. See also
    Constipation.
Anemia, dyspnea and, 298
  fatigue and, 156t
  hemolytic, 25
Aneurysm, aortic, 13, 16t
Angina, Prinzmetal's, 66, 70t
  Vincent's, 338, 341t
Angina pectoris, 63–65, 68, 70t, 284. See
    also Chest pain.
Ankle reflex, 36i
Ankylosing spondylitis, 29, 38–39
Anorexia. See Weight loss.
Anorexia nervosa, 235, 240
Antiarrhythmic drugs, 291–292
Antihypertensive drugs, 292
Anxiety. See also Emotional stress.
  dyspnea and, 303t
  palpitations and, 293t
Aortic aneurysm, 13, 16t
Aortoiliac disease, 252
Apnea, sleep, 196, 199t
Apophysitis, calcaneal, 243, 249t
Appendicitis, 3, 10, 14t
  children with, 22–23, 26t
Arm, contact dermatitis on, 325t
  pain in, 267, 287t. See also Shoulder
    pain and constituent parts.
  angina and, 284
Arrhythmia, 289–296. See also
    Palpitations.
  drugs for, 291–292
Arterial insufficiency, leg pain and, 253,
    261, 263t

Arteriovenous fistula, leg edema with, 344
Arteritis, cranial, 162
  of great vessels, 284–288
  temporal, 147t, 174t, 183t
Arthritis. See also *Degenerative joint
  disease (DJD, osteoarthritis)*.
  cervical, 169, 183t
  cervicodorsal, 65, 71t
  gouty, 256–257
  lumbosacral, 30, 41t
  of shoulder, 279
  patellofemoral, 268
  pyogenic, 256
  rheumatoid, fatigue and, 159
    in elbow, 282
    leg edema with, 344
    leg pain and, 261
    of fingers, 283
    of wrist, 282
    temporomandibular joint dysfunction
      and, 138
  septic, 281
  sternoclavicular, 283
Ascites, diagnostic studies for, 301
  weight gain from, 383t
Asherman's syndrome, 223
Asthma, 297–298, 302t
  bronchitis with, 300
  cough with, 95, 97, 101t
  diagnostic studies for, 301
  dyspnea and, 300
  nocturnal, 195
Astigmatism, headache from, 170
Athlete's foot, 323i–324i, 330t
Atopic dermatitis, 307, 309i–310i
  diagnosis of, 326t
Atrial fibrillation, 290, 296
Atrial tachycardia, 296
Axilla, contact dermatitis on, 325t

Babinski's sign, 284
Backache, 29–44
  associated symptoms with, 32–33
  children with, 29
  diagnostic studies for, 38
  differential diagnosis of, 40t–43t
  factors in, 33–34
  from infections, 29, 39
  from prostatitis, 33, 43t, 354–356
  herpes zoster and, 33, 43t
  in elderly, 30
  Paget's disease and, 38
  patient characteristics and, 29–30
  physical findings in, 34, 36i
  postural, 30, 41t
  rarer causes of, 38–44
  symptoms of, 30–32
Bacteriuria, 352
Baker's cyst, 255, 259, 261

Baker's cyst *(Continued)*
  in children, 269
  leg edema with, 347t
  rupture of, 344, 348
Balanitis, 360
Barlow's syndrome, 292
Barotrauma, otitic, 129–130, 134t
Basal cell carcinoma, 307, 331t
Belching, 45–47
  diagnostic studies for, 46
  differential diagnosis of, 50t
  factors in, 46
  indigestion with, 188
  patient characteristics and, 45–46
  rarer causes of, 47
  symptoms of, 46
Benign prostatic hypertrophy, 371–372,
  374t. See also *Prostatism*.
Beta blockers, 292, 293t, 299
Bicipital tendinitis, 276, 281, 285t
Bleeding, anovulatory, 203–206, 206t, 213
  estrogen-breakthrough, 204–205, 219t
  estrogen-withdrawal, 204, 219t
  from intrauterine device, 221t
  ovulatory, 205
  postmenopausal, 213
  progesterone-breakthrough, 205, 220t
  progesterone-withdrawal, 205, 220t
  uterine, 203, 219t–220t
  vaginal, 203, 205–207, 209t. See also
    Menstruation.
    before puberty, 213
    pregnancy and, 211, 213
Bloating, 47–52
  diagnostic studies for, 49
  differential diagnosis of, 50t–51t
  factors in 48–49
  physical findings in, 49
  rarer causes of, 49–52
  symptoms of, 48
Botulism, diarrhea with, 108
Bowel tumors, 85, 91t
Bradycardia, 296
Bragard test, 36i
Brainstem, dysfunction of, vertigo from,
  124t
Breast cancer, differential diagnosis of, 57t
  frequency of, 53
  mammography for, 58
  pain from, 54–55
  physical examination for, 55–58
  risk factors of, 54
Breast lumps, 53–59. See also
  Gynecomastia.
  benign, malignant vs., 55–58
  characteristics of, 53–54
  diagnostic studies for, 58
  differential diagnosis of, 56t–57t
  factors in, 55
  pain from, 54–55

Breast lumps *(Continued)*
    physical examination for, 55–58
    rarer causes of, 58–59
    symptoms of, 54–55
Bronchial adenoma, diagnostic studies for, 301
Bronchiolitis, 297
Bronchitis, asthmatic, 300
    chronic, 102t, 305t
    cough with, 100t
    diagnostic studies for, 301
    viral, 95
Buerger's disease, 282
Bulimia, 235
Bunions, foot pain from, 245
Burping. See *Belching.*
Bursitis, calcific, 276
    of elbow, 282, 287t
    of shoulder, 276
    subacromial, 275, 278–279, 285t
    trochanteric, 31t, 261–264
Buttock pain, 255, 262t
    in children, 269

Caffeine, palpitations and, 289–290, 293t
Calcaneal apophysitis, 243, 249t
Calcaneal periostitis, 245
Calcaneal spur, 243–244, 249t
Calcific bursitis, 276
Calcific tendinitis, 276, 285t
    physical findings in, 281
Calcium channel blockers, 292–293t, 299
Calf pain, 252, 263t. See also *Leg pain.*
    causes of, 255
    from cellulitis, 260
    from spinal stenosis, 254
    from varicose veins, 255–256
    from venous claudication, 253–254
Cancer. See also specific types.
    anorexia and, 385t
    basal cell, 307, 331t
    bladder, 360, 373
    bone, 260
    bowel, 85, 91t
    breast. See *Breast cancer.*
    cervical, 221t
    colon, 85–86, 91t
    dysmenorrhea and, 211
    dyspnea and, 298
    endometrial, 221t
    fatigue from, 158t
    gynecologic, 344
    hypothalamic, 386
    lung. See *Lung cancer.*
    of ampulla of Vater, 9
    palpitations and, 296
    pancreatic, 13
    rectal, 85, 91t
    skin, 307, 331t

Cancer *(Continued)*
    spinal, 39, 43t, 284
    squamous cell, 307, 331t
    urinary tract, 354
    uterine, 212
Candidiasis, 357, 365t
    diagnosis of, 330t, 366
    factors in, 337, 364
    in diabetics, 358t
    in infants, 322i
    of groin, 322i
    of throat, 334, 336t
    physical findings in, 338–339
    pseudohyphae of, 321i
    sore throat from, 341t
    vaginal discharge and, 361, 367t
Carbohydrate craving, 380
Cardiac disease, 290, 292, 295t. See also
        specific types, e.g., *Congestive heart
        failure.*
Carpal tunnel syndrome, 279, 280t, 282, 287t
Cauda equina claudication, 254t, 254–255, 261
Cauda equina syndrome, 30, 33
Cellulitis, calf pain with, 260
    leg edema with, 344
Cerumen, impacted, 129, 134t
Cervical disc syndrome, 279, 280t, 284
Cervicitis, 356, 361, 365
Chandelier sign, 365
Chest pain, 61–73
    aggravating factors in, 66–68
    ameliorating factors in, 65–66
    associated symptoms with, 64–65
    characteristics of, 62i–64i
    diagnosis of, 67t, 68–69
    differential diagnosis of, 70t–72t
    from angina, 63–65, 68, 70t, 284
    location of, 64i
    nausea and, 235–236
    noncardiac causes of, 62t
    patient characteristics and, 61–62
    physical findings in, 68
    precipitating factors in, 66–68
    rarer causes of, 69–73
    vomiting and, 235–236
Chest wall syndrome, 66, 67t, 68, 72t
Chicken pox, 307, 336t
Child abuse, dysuria and, 352
    gonorrhea and, 362
    vaginal discharge and, 362
Chills, fever with, 163
Chlamydial infections, 352–353, 355t
    diagnosis of, 357, 359t, 368t
    gonorrhea and, 365
    physical findings in, 365
    vaginal discharge from, 361
Cholecystitis, 3–5, 10–11, 14t
Cholelithiasis, 3–5, 14t

Chondromalacia patellae, 252, 260
  in children, 268, 270t
Choriocarcinoma, 212
Chronic obstructive pulmonary disease
    (COPD), cough with, 98–99, 102t
  diagnosis of, 301, 304t
  dyspnea from, 297
  emphysema and, 300–301, 305t
Cirrhosis, diagnosis of, 346t
  leg edema with, 343–344
  nausea and, 236
  weight gain from, 383t
Claudication, cauda equina, 254t, 254–
    255, 261
  intermittent, 252, 263t
    associated symptoms with, 256
    physical findings in, 258–259
  neurogenic, 261
  venous, 252–254, 254t, 263t
    physical findings in, 259
Cluster headaches. See Headache, cluster.
Coccidioidomycosis, cough with, 103
Colds, common, 75–77, 78t–80t. See also
    Respiratory infections.
  diagnosis of, 78t
Colitis, amebic, 110
  ulcerative, 108, 110
Colon, cancer of, 85–86, 91t
  irritable, abdominal pain in, 5, 9, 12, 16t
    backache from, 32, 43t
    constipation from, 86
    diarrhea with, 105–107, 115t
Comedones, 307, 308i
Compartment syndrome, 251, 264, 343
  leg edema with, 344
Congestive heart failure, chest pain from,
    68
  cough with, 96, 99, 102t
  diagnosis of, 346t
  dyspnea from, 298–299, 305t
  fatigue from, 153, 158t
  insomnia and, 195
  leg edema with, 343
  weight gain from, 383t
Conjunctivitis, glaucoma vs., 141–143
Constipation, 83–93. See also Laxative
    overuse and Obstipation.
  abdominal pain from, 9, 21, 24
  associated symptoms with, 86–87
  bloating and, 48
  diagnostic studies for, 92
  differential diagnosis of, 88t–91t
  factors in, 87
  from anal fissure, 84, 89t
  in children, 26t
  patient characteristics and, 84–85
  physical findings in, 87–92
  psychiatric causes of, 93
  rarer causes of, 92–93
  symptoms of, 85

Contact dermatitis. See Dermatitis,
    contact.
COPD. See Chronic obstructive pulmonary
    disease (COPD).
Coronary artery disease, 295t
Costochondritis, 66
Cough, 95–104
  asthma with, 95, 97, 101t
  common causes of, 95
  diagnostic studies for, 99
  differential diagnosis of, 100t–102t
  factors in, 97–98
  in children, 95
  incontinence and, 373
  physical findings with, 98–99
  rarer causes of, 99–103
  recurrent, 95
  smoking and, 96–98
  symptoms of, 96–97
  viral infections with, 95
Cremasteric reflex, 36i
Crohn's disease, 27
Croup, 297
Cushing's disease, 381, 383t, 386
Cystitis, 351, 356
  ameliorating factors in, 376
  diagnosis of, 358t
  recurrent, 373
  symptoms of, 352, 354t
Cystometry, 377
Cystoscopy, 377

De Quervain's disease, 282, 287t
Defecation, disorders of, 84. See also
    Constipation; Diarrhea.
Degenerative joint disease (DJD,
    osteoarthritis), 34, 252–253, 256, 262t,
    284. See also Arthritis.
  backache from, 37
  obturator hernia vs., 260–261
  of hip, 31t
  of lumbar spine, 32
  physical findings in, 257
Dementia, voiding disorders with, 375t
Dental abscess, facial pain with, 138, 147t
  fever with, 162
Depigmentation, 307, 328t
Depression. See also Emotional stress.
  backache from, 32, 43t
  fatigue and, 149–150, 154t–156t
  headaches and, 171
  in children, 150
  insomnia and, 195, 198t
  obesity and, 380
  seasonal, 380
  socioeconomic class and, 151t
  vomiting and, 235
  weight loss from, 380, 384t
Dermatitis. See also Skin problems.

Dermatitis *(Continued)*
  atopic, 307, 309i–310i, 326t
  contact, 317i
    causes of, 325t
    chronic, 318i
    diagnosis of, 328t
    edema from, 318i
    location of, 325t
  eczematous, 307
  nummular, 326t
  occupational, 307
  seborrheic, 307
    diagnosis of, 327t
    location of, 315i
    of ear, 315i
Dermatomes, of leg, 35i
Dermatosis, 307–332. See also *Skin problems.*
  plantar, 331t
"DES daughter," 215
Detrusor instability, diagnosis of, 374t
  stress incontinence vs., 373t
Diabetes mellitus, acidosis from, 21–22, 24
  diarrhea with, 105–106, 115t
  dizziness and, 121–122
  gastroparesis from, 239t
  leg edema in, 344
  peripheral neuropathy from, 260
  retinopathy from, 68
  urinary frequency with, 351
  vaginitis and, 364
  voiding disorders and, 377
Diaper rash, 317i
Diarrhea, 105–116
  acute, chronic diarrhea vs., 107
    differential diagnosis of, 112t–114t
  associated symptoms with, 107–109
  bloating and, 48
  chronic, 111–116, 115t
    acute diarrhea vs., 107
  diagnostic studies for, 110
  drug-induced, 109, 113t
  factors in, 109
  fever with, 109
  from laxatives, 113t
  in children, 111–116, 115t
  infectious, 108
  nature of, 107
  patient characteristics and, 105–107
  physical findings in, 109
  rarer causes of, 110–111
  toxin-mediated, 107–108, 114t
Diethylstilbestrol, 215
Digitalis, arrhythmias from, 291, 293t
Disc disease, 37. See also *Herniated disc syndrome.*
  backache from, 29–30, 34
  cervical, 279, 280t, 284
  degenerative, 31t
  lumbar. See *Sciatica.*

Diverticulitis, abdominal pain in, 14t
  acute, 12
  bloating from, 48
Diverticulosis, bloating from, 48
Dizziness, 120–126. See also *Vertigo.*
  associated symptoms with, 121
  common causes of, 120
  drug-induced, 120, 125t
  factors in, 121–122
  hypoglycemia with, 121, 125t
  in elderly, 120–121
  physical findings with, 122
  psychogenic, 120–121, 124t
  rarer causes of, 122
DJD. See *Degenerative joint disease (DJD, osteoarthritis).*
Drug abuse. See *Substance abuse.*
JD
Duodenal atresia, abdominal pain in, 25
Dupuytren's contracture, 282, 287t
Dysentery syndrome, 108, 114t
Dyshidrotic eczema, 330t
Dysmenorrhea, 225–231. See also *Amenorrhea* and *Menstruation.*
  diagnostic studies for, 230
  differential diagnosis of, 228t–229t
  endometriosis and, 227, 229t
  factors in, 227–230
  patient characteristics and, 226
  pelvic inflammatory disease and, 227, 229t
  physical findings in, 230
  premenstrual syndrome vs., 225
  primary, 225, 228t
  rarer causes of, 231
  secondary, 228t
  symptoms of, 226–227
Dyspareunia, 363–364
Dyspnea, 297–306
  acute, 298–299
  associated symptoms with, 298–299
  chronic, 298, 299
  common causes of, 297
  cough with, 96
  diagnostic studies for, 301
  differential diagnosis of, 302t–305t
  factors in, 299–300
  in children, 297–298
  patient characteristics and, 297–298
  physical findings in, 300
  rarer causes of, 306
  symptoms of, 298
Dysuria, 351–360. See also *Urethral discharge, Vaginitis,* and *Vulvar itching.*
  associated symptoms with, 354–356
  child abuse and, 352
  common causes of, 352
  diagnostic studies for, 357
  differential diagnosis of, 358t–359t

Dysuria *(Continued)*
    factors in, 356–357
    from cystitis, 352–354, 354t
    from herpes simplex, 360
    from meatal stenosis, 352, 359t
    in children, 352
    rarer causes of, 360
    symptoms of, 352, 354t
    vaginal discharge with, 363, 367t–369t
    with fever, 354

Eagle's syndrome, facial pain with, 144
Ear, contact dermatitis on, 325t
    nerve supply to, 127–128, 128i
    seborrheic dermatitis of, 315i
Earache, 127–135
    common causes of, 127
    diagnostic studies for, 130–135
    differential diagnosis of, 133t–134t
    factors in, 130
    from barotrauma, 129–130, 134t
    from temporomandibular joint dysfunc-
        tion, 129–130, 134t
    in children, 127–128
    physical findings in, 130–135
    rarer causes of, 135
    symptoms of, 129–130
ECG. See *Electrocardiography (ECG).*
Ectopic pregnancy, 13, 15t, 211, 220t
    diagnostic studies for, 214–215
Eczema, diagnosis of, 326t
    dyshidrotic, 330t
    nummular, 311i, 326t–327t
Eczematous dermatitis, 307
Edema. See also *Weight gain.*
    leg. See *Leg edema.*
    physical findings in, 381
    premenstrual, 380
    weight gain from, 380, 383t
Elbow, pain in, 282, 287t
    tennis, 282, 287t
Electrocardiography (ECG), for chest pain,
        68–69
    palpitations and, 289, 291–292
Embolism, leg pain and, 259
    pulmonary. See *Pulmonary embolism.*
Emotional stress. See also *Anxiety* and
        Depression.
    abdominal pain from, 20, 26t
    dyspnea from, 298
    enuresis and, 371, 375t
    fatigue and, 149–150, 155t, 158t
    hyperphagia and, 381, 382t
    indigestion from, 186
    insomnia and, 195–197, 199t
    nausea from, 235, 239t
    palpitations and, 293t

Emphysema, 300–301, 305t. See also
        *Chronic obstructive pulmonary disease
        (COPD).*
Endocarditis, fever with, 162
Endometriosis, 211, 215, 221
    dysmenorrhea and, 227, 229t
Enterocolitis, necrotizing, abdominal pain
        in, 25
Entrapment syndrome, neural, 282–284
Enuresis, 371–372. See also *Urination,
        disorders of.*
    diagnosis of, 375t
    nocturnal, 195, 198t
Epiglottitis, 297. See also *Sore throat.*
    physical findings in, 338
Epiphysitis, of hip, 267–270
    of knee, 268, 270t
Eructation. See *Belching.*
Erythrasma, 330t
Erythromelalgia, 250
Esophageal atresia, 233
Esophagitis, abdominal pain in, 16t
    chest pain from, 64–66, 70t
    peptic, 188
    reflux, 186, 188, 190t
Exanthems, pediatric, 307
Exocervicitis, 361
Eye pain, causes of, 148
Eyelids, dermatitis on, 325t

Face, contact dermatitis on, 325t
    scaling of, 331t
Facial pain, 137–148
    associated symptoms of, 140
    atypical, 147t
    diagnostic studies for, 143
    differential diagnosis of, 145t–147t
    drugs for, 141
    factors in, 140–141
    patient characteristics and, 137–138
    physical findings of, 141–143
    rarer causes of, 144–148
    symptoms of, 138–139
Fasciitis, heel, 245
    plantar, 244, 249t
Fat necrosis, in breast, 53, 57t
Fatigue, 149–160
    arthritis and, 159
    associated symptoms with, 152
    depression and, 149–150, 154t–156t
    diagnostic studies for, 159
    differential diagnosis of, 154t–158t
    drug-induced, 149, 155t, 158t
    factors in, 152–153
    fever and, 153
    in children, 150
    in elderly, 150
    patient characteristics and, 150–151,
        151t

Fatigue *(Continued)*
  physical findings in, 153–159
  physiologic, 149, 154t
  rarer causes of, 159
  symptoms of, 151–152
  tuberculosis and, 153
  types of, 149
Fecal impaction. See *Obstipation.*
Feet, dermatitis on, 325t
  edema of, 344
  pain in. See *Foot pain.*
  flat, 271
  pain in. See *Foot pain.*
  scaling of, 330t–331t
Female urethral syndrome, 358t
Fever, 161–168
  aggravating factors in, 164
  chills with, 163
  diagnostic studies for, 165
  diarrhea with, 109
  differential diagnosis of, 166t–167t
  drug-induced, 162, 166t
  dysuria and, 354
  factitious, 162, 167t
  factors in, 164
  fatigue and, 153
  of unknown origin, 161, 165t
  patient characteristics and, 162
  physical findings in, 164
  rarer causes of, 165–168
  sore throat with, 334, 335t
  symptoms of, 162–163
Fibrillation, atrial, 290, 296
Fibroadenoma. See also *Breast lumps.*
  diagnosis of, 56t
  in breast, 54–55
Fibrocystic disease, 55, 56t. See also
    Breast lumps.
Fibrosis, pulmonary, 306
Fibrositis syndrome, 277, 279i
Flatfoot, in children, 271
Flatulence, 47–52. See also *Bloating.*
  chest pain and, 66
  differential diagnosis of, 50t–51t
  foods causing, 49
  indigestion and, 186, 191t
Foot pain, 243–250
  diagnostic studies for, 246
  factors in, 244–245
  gout and, 243–244, 249t
  in children, 243
  patient characteristics and, 243–244
  physical findings in, 245
  rarer causes of, 246–250, 246t, 247i
  Raynaud's disease and, 247–250
  symptoms of, 244
Foreign body aspiration, 298, 300, 303t
Fractures, stress, 251, 264
Frozen shoulder, 276–277, 281, 286t. See
    also *Shoulder pain.*

Fungal infections, 307, 329t. See also *Skin
    problems.*
Fusospirochetal infections, 334, 336t
  diagnosis of, 341t
  physical findings in, 338–339
  trench mouth and, 338

Gait, examination of, 271
Gallbladder disease, 191t. See also
    Cholecystitis; Cholelithiasis.
Gas entrapment syndrome, 48, 51t
  chest pain from, 66, 69, 72t
  indigestion with, 191t
Gastritis, abdominal pain from, 14t
  diagnosis of, 190t
  nausea and, 234, 238t
Gastroenteritis, 14t, 21
  diarrhea with, 105–106, 112t
  fever with, 162, 166t
  in children, 26t
  nausea with, 234, 236, 238t
Gastroesophageal reflux, 102t
Gastroparesis, diabetic, 239t
German measles, 307
Giardiasis, bloating from, 51t
  diarrhea from, 106, 108, 115t
Giddiness, 120
Gingivitis, 338
Glaucoma, diagnosis of, 146t, 183t
  facial pain from, 138–139
  headache with, 169, 178, 183t
  physical findings of, 141–143
Gonorrhea. See also *Dysuria.*
  associated symptoms with, 357
  chlamydial infections and, 365
  diagnosis of, 357, 368t
  in children, 362
  oropharyngeal symptoms of, 334
  urethritis from, 354, 355t
  vaginal discharge from, 361
Gout, arthritis and, 256–257
  diagnosis of, 257
  foot pain from, 243–244, 249t
  leg pain with, 252, 263t
Growing pains, 267–268, 270t
Gynecomastia, 54. See also *Breast lumps.*
  diagnosis of, 57t
  physical examination for, 58

Hair disorders, 307. See also *Skin
    problems.*
Hand, pain in, 282–283, 287t. See also
    Arm, pain in.
  thoracic outlet syndrome and, 279,
    280t, 282, 287t
  psoriasis on, 314i
Hand-foot-and-mouth disease, 336t

HCM. See *Hypertrophic cardiomyopathy (HCM)*.
Headache, 169–184
  associated symptoms with, 176–177
  brain disease with, 177
  cervical arthritis with, 183t
  cluster, 175, 178
    diagnosis of, 181t–182t
    facial pain with, 147t
    factors in, 174t
  depression with, 171, 182t
  diagnostic studies for, 179
  differential diagnosis of, 180t–183t
  factors in, 177–178
  fever with, 182t
  glaucoma with, 169, 178, 183t
  hypertension and, 169, 175
  in children, 170–171
  in elderly, 171–172
  increased intracranial pressure with, 183t
  location of, 172t
  migraine, 174t, 175, 181t
    children with, 25–28, 118, 170
    patterns of, 176
    symptoms of, 171
    tension headache vs., 170, 173t
    vomiting and, 235
  patient characteristics and, 170–172
  patterns of, 175–176
  physical findings in, 178–179
  rarer causes of, 179–184
  sinus, 178, 182t
    from neoplasm, 176
    in children, 170
  symptoms of, 172t–174t, 172–175
  temporal arteritis with, 183t
  tension, 170, 180t
    migraine vs., 170, 173t
    patterns of, 175
  trigeminal neuralgia with, 183t
  types of, 170
  vascular, diagnosis of, 180t
Heart failure, congestive. See *Congestive heart failure*.
Heartburn, 185–193
  associated symptoms with, 188
  diagnostic studies for, 192
  differential diagnosis of, 190t–191t
  drug-induced, 186
  factors in, 188–189
  in children, 185–186
  in elderly, 186
  patient characteristics and, 185–186
  physical findings in, 189–192
  rarer causes of, 192
  stress and, 186
  symptoms of, 186–187
Heel, fasciitis of, 245
  pain in. See *Foot pain*.

Heimlich maneuver, 300
Hematuria, 354, 357, 372–373
Hemorrhoids, constipation from, 86–87, 90t
Hemosiderosis, dyspnea and, 306
Hepatic flexure, bloating from, 51t
Hepatitis, fatigue from, 150, 153, 158t
  fever with, 162, 167t
  nausea in, 236
Hernia, hiatal, 186
  incarcerated, 16t
  inguinal, children with, 24
  obturator, 260–261
Herniated disc syndrome, 29–30, 32, 37, 284. See also *Disc disease*.
Herpangina, 334, 336t
  diagnosis of, 341t
  physical findings in, 338–339
  predisposing factors to, 337
Herpes genitalis, 366–370
  vaginal discharge from, 361
Herpes simplex, 307, 329t. See also *Skin problems*.
  dysuria from, 360
  physical findings in, 338–339
  predisposing factors to, 337
  sore throat from, 334, 336t, 341t
  vaginal discharge from, 361, 366
Herpes zoster, backache from, 33, 43t
  diagnosis of, 329t
  in children, 271
  physical findings in, 338–339
  sore throat from, 334
Hiatal hernia, 186
Hip, congenital dislocation of, 267
  epiphysitis of, 267–270
  osteoarthritis of, 31t
Hirschsprung's disease, 25, 89t, 92
Hodgkin's disease, 162
Holter monitoring, 289, 291–296
Homans' sign, thrombophlebitis and, 259
Horner's syndrome, 176–177
Horton's cephalalgia. See *Headache, cluster*.
Hydatidiform mole, 212
Hydralazine, 292, 293t
Hydrocephalus, headache from, 171
Hypermenorrhea, 205
Hyperphagia. See also *Weight gain*.
  reactive, 381, 382t
Hypersensitivity pneumonitis, 300
Hypertension, chest pain from, 68
  drugs for, 292
  headaches and, 169, 175
  pulmonary, 63, 73
Hyperthyroidism, dyspnea from, 306
  fatigue from, 153
  insomnia and, 195
  masked, 150
  palpitations and, 289, 294t

Hypertrophic cardiomyopathy (HCM), 65–66, 71t
  diagnosis of, 66–68
  electrocardiogram for, 69
Hyperventilation, 298, 303t
  dizziness from, 120, 125t
  palpitations and, 289, 292
Hypoglycemia, dizziness from, 121, 125t
  palpitations and, 289, 291, 293t
  reactive, 121, 289, 291, 295t
    dizziness from, 125t
Hypoproteinemia, 346t
Hypotension, orthostatic, 121–122, 125t
Hypothalamus, tumors of, 386
Hypothyroidism, fatigue from, 153, 156t
  physical findings in, 381
  sore throat from, 339–342
  weight gain from, 379–380

Impetigo, 308i, 326t
Impingement syndrome, in shoulder, 277, 278i, 281, 286t
Incarcerated hernia, 16t
Incontinence, 371–378. See also *Urination, disorders of.*
  cough and, 373
  diagnostic studies for, 376–377
  differential diagnosis of, 374t–375t
  drug-induced, 373
  physical examination for, 376
  rarer causes of, 377
  stress, 372, 374t
    detrusor instability vs., 373t
    Q-tip test for, 377
  symptoms of, 372
Indigestion, 185–193
  associated symptoms with, 188
  diagnostic studies for, 192
  differential diagnosis of, 190t–191t
  drug-induced, 186
  factors in, 188–189
  in children, 185–186
  in elderly, 186
  patient characteristics and, 185–186
  physical findings in, 189–192
  rarer causes of, 192
  stress and, 186
  symptoms of, 187
Inflammatory bowel disease, 20, 115t
Influenza, 75–80, 80t. See also *Respiratory infections.*
  fever with, 162, 166t
  signs of, 76
Inguinal hernia, 24
Insect bites, 316i, 328t
Insomnia, 195–201
  depression and, 195, 198t
  diagnostic studies for, 201
  differential diagnosis of, 198t–199t

Insomnia *(Continued)*
  drug-induced, 195, 199t
  factors in, 200–201
  from fibrositis syndrome, 277–278
  in children, 195–196
  in elderly, 196
  patient characteristics and, 195–196
  physical findings in, 201
  rarer causes of, 201
  symptoms of, 196–197
Intermittent claudication, 252, 263t
  associated symptoms with, 256
  physical findings in, 258–259
Intertrigo, seborrheic, 330t
Intestinal obstruction, 4, 11, 15t
Intestinal perforation. See *Peritonitis.*
Intracranial pressure, increased, headache with, 170–171, 183t
  nausea with, 234, 239t
Intrauterine devices (IUDs), dysmenorrhea from, 225
Intussusception, abdominal pain from, 24, 26t
Iritis, glaucoma vs., 141–143
Irritable bowel syndrome. See *Colon, irritable.*

Jogging injuries, 248t, 251
  in children, 268, 270t
Joint disease. See *Arthritis; Degenerative joint disease (DJD, osteoarthritis).*
Joint sprain, 259
Jumper's knee, 269

Keratosis, seborrheic, 307, 327t. See also *Skin problems.*
Ketoacidosis, diabetic, vomiting and, 236
Knee, epiphysitis of, 268, 270t
  jumper's, 269
  landmarks of, 258i
  pain in, 257, 260, 262t. See also *Leg pain.*
    children with, 268, 270t
Knee reflex, 36i
Kussmaul's respirations, 24
Kyphoscoliosis, 301

Labyrinthine disorders, nausea with, 236
Labyrinthitis, vertigo from, 123t
Lactose intolerance, abdominal pain from, 27
  bloating from, 47–48, 51t
  diarrhea with, 106, 109, 115t
Laparotomy, for abdominal pain, 12
Lasègue's test, 36i, 37–38
Laurence-Moon-Biedl syndrome, 386

Laxative overuse, 84, 90t, 113t. See also
    Constipation.
Lead poisoning, 28
Leg, contact dermatitis on, 325t
    nerve supply to, 35i
    physical examination of, 348
Leg edema, 343–349
    associated symptoms with, 345
    diagnostic studies for, 348–349
    differential diagnosis of, 346t–347t
    drug-induced, 345, 347t
    factors in, 345–348
    from cirrhosis, 343–344
    from congestive heart failure, 343–344
    from gynecologic cancer, 344
    from lymphedema, 343
    from nephrotic syndrome, 343–344
    from thrombophlebitis, 343
    in alcoholics, 344
    in children, 343
    patient characteristics and, 343–344
    rarer causes of, 349
    symptoms of, 344
    unilateral, 344
Leg pain, 251–265. See also Calf pain and
    Foot pain.
    ameliorating factors in, 256–257
    associated symptoms with, 256
    diagnostic studies for, 257–259
    differential diagnosis of, 251, 262t–263t
    from arterial insufficiency, 253, 261,
        263t
    from gout, 252, 263t
    from muscular strain, 251, 262t
    from sciatica, 253, 262t
    from trochanteric bursitis, 261–264
    in children, 267–271
    patellar causes of, 252
    patient characteristics and, 251–252
    physical findings in, 257–259
    precipitating factors in, 256
    rarer causes of, 259–264
    sports medicine and, 264
    symptoms of, 252–256
    varicose veins and, 255–256
Legg-Calvé-Perthes disease, 267, 270t
Leukemia, fever with, 162
    menstrual irregularities with, 215
Leukorrhea, 362
Lichenification, 309i, 326t
Ligamentous strains, 251, 257, 262t
Lightheadedness. See Dizziness.
Limp, in children, 267–271
Lipedema, 344, 347t, 349
Liver, cirrhosis of. See Cirrhosis.
    inflammation of. See Hepatitis.
Lumbar disc disease. See Sciatica.
Lumbosacral strain, 30, 37, 40t
Lung cancer, 298, 301
    chest pain from, 73

Lung cancer (Continued)
    cough from, 99
Lupus erythematosus, 282
Lymphedema, diagnosis of, 347t
    of leg, 344
    types of, 343

Malabsorption syndromes, bloating from,
        47, 51t
    diarrhea from, 111
    indigestion from, 186
Mammography, 58
Mastodynia, 54–55
Mastoiditis, 129, 131, 134t
Measles, 162, 307
Melanoma, malignant, 331t
Menarche, 207, 208t, 215
Meniere's disease, vertigo from, 118–119,
        123t
    vomiting and, 235
Meningeal tumors, 284
Meningitis, 77
Meniscal injuries, in children, 269
Menometrorrhagia, 205
Menorrhagia, 205, 206t, 211–213
Menstruation, absence of. See
        Amenorrhea.
    characteristics of, 209t
    drugs affecting, 210t
    irregular, 203–223
        associated symptoms with, 213
        diagnostic studies for, 214
        differential diagnosis of, 219t–222t
        leukemia and, 215
        patient characteristics and, 207–210
        physical findings in, 214
        precipitating factors in, 213
        rarer causes for, 214
        symptoms with, 210–213
        types of, 205–207
        von Willebrand's disease and, 215
    pain with. See Dysmenorrhea.
    patterns of, 205–207
    physiology of, 204i
Meralgia paresthetica, 31t, 260
Mesenteric adenitis, 15t, 21
    in children, 22–23
Mesenteric infarction, abdominal pain
        from, 16t
Metatarsalgia, 246t, 246–247
Metrorrhagia, 205, 206t, 212
Migraine. See Headache, migraine.
Minoxidil, 292, 293t
Mitral valve prolapse, 64–66, 68, 290, 292,
        295t
    chest pain from, 71t
    diagnosis of, 67t
Mittelschmerz, 13, 25, 213
Mole, hydatidiform, 212

Mondor's disease, 59
Moniliasis. See *Candidiasis*.
Mononucleosis, infectious, diagnosis of,
    339, 340t
    fatigue from, 150, 153, 158t
    fever with, 162, 167t
    physical findings in, 337–338
    sore throat with, 333–334
Monospot test, 339, 340t
Morning sickness, 239t
Morton's neuroma, 247, 247i
Motility disorders, 88t
Multiple myeloma, 38, 39
Multiple sclerosis, 137–138, 377
Muscle strain, 257
    of leg, 251, 255, 262t
Myalgia, in children, 268
Myocardial infarction, chest pain from, 72t
    dyspnea from, 298
Myositis, intercostal, 71t
    nonspecific, 66
Myxedema, pretibial, 344, 349

Nails, pitting of, 313i
    psoriasis of, 313i–314i
    tinea pedis of, 324i
Nausea, 233–241. See also *Indigestion* and
    Vomiting.
    associated symptoms with, 235–236
    diagnostic studies for, 237, 238t
    differential diagnosis of, 238–239
    drug-induced, 236, 238t
    dysuria with, 356
    factors in, 236
    patient characteristics and, 233–234
    physical findings in, 236–237
    rarer causes of, 237–240
    symptoms of, 234–235
Neck, contact dermatitis on, 325t
Neoplasm, occult, fever with, 162, 167t
Nephrotic syndrome, diagnosis of, 346t,
    383t
    leg edema with, 343–344
    weight gain from, 379
Neuralgia. See also *Trigeminal neuralgia*.
    factors in, 174t
    glossopharyngeal, 144, 145t
    sphenopalatine, 140, 144, 145t
Neuroma, acoustic, 118–119
    facial pain from, 137–138
    vertigo from, 124t
    Morton's, 247, 247i
    trigeminal, facial pain from, 137–138
Neuropathy, diabetic, 260, 377
    entrapment, 282–284
    peripheral, 256, 260
Neurosis. See *Emotional stress*.
Nightmares, insomnia and, 196, 198t
Nitroglycerin, 65–66

Norwegian pulseless disease, 284–288
Nutritional deficiency, fatigue from, 153
Nystagmus, nausea and, 236
    vertigo with, 119

Obesity, 303t. See also *Weight gain*.
    depression and, 380
    diagnostic studies for, 301
    dyspnea from, 297–298
    endogenous, 379, 381
    exogenous, 379
    familial, 380
    in children, 379
    leg edema with, 344, 349
    physical findings in, 381
Obstipation, 84–85, 89t. See also
    Constipation.
    abdominal pain from, 24
    from antidiarrheal drugs, 111
Obturator hernia, 260–261
Ornithosis, cough with, 103
Oropharyngeal ulcers, cause of, 334, 336t
    diagnosis of, 341t
    physical findings in, 338–339
Osgood-Schlatter disease, 268, 270t
Osteoarthritis (degenerative joint disease,
    DJD), 34, 252–253, 256, 262t, 284. See
    also *Arthritis*.
    backache from, 37
    obturator hernia vs., 260–261
    of hip, 31t
    of lumbar spine, 32
    physical findings in, 257
Osteochondritis, 269
Otalgia. See *Earache*.
Otitis externa, 127–128
    diagnosis of, 133t
Otitis media, 77, 127–129, 133t
    diagnosis of, 133t
    fever with, 162
    nausea and, 234, 238t
    vertigo from, 117–118, 123t
    vomiting and, 236
Otoscopy, pneumatic, 131i
Ovarian cyst, 211–212

Paget's disease, 38
Palpitations, 289–296
    associated symptoms with, 291
    differential diagnosis of, 293t–295t
    factors in, 291–292
    patient characteristics and, 289–290
    physical findings in, 292
    rarer causes of, 296
    symptoms of, 290–291
Pancoast's tumor, 283
Pancreas, cancer of, 13
Pancreatitis, 44

Pancreatitis *(Continued)*
abdominal pain from, 14t
fever with, 162
indigestion from, 189
nausea from, 234, 239t
Panic disorder, 298. See also *Emotional stress.*
Papanicolaou test, 214, 230
Papules, diagnosis of, 326t
inflamed, 327t–328t
pruritic, location of, 316i
Patella, bursitis of, 252
chondromalacia of, 252, 260
in children, 268–270, 270t
dislocation of, 269
osteochondritis of, 269
tendinitis of, 252
Patellar reflex, 36i
Patellofemoral problems, 251
Pediculosis, 307, 320i, 330t. See also *Skin problems.*
Pelvic inflammatory disease, 365
dysmenorrhea from, 227, 229t
Pelvic tilt, 269
Peptic ulcer, 4, 11, 15t
in children, 25
Pericarditis, 65, 72t, 73
Peritonitis, 10, 15t
Pes planus, 271
Pharyngitis, 333. See also *Sore throat.*
allergic, 338, 340t
gonococcal, 340t
physical findings in, 337
streptococcal, 77, 333–334, 337, 339, 340t
ulcers with, 334, 336t
viral, 340t
Pica, abdominal pain from, 27
Pityriasis rosea, 307, 312i. See also *Skin problems.*
diagnosis of, 326t
location of, 311i
Placenta previa, 213
Plantar fasciitis, 244, 249t
Plantar warts, 244, 248t
Plaques, 326t–327t. See also *Skin problems.*
Pleural effusion, 300–301
Pneumoconiosis, 301, 306
Pneumonia, abdominal pain from, 13
children with, 25
bacterial, 77, 95
chest pain from, 65
cough with, 95, 100t–101t
dyspnea from, 298
viral, 75
Pneumonitis, 300
Pneumothorax, 300
diagnosis of, 304t
dyspnea from, 298

Podagra, 256
Poisoning, 20, 250
lead, 28
Polycythemia, 250
Polymenorrhagia, 205–207, 210–211
Polyps, menorrhagia and, 212
Popliteal cyst, 255, 259, 261
in children, 269
rupture of, 344, 348
Postnasal drip, cough with, 97–98, 101t
from sinusitis, 143
sore throat from, 338, 341t, 342
Pott's disease, 284
Prader-Willi syndrome, 386
Pregnancy, dyspnea in, 306
ectopic, 13, 15t, 211, 220t
diagnostic studies for, 214–215
morning sickness in, 239t
thrombosis in, 349
weight gain during, 379, 382t
Premenstrual syndrome, 225, 228t
Prinzmetal's angina, 66, 70t
Prolactinoma, 222t
Prostatism, 371–372, 374t
ameliorating factors in, 376
physical examination for, 376
symptoms of, 372
ultrasonography of, 377
Prostatitis, 351, 354–356
backache from, 33, 43t, 354–356
diagnosis of, 358t
factors in, 356
fever with, 162, 166t
Pruritic papules, location of, 316i
Pseudohypoparathyroidism, 386
Pseudothrombophlebitis, 255, 255t, 261
Pseudotumor cerebri, headache from, 171
Psoriasis, 307. See also *Skin problems.*
diagnosis of, 327t
location of, 313i
nail pitting with, 313i
of toes, 314i
palm lesions with, 314i
Pulmonary edema, 300
diagnosis of, 301, 304t
dyspnea from, 298
Pulmonary embolism, 300
chest pain from, 61–62, 65
diagnosis of, 302t
dyspnea from, 297–298
Pulmonary fibrosis, 306
Pulmonary hemosiderosis, 306
Pulmonary hypertension, 63, 73
Pustules, diagnosis of, 326t
Pyelonephritis, 354, 356
abdominal pain from, 21
fever with, 163
Pyloric obstruction, nausea and, 234

Radial head, dislocation of, 282, 287t
Radiculitis, 283
Raynaud's disease, 247–250, 282
Rectosigmoid tumor, 91t
Rectum, cancer of, 85
Reflexes, root origin of, 36i
Regurgitation. See *Vomiting.*
Reiter's syndrome, backache from, 29
   urethritis with, 360
Renal colic, backache from, 32
Respiratory infections, 75–77, 78t–80t
   AIDS and, 76
   cough with, 95, 100t
   diagnostic studies for, 81
   differential diagnosis of, 78t–80t
   fever with, 161–162, 166t
   physical findings in, 77–81
   rarer causes of, 81
   viral, 76
Retinopathy, diabetic, 68
Retropharyngeal abscess, 338
Rheumatoid arthritis. See *Arthritis,*
   rheumatoid.
Rhinitis, allergic, 77, 79t, 96
   chronic, 76–77, 79t
Rhinitis medicamentosa, 76, 80t
Roseola, fever with, 162
Rotator cuff trauma, 275–276, 278–279,
   285t
   ameliorating factors in, 281
   physical findings in, 281
Rubella, 307
Rubeola, 162, 307
Runners' injuries, 251, 264
   in children, 268, 270t
   leg edema from, 347t

Sacroiliitis, 31t, 32
Salmonellosis, 108, 112t
Salpingitis, 211, 221t
   abdominal pain from, 11, 15t
Salpingo-oophoritis, 212
Sarcoidosis, 296, 301
Scabies, 307, 327t
Scaling plaques, 326t. See also *Skin*
   problems.
Scalp, patchy alopecia of, 329t–330t
   ringworm of, 319i
   scaling patches on, 327t
   seborrheic dermatitis of, 315i
Sciatic nerve stretch test, 36i
Sciatica, 253, 262t
   associated symptoms with, 256
   physical findings in, 258
Scleroderma, 282
Scrotum, contact dermatitis on, 325t
Seasonal affective disorder, 380. See also
   Depression.

Seborrheic dermatitis, 307. See also *Skin*
   problems.
   diagnosis of, 327t
   location of, 315i
   on ear, 315i
Seborrheic intertrigo, 330t
Seborrheic keratosis, 307, 327t. See also
   Skin problems.
Sepsis, bacterial, 166t
Sex characteristics, development of, 208t
Sexually transmitted diseases, 352, 356–
   357. See also specific types, e.g.,
   Gonorrhea.
   vaginitis and, 361, 368t
Shin splints, 251
Shortness of breath. See *Dyspnea.*
Shoulder, anatomy of, 273i–274i
   bursitis of, 276
   dislocation of, 275, 277
   frozen, 276–277, 281, 286t
Shoulder pain, 273–281, 285t–287t
   diagnostic studies for, 283
   factors in, 281
   from angina pectoris, 284
   from cervical disc syndrome, 279, 280t
   location of, 277
   patient characteristics and, 275
   physical findings in, 281
   rarer causes of, 283
   symptoms of, 275–279
   types of, 273–274
Sick sinus syndrome, 289–291, 295t
Sickle cell crisis, 13, 20
Sinusitis, 76–77, 81
   cough with, 96, 98
   diagnosis of, 79t–80t, 145t
   facial pain with, 138
   fever with, 162
   headaches from, 169
   pharyngitis with, 333
   physical findings in, 143
   sore throat from, 338, 341t
Skiers' injuries, 251, 268, 270t
Skin problems, 307–332. See also specific
   types, e.g., *Dermatitis.*
   differential diagnosis of, 326t–331t
   in children, 307
Skin tumors, 307
   diagnosis of, 331t
Sluder's syndrome, 144
Smoking, cough from, 96–98
   dyspnea from, 297, 299
Sore throat, 333–342
   cultures for, 333t–335t
   diagnostic studies for, 339
   differential diagnosis of, 340t–341t
   fever with, 334t–335t
   from candidiasis, 334, 336t
   from fusospirochetal infection, 334, 336t
   from hand-foot-and-mouth disease, 336t

Sore throat *(Continued)*
  from herpangina, 334, 336t
  from herpes simplex, 334, 336t, 341t
  from herpes zoster, 334
  from mononucleosis, 333
  from pharyngitis, 333
  from syphilis, 336t
  from tonsillitis, 333
  from varicella, 336t
  infectious causes of, 336t
  patient characteristics and, 334
  physical findings in, 337–339
  predisposing factors in, 337
  rarer causes of, 339–342
  symptoms of, 334
Spinal stenosis, 254t, 254–255
  precipitating factors in, 256
  rarer causes of, 261
Spine, cancer of, 39, 43t, 284
  infections of, 29, 39
Splenic flexure, bloating from, 51t
Spondylolisthesis, 29, 44
Spondylolysis, 29, 44
Spondylosis, cervical, 283–284
Sports medicine, 264
Squamous cell carcinoma, 307, 331t
Steatorrhea, 108
Sternoclavicular arthritis, 283
Stimulants, palpitations and, 289–290, 293t
Stomatitis, 334. See also *Sore throat.*
Strabismus, headache from, 170
Strain, muscle, 257
  of leg, 251, 255, 262t
Strangury. See *Dysuria.*
Stress. See *Emotional stress.*
Stress fractures, 251, 264
Stress incontinence, 372, 373t, 374t, 377.
  See also *Incontinence.*
Subacromial bursitis, 275, 278–279, 285t
Substance abuse, fatigue from, 150
  fever and, 162
  indigestion from, 186
  insomnia and, 199t
  leg edema and, 344
  nausea and, 235, 239t
  palpitations and, 289–290, 293t
  septic arthritis from, 281
Supraspinatus tear, 275
Supraspinatus tendinitis, 274–275, 285t
  physical findings in, 281
Syphilis, sore throat from, 336t
  voiding disorders and, 377
Syringomyelia, foot pain and, 250

Tachycardia, 290, 296
Temporomandibular joint dysfunction,
    arthritis and, 138
  diagnosis of, 146t

Temporomandibular joint dysfunction
    (Continued)
  earache with, 129–130, 134t
  facial pain with, 138–139
  headache with, 169, 183t
  referred pain from, 131
Tendinitis, Achilles, 243–244, 249t
  bicipital, 276, 281, 285t
  calcific, 276, 281, 285t
  supraspinatus, 274–275, 281, 285t
  tricipital, 276
Tendo Achillis reflex, 36i
Tennis elbow, 282, 287t
Tenosynovitis, of wrist, 282, 287t
Thoracic outlet syndrome, 279, 280t
  and hand pain, 279, 280t, 282, 287t
Throat pain. See *Sore throat.*
Thrombophlebitis, 255, 263t
  cellulitis vs., 260
  leg edema with, 343–344, 346t
  physical findings in, 259
Thrombosis, 348–349
Thyroiditis, sore throat from, 338–339
Tic douloureux. See *Trigeminal neuralgia.*
Tietze's syndrome, 66
Tinea, hyphae of, 317i, 321i
Tinea capitis, 319i
Tinea cruris, 323i, 330t
Tinea pedis, 323i, 330t–331t
  of nails, 324i
Tinea versicolor, 316i–317i, 328t
Tinnitus, vertigo with, 118
Tonsillitis, 333. See also *Sore throat.*
  fever with, 162
Trench mouth, 338
Trichomoniasis, 357, 365t
  diagnosis of, 359t, 366, 368t
  vaginal discharge from, 361
Tricipital tendinitis, 276
Trigeminal neuralgia, 137–139, 144, 145t, 169
  headache with, 175, 183t
Trochanteric bursitis, 31t, 261–264
Tuberculosis, fatigue and, 153
  fever with, 162, 167t
  of urinary tract, 353, 357, 360
  vulvovaginitis from, 366
Tympanometry, 132i

Ulcer, peptic. See *Peptic ulcer.*
Uremia, nausea and, 239t
Ureterolithiasis, 12, 16t
Urethral discharge, 351–360. See also
    Dysuria.
  diagnostic studies for, 357
  differential diagnosis of, 358t–359t
  factors in, 356–357
Urethral syndrome, 353, 354t, 358t
Urethritis, 351–352

Urethritis *(Continued)*
  diagnostic studies for, 357
  gonorrheal, 354, 355t, 357, 359t
  mechanical, 352, 359t
  nongonorrheal, 353, 355t, 359t
  rarer causes of, 360
  symptoms of, 353, 355t
  with Reiter's syndrome, 360
Urinary tract infections, fever with, 162,
    166t
Urination, disorders of. See also *Enuresis;*
    Incontinence.
  diagnostic studies for, 376–377
  differential diagnosis of, 374t–375t
  drug-induced, 373–376
  enuresis and, 371–372
  overflow, 375t
  physical examination for, 376
  frequent, 351
    psychogenic cause of, 356
    rarer causes of, 360
  painful. See *Dysuria.*
Urolithiasis, 21

Vaginal discharge, 361–370
  child abuse and, 362
  common causes of, 361
  diagnostic studies for, 365–366
  differential diagnosis of, 367t–369t
  factors in, 364
  in children, 361–362
  in elderly, 362–363
  patient characteristics and, 361–362
  physical findings with, 364–365
  rarer causes of, 366–370
  symptoms of, 363–364
Vaginitis, atrophic, 363–365, 365t, 369t
  cervicitis vs., 361
  chemical, 352, 356, 358t
    in children, 362
    precipitating factors in, 364
  classification of, 365t
  diabetes and, 364
  diagnosis of, 358t
  rarer causes of, 366–370
  symptoms of, 363
  vaginal discharge with, 367t–369t
Vaginosis, bacterial, 368t
Varicella, 307, 336t
Varicose veins, 255–257
Venereal diseases. See *Sexually*
    transmitted diseases.
Venography, 348
Venous claudication, 252–254, 254t, 263t
  physical findings in, 259
Venous insufficiency, leg edema with,
    343–344, 346t
Ventricular tachycardia, 290
Vertigo, 117–120. See also *Dizziness.*

Vertigo *(Continued)*
  associated symptoms with, 118–119
  diagnostic studies for, 119–120
  differential diagnosis for, 123t–124t
  drug-induced, 124t
  factors in, 119
  patient characteristics and, 117–118
  physical findings in, 119
  rarer causes of, 120
Vesicles, 326t, 328t–330t. See also *Skin*
    problems.
Vincent's angina, 338, 341t
Vitiligo, 307, 328t. See also *Skin problems.*
Vocal cord, paralysis of, 298
Voiding disorders. See *Urination, disorders*
    of.
Volvulus, abdominal pain in, 25
Vomiting, 233–241. See also *Nausea.*
  abdominal pain with, 9
  associated symptoms with, 235–236
  diagnostic studies for, 237, 238t
  differential diagnosis of, 238–239
  drug-induced, 236, 238t
  dysuria with, 356
  factors in, 236
  in children, 234
  in elderly, 234
  in infants, 233–234
  patient characteristics and, 233–234
  physical findings in, 236–237
  postprandial, 235
  projectile, 234
  psychogenic, 235
  rarer causes of, 237–240
  regurgitation vs., 233
  self-induced, 234
  symptoms of, 234–235
von Willebrand's disease, 215
Vulvar itching, 361–370
  differential diagnosis of, 367t–369t
  factors in, 364
  physical findings with, 364–365
  rarer causes of, 366–370
  symptoms of, 363
Vulvovaginitis, 361–362
  chemical, 362
  physical findings with, 364–365
  rarer causes of, 366–370
  symptoms of, 363

Warts, 307. See also *Skin problems.*
  plantar, 244, 248t
Weight gain, 379–387. See also *Edema*
    and Obesity.
  carbohydrate craving and, 380
  differential diagnosis of, 382t–383t
  drug-induced, 379, 381, 383t

Weight gain *(Continued)*
 rarer causes of, 381–386
 symptoms of, 380
Weight loss, 386
 differential diagnosis of, 384t–385t
 drug-induced, 385t
 in elderly, 384t, 386
Wheezing, cough with, 97

Wolff-Parkinson-White syndrome, 289,
 295t
 dizziness from, 120, 125t
Wrist, contact dermatitis on, 325t
 pain in, 282–283, 287t

Xanthomas, 68